Animal Health Economics

NIPA® GENX ELECTRONIC RESOURCES & SOLUTIONS P. LTD.
New Delhi-110 034

About the Author

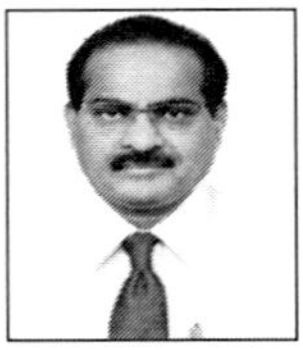

Dr. M. Thirunavukkarasu is the former Professor and Head, Dept. of Livestock Business Management, Madras Veterinary College, Tamil Nadu Veterinary and Animal Sciences University (TANUVAS), Chennai, Tamil Nadu (India). He graduated from Madras Veterinary College in the year 1986, did his post-graduation in Agricultural Economics at Tamil Nadu Agricultural University (1987 - 90), Coimbatore and doctorate in Animal Husbandry Economics (1993 - 96) at TANUVAS, Chennai. He joined the TANUVAS, Chennai in 1989 as Assistant Professor and was promoted as Associate Professor in 1997. He was elevated as the Professor of Animal Husbandry Statistics and Computer Applications in 2000. Considering his eminent achievements in education, research, extension, administration and institution building, he was then raised up as the Professor (Higher Grade) in 2011. His laudable accomplishments have also enabled him to hold the coveted posts of the Controller of Examinations, TANUVAS during 2012 – 15 and the Dean, Veterinary College and Research Institute, Tirunelveli (2016 - 18), besides holding the post of the Registrar, TANUVAS for a brief period from April to August, 2018.

He underwent advanced training programmes on Livestock Economics and Planning, and Quantitative Methods in Livestock Health and Production at the University of Reading, UK, in 1998 and training on Instructional Technology – eLearning guidelines, standards and protocols at Michigan State University, USA in 2009. He has also visited Uganda and Malawi for research and consultancy works. He has published 117 research papers in International and National journals, organised 3 International Conferences, presented more than 65 research papers (including 5 lead / invited papers) in International and National Conferences / Seminars, edited 11 books and authored 19 books, teaching manuals and booklets. He has been bestowed with 20 awards including the Best PG Student Award, Best Teacher Award, Best Scientist Award and Lifetime Achievement Award in his professional career spanning more than 33 years. He has implemented 21 Research Projects funded by National and International agencies including ICAR, NAIP, FAO, USDA, GoI, GoTN, AWBI, etc. He has started four new post graduate programmes – MVSc, MFSc and MSc in Biostatistics (2011-12) and PG Diploma in Animal Health Economics (2019-20). He has contributed significantly in the areas of Livestock Economics, Animal Health Economics, Bio-statistics, IT Applications in Animal Sciences and Development of e-Courses for Veterinary Education.

Animal Health Economics Principles and Methods

M. Thirunavukkarasu
BVSc, MSc (Ag), PhD
Former Professor and Head
Department of Livestock Business Management
Madras Veterinary College
Tamil Nadu Veterinary and Animal Sciences University
Chennai – 600 007, Tamil Nadu, India

NIPA® GENX ELECTRONIC RESOURCES & SOLUTIONS P. LTD.
New Delhi-110 034

NIPA® GENX ELECTRONIC RESOURCES & SOLUTIONS P. LTD.

101,103, Vikas Surya Plaza, CU Block
L.S.C. Market, Pitam Pura, New Delhi-110 034
Ph : +91-11-43860225, Mob.: +91 9717133558, 9540816132
E-mail: newindiapublishingagency@gmail.com
Website: www.nipaersources.com

Print ISBN: 978-93-58877-83-0
ebook ISBN: 978-93-58871-85-2

Composed and Designed by NIPA®.

Preface

Livestock and poultry play a vital role in the upliftment of the rural poor farmers by improving their income and employment. Expanding urbanization and increasing per capita incomes, especially in countries like India, are continuously pushing up the demand for protein rich livestock and poultry products, which in turn resulted in increasing intensification and commercialization of these subsectors to augment output. Together with the paradigm shift in the farming system, the genetic makeup of the animals and birds has undergone a laudable shift, thus improving the production and productivity of livestock industry.

Despite the tremendous increase in livestock and poultry output in the last six decades, this rosy picture is not without any issues. When the country started importing improved germplasms, the exotic pure and crossbreds could not withstand the hardships and contingencies peculiar to Indian agroclimate and started suffering from many new diseases / disorders, which started affecting the profitability of the farm business. Further, a disease in livestock not only brings down the attainable revenue within the farm, but also has serious negative effects on the related industries like feed and products processing businesses. Most importantly, the presence of contagious diseases like Foot and Mouth Disease has adverse havoc on the export markets.

Unfortunately, there are no adequate reading materials on the economics of animal diseases and their control. Although developed countries had started working on estimating animal disease costs and disease control and prevention costs in the early 1970s, developing countries like India initiated research works in this field only in 1990s, that too sporadically. This book has been written with the basic purpose of documenting the principles and methods of animal health economics, relatively a newer discipline for the country, to propagate the knowledge of the concepts and procedures in measuring animal disease frequencies, disease loss estimation methods, and economics of disease control programmes to help the practicing veterinarians, academicians, research workers, planners and administrators of livestock and poultry sectors.

There is hardly any branch of discipline nowadays, be it science, education, research, health, space or weather, one may care to mention, which does not use economics for its growth and development. Even if economics is not the veterinarian's primary field of study, it has now become essential for a veterinarian to know the basic principles of economics as applied to veterinary epidemiology and animal disease control and prevention. In this context, this book, probably the first of its kind in the country, will be of exceptional help to all those working in livestock and poultry subsectors.

M. Thirunavukkarasu

Contents

1

Diseases in Livestock and Poultry An Economic Insight

Human life on the earth has been intertwined with the fabric of crops and livestock for its sustenance, since time immemorial, for food and protection against the vagaries of nature. When agricultural and livestock production systems began to change in the 1950s, from traditional extensive systems to semi-intensive and intensive production systems, diseases of rural farm enterprises became challenging. Especially, the emerging diseases in livestock continued to demand more and more investments for ensuring food safety and security. Despite significant progress made in the recent past in reducing the prevalence of animal diseases, there is still an increasing concern over the losses associated with diseases of economic importance that result in production inefficiency. The scientific foundation for the discipline of animal health economics was laid by Morris (1969) and further steps were taken by Ellis (1972) to economically evaluate the Swine Fever eradication programme in Great Britain using cost-benefit analysis, Martin Hugh-Jones (1975) to specialize in GIS to model diseases and assessed the economic impact on production by infectious diseases, James and Ellis (1978) to use the same tool for FMD control programme, Renkema and Stelwagen (1979) to evaluate the replacement rates in dairy herds, Renkema (1980) to analyze the economic aspects of diseases in animals, Ellis and Putt (1981) to suggest the epidemiological and economic implications of FMD vaccination programme in Kenya, and McInerney (1983) to analyze the economics of animal diseases in dairy cattle, the multidisciplinary field of animal health economics was not amply exploited especially in developing countries to assess the extent of livestock disease losses (Ngategize and Kaneene, 1985).

With the increasing intensification and commercialization of livestock and poultry industries, the economic implications of livestock and poultry diseases became more important (McInerney, 1988), as animal diseases led to avoidable waste of scarce resources because animal diseases destroy the basic resources, reduced the attainable output and or dwindled the resource use efficiency (McInerney, 1995). Schepers and Dijkhuizen (1991) critically analyzed the past estimates to work on the economics of mastitis and mastitis control in dairy cattle. Perry *et al.* (2001 and 2002) cooperated with McDermott and Randolph in the field of economics of animal diseases, with Bennett (2003) also contributing. Acknowledging the importance of investigating the economic impacts of health problems in animal populations, veterinary epidemiologists then started to evaluate the causal relationships, predict and measure the levels of association, and prescribe the optimal preventive and/or control measures for animal diseases. However, despite the significant progress in this area of animal health economics, the tendency to overlook the need to correct the definition and interpretation of the economic concepts and relationships used had been recognized (Howe and Christiansen, 2004).

1.1 ANIMAL HEALTH ECONOMICS

The increasing concern over the enormous economic losses associated with animal diseases, estimation of disease losses, and assessment of relationships between the disease and the environment have become important for understanding the ill effects of livestock diseases and determining research priorities. This had given birth to relatively a new discipline namely 'Animal Health Economics' to assess the economic implications of animal diseases. Animal health economics came to be recognized as an area that applies the principles and methods of economics to animal health problems.

Research in this field primarily started to deal with three interrelated aspects: (1) quantifying the financial effects of animal disease, (2) developing methods for optimizing decisions when individual animals, herds, or populations are affected, and (3) determining the costs and benefits of disease control measures (Dijkhuizen, 1983). Accordingly, animal health economics is now described as a discipline that aims to provide a framework of concepts, procedures, and data to support the decision-making process in optimizing animal health management (Dijkhuizen, 1992), even though there existed some issues and problems in extrapolating the farm-level and village-level estimates of the economic benefits of livestock disease control to the national level, with the main problem being the possibility that aggregation or extrapolation of micro-data would fail to account for externalities, market changes dependent on aggregate production, such as variations in market price, and changes in access to markets, such as export markets (Tisdell, 1994). Animal health economics was then progressively developing a framework of concepts, procedures, and data to support the decision-making process in optimizing animal health management (Dijkhuizen, *et al.,* (1995).

McLeod and Leslie (2001) discussed various socioeconomic impacts of livestock diseases and export promotion in developing countries in a policy paper of FAO. To estimate the potential revenue impacts of an outbreak of FMD in the United States, Paarlberg *et al.* (2002) carried out an analysis, by incorporating quarantine and slaughter of animals, export ban, and consumer fears about the disease, to determine the combined impacts. The impacts of diseases needed to be separated into two components: (1) direct losses due to reduced production and changes in herd structure; and (2) indirect losses caused by costs of disease control, poor access to markets, and limited use of improved production technologies.

The losses arising from diseases in livestock may be direct and or indirect, with direct losses arising from destroying the basic resource (the animal itself), by lowering the efficiency of the production process or by reducing the quantity or the quality of the output and indirect losses arising from additional costs incurred to avoid or reduce the prevalence of diseases like deworming, vaccination, etc., or affecting even human health through zoonosis. A system of categorization of the direct costs and consequential losses was suggested by Horst *et al.* (1999a) for calculating the costs and losses incurred during outbreaks, besides providing a basic framework for the economic evaluation of animal diseases at different economic levels. McDermott *et al.* (2013) focussed on estimating the economic burdens of brucellosis in low-income countries in tropical Asia and Africa and found that the prospects for technically feasible, and economically viable national brucellosis control programmes in most low-income countries are limited, while some targeted control programmes could be beneficial and be feasibly managed to provide good economic returns.

1.1.1 Economic Impact of a Disease

A disease's economic impact can be measured at several levels: on an animal, a farm or herd, the whole sector including the related supply and processing industry, and the consumer. At the national level, the aggregated losses will be generally lower than those at the production level, due to the activities undertaken through veterinary services. A contagious disease outbreak in a country may lead to trade restrictions among importing countries. However, measuring the economic impacts of animal diseases is not that simple, because many diseases are not always noticeable, having been influenced by other factors such as management (e.g., nutrition and housing) and environment, having a temporal dimension adding to the complexity of evaluating the impacts at different times, and manifesting themselves with other diseases.

The direct or indirect consequences of a disease can be described and analyzed by listing the disease loss components, *viz.*, mortality and abortions, cost of treatments, cullings, decrease in selling prices; discarded products and slaughter refusals, trade restrictions; costs of preventive interventions; reduction in productivity, increase in culling rate; and decrease in genetic improvement and additional labour costs. These components need to be aggregated to obtain the whole cost of a disease.

1.1.1.1 Assessment of the Economic Impact of a Disease

1. **Determination of Reduction of Outputs:** Identifying different forms of the disease that occur and measuring the incidence and prevalence of each of the diseases are the first steps. Modelling can be done to express the quantitative deviation in the production of the herd due to a disease. There are some theoretical approaches too, based on programming and simulation methods, using the existing knowledge about the disease and the anticipated revenues and expenditures, had the disease not occurred. Meuwissen, *et al.* (1999) developed a simulation model to calculate the financial consequences of a Classical Swine Fever (CSF) outbreak on the affected stakeholders, including governments, farms, and related industries in the production chain and applied that model to the 1997-98 outbreak of CSF in the Netherlands, which indicated that the total financial consequences of the outbreak were US $2.3 billion, including the losses to the farmers (US $423 million) and related industries (US $596 million). This model could be adapted easily to other diseases and countries.
2. **Measurement of Inputs Wasted and the Expenditures due to Interventions:** Though necessary data can be obtained from the disease monitoring systems, the validity of the results obtained from these systems is generally low because the economic characteristics of a disease may differ between farming systems. Further, the components taken from a particular disease monitoring system may vary from that of the other. Also, the economic indicators assessed may be an underestimation of the losses due to farm variability. Most importantly, the transboundary livestock diseases have serious economic and international trade consequences, posing a grave threat to world food security, by spreading rapidly and causing heavy drops in the production of milk, meat, and other products. Hence, the importance of minimizing the impact of transboundary livestock diseases through enhanced emergency preparedness with well-coordinated national, regional, and global disease control and eradication needed to be brought to the attention of the World Food Summit (FAO, 1997).

1.2 ECONOMIC WORTH OF INTERVENTIONS TO CONTROL ANIMAL DISEASES

Although most of the economic benefits of animal disease control can be expressed in monetary terms (like availability of more animal products for sale, a higher price per unit of product, lower production costs, etc.), some elements (e.g., reduced risk of human infection through zoonoses and increased work capacity of animals for crop production) cannot be valued so easily in monetary terms. Farmers' perceptions of risk and attitudes towards the risks predisposing to health problems may also differ. Hence, the farmers' strategies towards disease control interventions may be elimination of disease, limitation of disease occurrence by reducing the exposure to risk factors, and limitation of the consequences of disease by treatments. The choice of strategies and related interventions by the farmers to bring down the disease losses will be based on their economic worth. The economic worth of disease prevention and or control is established using two approaches:

Positive (or observational) studies: 'With vs without' designs ('after vs before' or 'program vs control') are mostly used in field experiments to evaluate the economic worth of interventions. These studies are often time-consuming and expensive and provide only ex-post information.

Theoretical (or normative) studies: These are mostly used to study the intervention on enzootic diseases, e.g., decision trees, partial budgeting, and simulation models, which provide relevant ex-ante information when sufficient previous knowledge exists.

A dynamic optimization model was developed and used by Kobayashi *et al.* (2007a and 2007b) to evaluate alternative FMD control strategies. To adequately allocate resources for the control of Contagious Bovine Pleuro Pneumonia (CBPP) in sub-Saharan Africa, Onono *et al.* (2014) estimated the impact of CBPP on pastoralists, using a stochastic spreadsheet model, to identify a control strategy with minimum cost from both expenditures on control strategies and output losses. The impact of CBPP on the nation was estimated to be US$ 7.6 million per year. The control strategy with a minimum cost per herd was preventive vaccination with an estimated cost of US$ 193 per 100 cows per year, while the slaughter of clinical cases had an estimated cost of US$ 912 per 100 cows per year, indicating that the control of CBPP was more profitable through preventive vaccination.

1.3 GROWTH OF ANIMAL HEALTH ECONOMICS ACROSS THE WORLD

Zhukovsky and Nedosekov (source unknown) in their paper on *'Introduction to the economics of animal health in Ukraine'* and later Rushton *et al.* (2007) have given detailed notes on the history of animal health economics. The eminent scientists with their affiliations to the institutions (some of them might have changed their affiliation from time to time) who quantified animal disease losses and also the costs of disease control (not necessarily by their prominence, may not be in chronological order too, besides being the list not exhaustive) include:

- Ellis, Morris, Hugh-Jones, Putt, James, Bennett, and Shaw at the University of Reading, UK
- Carpenter at the University of California, Davis, USA
- Mclnerney and Howe at the University of Exeter, UK
- Dijkhuizen at the Wageningen Agricultural University, The Netherlands
- Tisdell, Harrison, and Ramsay at the University of Queensland, Australia
- Perry at the International Livestock Research Institute (ILRI), Kenya

Ellis was the founder of the Veterinary Epidemiology and Economics Research Unit (VEERU) at the University of Reading, the UK and in many ways, was a pioneer in the subject of animal health economics. His interest in economics evolved from his work on FMD in South America where he discovered that the epidemiology of FMD could not be separated from livestock prices and farm management systems. Moving to the University of Reading where he began analyzing Classical Swine Fever eradication in the UK, he was the first to apply the principle of cost-benefit analysis to appraise an animal disease and its effects. At this point, Martin Hugh-Jones also went to Reading to work on this project.

During these early works on animal health economics in the UK, Roger Morris was working at the University of Melbourne on the economics of animal production diseases. Morris after a meeting with Ellis at WHO in 1970 in Geneva to discuss the approaches to evaluate the control of zoonoses, went to Reading on a sabbatical in 1972, where Ellis and Morris consolidated their views, which were presented at a follow-up workshop for WHO at Reading, UK. This workshop produced a working document, which was widely distributed as a guideline for international disease cost evaluations.

Demand for help from the European Economic Council/European Union and support for research from the Overseas Development Administration (ODA) of the British Government, now DFID, resulted in the development of an interdisciplinary team designated as VEERU in 1975. The early contributors to this group were Andrew James (economist), Nick Putt (veterinarian), Alexandra Shaw (economist), Lindsay Tyler (veterinarian), Dick Esselmont (farm management specialist), Tony Woods (statistician), Andrew Stephens (veterinarian), Richard Matthewman (animal production specialist), Howard Pharo (veterinarian), and later James Hanks (animal production specialist), Anni McLeod (economist) and Jackie Leslie (economist).

In 1976, Ellis invited all the professionals who were interested in veterinary epidemiology and economics to Reading for an exchange of ideas. About 80 experts attended the meeting and the proceedings provided a reference document. The main result of that meeting was the creation of the International Society of Veterinary Epidemiology and Economics (ISVEE). Shortly after this meeting, the Society for Veterinary Epidemiology and Preventive Medicine (SVEPM) was founded in the UK and similar societies were created in France and other countries too.

A few of the key experts who worked at VEERU, UK, apart from Ellis, were/are:

- Martin Hugh-Jones, who specialized in GIS, and modeling diseases, worked on the study of the economics of Brucellosis eradication in England and Wales.
- Roger Morris worked on the economics of livestock diseases in Australia at the same time, as Ellis began working on this subject in the UK. He did his PhD supervised by Ellis in which he explored complementary methodology including the applications of risk analysis.
- Nick Putt worked on the epidemiology and economics of Trypanosomiasis in Nigeria and Zambia.
- Alexandra Shaw, who specialized in the economics of Trypanosomiasis and its control, used her experiences from western Africa to explore not just the impact of the disease at the herd level, but also its impact on land use and the general economy.
- Andrew James worked on the early assessment of FMD costs and their control, first in general terms and then with examples from India and later concentrated on East Coast Fever, and tick and tick-borne disease economics.

Their major contributions were the early use of scientific studies of cost-benefit analysis techniques, the development of herd models (like CUPPER and LPEC), herd monitoring systems (like DAISY, EVA, MONTY, and INTERHERD), and examining the economic impacts of animal diseases across different levels of the society.

- Erb and Martin (1978) measured the age, breed and seasonal patterns in the occurrence of 10 dairy cow diseases and Erb and Grohn (1988) observed the epidemiology of metabolic disorders in periparturient dairy cows.
- Tim Carpenter (University of Davis, California) was another pioneer in the field of animal health economics during the 1970s.
- Kauppinen (1983) observed the prevalence of bovine ketosis in relation to the number and stage of lactation.
- McInerney and Howe at Exeter University, UK began research on the theoretical economics of livestock disease, developing largely conceptual models of farmers' behaviour towards animal diseases. They continued this approach with Richard Bennett at the University of Reading, to teach their veterinary colleagues.
- Dijkhuizen began investigations into the costs of animal diseases with Renkema at the Wageningen Agricultural University, The Netherlands in the 1970s. Dijkhuizen worked particularly on mastitis and diseases that affect dairy cattle. Dijkhuizen and his team, in particular, Jalvingh and Huirne worked on various disease problems like CSF, Porcine reproductive and respiratory syndrome, disease problems in bovines like reproductive economics, lameness, respiratory diseases, Mastitis, Paratuberculosis, Leptospirosis, viral diarrhoea, BSE, Herpes virus, and FMD.
- Tisdell, Harrison, and Ramsay at the University of Queensland, Australia worked on an animal health project in Thailand during the 1990s. They examined the use of cost-benefit analysis for assessing animal disease programmes.
- Bennett at the University of Reading, UK made contributions with works on how to use the data on animal health decisions and decision-making for Leptospirosis in cattle.
- Brian Perry, Mukhebi, Young, Tom Randolph, John McDermott and Karl Rich were at the Epidemiology and Disease Control Unit at ILRI, Nairobi, Kenya, working on the epidemiology and economics of parasitic diseases and FMD.
- Yang *et al.* (1999) reported the economic consequences of a devastating outbreak of FMD, serotype O, that occurred in pigs in Taiwan, during March - July 1997.
- Awa *et al.* (2000) found that PPR and gastrointestinal helminthiasis are important causes of economic losses in small ruminants in Cameroon.

Because of these significant efforts made by these experts, the discipline of animal health economics was progressively developing. The key achievement of this discipline is the establishment of epidemiological and economic techniques, offering a distinctive and successful method of investigation and resolving animal health problems. In short, the discipline of animal health economics started to compare the cost of tolerating a disease with the cost of controlling it to allow animal health improvement strategies to obtain maximum benefit from available scarce resources. Lots of conceptual refinements were made by these pioneers and now the discipline of animal health economics has come to remain as a multidisciplinary field encompassing the fields of animal science, epidemiology, statistics, and economics.

1.3.1 Growth of Animal Health Economics in India

Though there have been several studies undertaken in this field in the UK (University of Reading), the Netherlands (Wageningen Agricultural University), New Zealand (Massey University), and Australia (University of Queensland), this field was yet to be amply exploited in developing countries like India, although a few attempts have been made in this emerging field in the recent past. For e.g., a total of Rs.1607.20 crores was estimated to be lost due to bovine mastitis in India through a descriptive study based on the secondary data by Singh and Singh (1994). Saxena (1994) estimated the economic value of milk loss caused by FMD in India. Later, Jadhav *et al.* (1995) and Jadhav *et al.* (1996) worked out the economics of health disorders in crossbred cows.

Thirunavukkarasu (1996) undertook a study in India in the field of animal health economics, using relatively newer analytical tools like discriminant analysis and logistic regression analysis, at the Tamil Nadu Veterinary and Animal Sciences University (TANUVAS), Chennai (India) to estimate the economic losses due to mastitis in bovines, based on the primary data collected across the State of Tamil Nadu from 1993 to 1996. Many such studies then followed to be conducted by the research students under the guidance of Prabaharan and Thirunavukkarasu (1993 - 2010) and the research fraternity of TANUVAS to analyze the economic consequences of diseases in layer farms (Selvam, 2000), post-partum reproductive disorders in bovines (Jeyakumari, 2000), conception failures in artificially inseminated bovines (Thirunavukkarasu, 2003a), sheep pox and enterotoxaemia in sheep (Senthilkumar, 2003), FMD in ruminants and pigs (Thirunavukkarasu, 2004), and metabolic disorders in female bovines (Thirunavukkarasu, 2008). Further, John Christy and Thirunavukkarasu (2006) outlined the emerging importance of animal health economics.

Thirunavukkarasu and Prabaharan (1998a and 1999a) observed the prevalence of clinical mastitis in bovines in Tamil Nadu and analyzed the factors influencing the same. The estimates of Risk Ratio (RR), Odds Ratio (OR), Attributable Rate (AR), and Attributable Fraction (AF) for various factors predisposing to Mastitis in female bovines both for the sample and the population by Thirunavukkarasu and Prabaharan (1998b) are the firsts of their kind in India. Thirunavukkarasu and Prabaharan (1999c) used a logistic regression model to predict whether a female bovine would pick up mastitis or not in the future, based on the animal and environmental characteristics like species, breed, milk yield, stage of lactation, age, order of lactation and season of calving. During the same period, Thirunavukkarasu and Prabaharan (1999b and 2000) estimated the economic impact of mastitis in dairy farms and identified the factors determining mastitis losses through a regression analysis, respectively. Thirunavukkarasu (2003b) developed a discriminant model to discriminate between mastitic and non-mastitic milch animals based on certain animal and environmental attributes/factors. While Jeyakumari *et al.* (2003a) assessed the epidemiological measures of association between the incidence of post-partum disorders in dairy animals and their predisposing factors, Jeyakumari *et al.* (2003b) estimated the economic Impact of postpartum reproductive disorders on dairy farms and Jeyakumari *et al.* (2004) assessed the prevalence of postpartum reproductive disorders in bovines in Tamil Nadu. In the forward given for the book released by the Indian Council of Agricultural Research (ICAR), New Delhi, Yadav (2003) indicated that FMD caused substantial monetary losses by reducing milk yield and working ability of draught animals.

Selvam *et al.* (2000) attempted to identify the factors influencing loss due to diseases in layer farms. Selvam *et al.* (2003) measured the disease frequencies in commercial layer farms and Selvam *et al.* (2004) estimated the economic losses due to infectious bursal disease and Ranikhet diseases in layers. Further, Thirunavukkarasu and Kathiravan (2006a) estimated the economic losses due to mortality and culling of FMD-affected livestock, assessed the factors influencing the economic losses due to conception failures in the artificially inseminated bovines (Thirunavukkarasu and Kathiravan, 2006b) and estimated the monetary losses due to reproductive failures in FMD-affected bovines (Thirunavukkarasu and Kathiravan, 2007).

Thombre *et al.* (2009) conducted a cross-sectional sample survey across six villages severely affected by PPR to assess the extent of loss in small ruminants. The total losses due to disease were found to range between Rs.918 in sheep to Rs.945 in goats. Reduction in the market value of animals was the major loss component, costing Rs.404 (44 percent) in sheep and Rs.408 (43 percent) in goats. Expenditure on medicine and infertility was found to cause more than 80 percent of the total cost.

While Thirunavukkarasu *et al.* (2010a) assessed the prevalence of ketosis in dairy farms through a survey in Tamil Nadu, Thirunavukkarasu *et al.* (2010b) estimated the economic losses arising out of milk fever in dairy farms bovines, Thirunavukkarasu *et al.* (2010c) reported the factors influencing the economic losses due to milk fever in dairy animals, and Thirunavukkarasu *et al.* (2010d) worked out the epidemiological measures of association between the factors predisposing and prevalence of milk fever among dairy animals. Further, Thirunavukkarasu *et al.* (2011a) measured the epidemiological measures on the prevalence of ketosis in dairy farms and Thirunavukkarasu *et al.* (2011b) estimated the economic losses due to ketosis in dairy farms. A few studies have also been undertaken at the National Centre for Agricultural Economics and Policy Research (NCAP), now called as National Institute for Agricultural Economics and Policy Research (NIAP), of ICAR to estimate the economic losses due to PPR and FMD in livestock.

Sinha *et al.* (2017) collected data from 2006-07 from 60 small farmers in the Pune region and analyzed them to assess the economic impacts of FMD. The loss in terms of reduced revenues and cost as extra resources used for treatment were quantified and aggregated. The estimated production loss was Rs.3,184 in crossbred cows and Rs.3062.50 in buffaloes. The major loss component was the reduction in milk yield, which accounted for Rs.894.60 and Rs.510, representing 20.88 and 13.60 percent of the total loss in crossbred cows and buffaloes, respectively. The cost of treatment was worked out to be Rs. 1313.80 in crossbred cows and Rs. 645.63 in buffaloes. The cost of medicine alone constituted around 50 percent of the total cost component.

2

Basic Statistics for Animal Health Studies

Statistics is defined as a discipline that includes procedures and techniques used to collect, process, and analyze numerical data to make inferences about the data. The word statistic is used as a singular, denoting the numerical data. Statistics are the numerical quantities calculated from sample observations. Here, the word statistics hence is plural. Basically, statistics is defined as the statistical data (in the plural sense) and also as statistical methods (in the singular sense). A clearer and more precise definition is that 'statistics is the study of methods and procedures for collecting, classifying, presenting, analyzing, and interpreting data to make scientific inferences from it'. Bio-statistics is the science dealing with the application of statistical methods to the problems of biological sciences.

2.1 FUNCTIONS OF STATISTICS

a) **To present the facts in a definite form:** If the data or results are given in numbers, rather than in qualitative statements, they will be more useful. The statements like 'there is a considerable amount of unemployment in a country or the human population in a state is increasing at a faster rate' are not in definite forms. The statements should be in definite form like there is a 15 percent unemployment in 2023 or the population is increasing by 5 percent every decade.

b) **To simplify the mass of figures:** Once the data are presented in definite forms, they need to be condensed into simple figures, like averages. The original data are thus presented as a table, graph, or diagram after converting them into averages.

c) **To facilitate comparison of data:** After simplifying the data, they are compared or correlated. Quantities like averages can represent the relationship between the two population groups. Comparison is one of the main functions of statistics, as presenting absolute data may not convey any meaning to the data presented.

d) **To formulate and test hypothesis:** Statistical methods help to formulate a hypothesis about the data gathered from the field or laboratory and test the same for their validity. A hypothesis is a tentative and unproved assumption about a phenomenon, proposed for the sake of argument so that it can be tested to see if it is true. E.g., the statement "Smoking causes lung cancer" can be a hypothesis. Simply, a hypothesis is a statement that is consistent with known data, but not tested to be true or false.

e) **To help in prediction or forecasting:** Statistics can be used to predict the future course of an event or phenomenon based on past data. We can predict the supply of and / or demand for milk in 2030, based on the past data on milk and the growth of the human population.

f) **To help in the formulation of policies:** Through prediction or forecasting, Government agencies make policies for future growth and individual farmers / producers can exploit the market situation profitably if they know the trends in the market. The government can plan how much milk is to be produced in 2030 to export, besides fulfilling domestic demand.

Applications of Statistics

There is hardly any branch of science today that does not make use of statistics. Any greatest victory of mankind from computers to cloning, landing on the moon to heart transplantation could not have succeeded without the help of statistics. The broader areas where statistics is increasingly used today include science, production, education, health, transport, economics, marketing, finance, commerce and trade, weather, diseases, sports, and any subject we may care to mention.

2.2 CLASSIFICATION OF STATISTICS

Descriptive statistics deals with collecting, organizing, summarizing, analyzing and presenting data in a convenient form. E.g., a shopkeeper may wish to compare the weekly sales in the last year at two of his outlets. Whereas, inferential statistics consists of methods and procedures for drawing conclusions about the characteristics of a population based on the information available in the sample taken from a population. The broad classification of statistics, in particular bio-statistics, is as below:

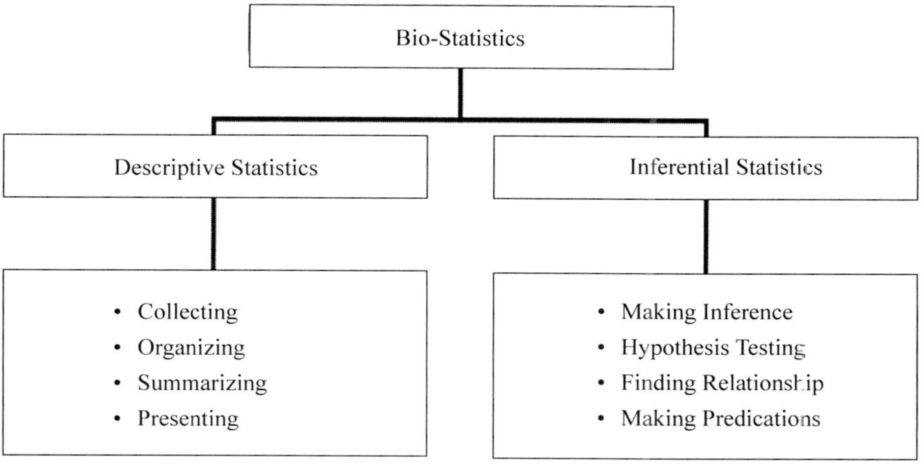

2.3 STATISTICS AS A TOOL OF MEASURING DISEASE IMPACTS

The methods used for assessment of the economic impacts of animal diseases can be categorized into two groups *viz.*, (i) statistical or epidemiological methods and (ii) economic methods. Statistical or epidemiological methods are primarily used to identify the factors that contribute to the development of the disease conditions, the magnitude and direction of their contributions, and their relationships with the diseases. In these methods, first, the cause(s) of a disease is (are) identified, then they are disaggregated for quantifying them, and in the next step, the quantified impacts are expressed in monetary terms.

Economic methods of disease loss estimation include the Equi-marginal principle, Partial budgeting, Cost-benefit analysis, Decision analysis, Linear programming, Markov chains, Systems simulation, Dynamic programming, etc.

2.3.1 Statistical Methods

2.3.1.1 Concepts and Terms

- **Population** - A set of individuals studied through an enquiry is referred to as the universe or population. E.g., all animals in a farm.
- **Sample** – A small group of a population selected for conducting an investigation and collecting data is called a sample. E.g., animals of a particular species or breed in a farm.
- **Variable** - The quantitative (numerical) or qualitative (categorical) characteristic of the data is called a variable. The value of a variable is termed a variate or variate value. E.g., the age of an animal or the breed of the animal.

- A **quantitative variable** is a characteristic of a sampling unit, which can be either discrete (1, 2, 3, ...) or continuous (1.1., 1.2, 1.3, ...), that is measured in some units. E.g., age, weight, length, etc.
  - **Discrete or discontinuous variable** - If a quantitative variable takes only integral values, then it is called a discrete (or) discontinuous variable. E.g., no. of animals in a farm.
  - **Continuous variable** - If a quantitative variable takes intermediate values between any integral values, then it is called a continuous variable. E.g., the weight of an animal.
- A **qualitative variable** is a qualitative characteristic of a sampling unit that cannot be measured, but expressed only in qualities called attributes. E.g., the breed of the animal, colour of the skin, etc.
- A **constant** is a numerical value, which does not vary from one individual to another in the population. E.g., no. of legs in cows.
- A **parameter** is the descriptive measure of a population. E.g., mean, standard deviation, etc. of the population.
- A **statistic** is the descriptive measure of a sample is called as a statistic. E.g., mean, standard deviation, etc. of the sample.
- **Data** are the observations with which the investigators deal. E.g., body weight, milk yield, etc.

2.3.1.2 Primary Data and Secondary Data

Primary Data

The data collected from the sample or population are called the primary data. They are collected through personal surveys using interview schedules by the investigator himself or by distributing the questionnaires either to the respondents directly or to the field data collectors and getting the filled-in questionnaires back by post or by special messengers. The source of primary data is called the primary source.

Methods of Collecting Primary Data

1. **Direct Personal Observation:** This method consists of the collection of data personally by the investigator himself from the primary sources. An interview schedule (containing a set of questions to be asked to the respondents) is framed by the investigator for use during data collection and the details obtained from the chosen respondents are filled in directly in the schedules. For every respondent, there is a separate schedule, and hence, at the end of the data collection process, there will be as many number of filled-in schedules, as the number of respondents.

2. **Indirect Observation:** This is similar to direct observation, but here the investigator collects the data through the field investigators, selected and trained for data collection. Interview schedules framed by the investigator will be used by the field investigators or enumerators for data collection from the respondents chosen by the investigator. The enumerators will fill in the schedules by personal interview and submit the schedules to the investigator for further statistical analysis.
3. **Data Collection through Questionnaires:** Here, the investigator prepares the questionnaires and sends them to the respondents through post or other modes to collect data from them. A letter explaining the aim and purpose of collecting the data is also sent along with the questionnaire. The letter will also highlight that the data collected from the respondents will be used for research purposes only and will be kept confidential. This will take the respondents into confidence and ensure a quick and better response from them. Necessarily, the return postage expenses are to be borne by the investigator by sending a stamped envelope. Since the investigator is not going to meet the respondents in person, the questionnaire should be prepared with utmost care so that the respondents are not misled by any of the questions asked. Hence, the investigator will frame the questionnaire by following certain good principles, as below:
   a) The questions put in the questionnaire should be simple, small, and easy to understand even by the less literate respondents.
   b) All the questions should be designed in such a way that the respondents need to give only short and objective answers, not requiring much of their time.
   c) The questions should be arranged in a logical sequence so that the respondents are not misled or carried away to give particular answers.
   d) The investigator should avoid any kind of leading or misleading questions.
   e) The questions which are likely to hurt the respondents' feelings and sentiments should be avoided.

4. Merits and Demerits of Different Methods of Primary Data Collection

Method of Data Collection	Merits	Demerits
Direct personal observation	1. Data are first-hand and hence are reliable and accurate. 2. Respondents are contacted personally and hence, the response is generally good. 3. Can be used even if the respondents are illiterate.	i. Expensive in terms of time and money. ii. Not suitable for big surveys involving large numbers of respondents.
Indirect personal observation	1. Saves time. 2. Useful in large-scale surveys. 3. Yields reliable results, as data are recorded by trained enumerators. 4. Can be used even if the respondents are illiterate.	i. Enumerators should possess thorough knowledge of what is being investigated. ii. Requires more money and time.
Data collection through questionnaires	1. Most economical in terms of time, money, and manpower. 2. Good for extensive enquiry covering a wide area. 3. Fewer errors due to the personal biases of investigators.	i. Poor response. ii. Possibility for incomplete /vague / inaccurate data. iii. Not suited for illiterate respondents.

Secondary Data

The secondary data include the data collected from the already available print and non-print sources like published reports, documents, journals, websites, etc. The sources from which the secondary data are collected are called secondary sources of data. These sources include published sources (e.g., publications and documents of national and international government and non-government agencies, research institutes, academic institutions, books, journals, newspapers, periodicals, etc.) and unpublished sources (private societies, private firms, business enterprises, etc.). While the primary data are specially collected to achieve a particular objective, the secondary data are the ones that were collected for some other purposes.

Advantages of Secondary Data

a) Easier and quicker to obtain than primary data, as they are already available.

b) More convenient to use, as they are already available in some published form.

c) Requires less time, labour, and money than primary data.

d) At times, secondary data are the only possibility, as it may be less feasible to collect primary data all the time. E.g., the livestock census data cannot be collected as and when required from the primary sources, but are obtained only from Government publications.

Disadvantages of Secondary Data

a) Accuracy of the secondary data may not be always precise and it depends on the type of agencies that collected the data and the purpose for which they were collected.
b) Not all the data required for an investigation may be available in secondary sources.
c) At times, the secondary data available may not be reliable. The reliability of the data would depend on who or which agency collected the data, which method was used for data collection, and for what purpose the data were collected.

2.4 CLASSIFICATION OF DATA

Classification of data is the next step after the collection of data. It is the process of arranging the data in a definite pattern and presenting it in a systematic way. When the data are collected from an experiment or a survey, they may be in a crude and unorganized form. The data in this form are called ungrouped data. It is difficult to study and draw inferences from ungrouped data. Also, sometimes the original data collected may be so large which may be difficult to present in a suitable form. Hence, it is essential to classify and present data in a convenient form to understand.

2.4.1 Objectives of Classification of Data

a) To remove unnecessary details
b) To better understand the data
c) To detect errors in the data
d) To bring out explicitly the significant features in the data
e) To make quick comparisons and draw inferences

2.4.2 Types of Classification of Data

Numerical classification (Classification by size) - Classification of data according to quantitative characters. e.g. classification of animals according to their weights.

Descriptive classification (Classification by attribute) - Classification of data according to qualitative characters (attributes). e.g., classification of animals according to breeds.

Spatial classification (Classification by space) - Classification of data according to location of data. e.g., district-wise livestock population.

Temporal or chronological classification (Classification by time) - Classification of data according to time. e.g., livestock population in different years.

2.5 TABULATION OF DATA

2.5.1 Objectives of Tabulation

a) To simplify the complex data
b) To economize the space
c) To depict the trend
d) To facilitate comparison of data
e) To facilitate statistical analysis of data

2.5.2 Parts of a Table

Generally, a table has a few important parts *viz.*, table number, title of table, caption (column heading), stub (row heading), body of the table, head note, and footnote.

Table number: A table must be numbered (say 1, 2, 3, 4, etc.) whenever more than one table is prepared.

Title: The title of the table should be brief and self-explanatory, giving complete information about the contents of the table.

Captions and stubs: Headings given to columns and rows are called captions and stubs, respectively. There could be sub-captions and sub-stubs also.

Body of the table: It contains the data.

Head note: It is a description, given below the title to explain the contents of the table. E.g., in million tons.

Footnote: It is a description given below the table to give some specific information about some contents in the body of the table.

General Structure of a Table

Stub Heading	**Main Caption**[a]	
	Sub-caption No. 1[b]	
	Tertiary No.1	**Tertiary No.2**
Stub No. 1[c]	Field item No.1	Field item No.2
Stub No. 2	Field item No.3	……

[a,b,c,]*Footnotes, if any, given horizontally*

Types of Tables

Based on construction, tables are classified as follows:

a) *Simple table:* This is made based on just one characteristic. Hence, it is called a one-way table.

One-Way Table

Milk Yield in Kg	Number of Cows
1 – 10	
11 – 20	
21 - 30	
> 30	
Total	

b) *Complex table:* This is formed based on more than one characteristic – e.g., distribution of animals based on sex, body weights, etc. If the complex table is based on two characteristics, it is called a two–way table and if it is based on three characteristics, it is named a three-way table. If there are more than three characteristics, it is called a manifold – table.

Two-Way Table

Body Weights in Kg	Number of Cattle		
	Male	**Female**	**Total**
< 200			
200 – 300			
301 – 400			
401 - 500			
> 500			
Total			

Three-Way Table

Body Weights in Kg	Number of Cattle and Buffaloes					
	Male		**Female**		**Total**	
	Cattle	**Buffaloes**	**Cattle**	**Buffaloes**	**Cattle**	**Buffaloes**
< 200						
200 – 300						
301 – 400						
401 - 500						
> 500						
Total						

2.5.3 Essentials of a Good Table

- A table should be designed according to the objective of the statistical investigation.
- A table should not be overloaded with details.
- A table should be well-balanced. Care should be taken in deciding the size of a table and the proportion of columns and rows.
- A table should be complete in itself, having all the explanations necessary to make the meaning of items clear.
- Units of measurement in a table must be clearly stated such as "price in Rs." or "weight in kg".
- The size of the table should not be too big or too small.
- As far as possible, a table should be typed vertically. However, in exceptional cases, the horizontally typed table is also accepted.

2.6 CLASSIFICATION OF DATA USING CLASS INTERVAL (FREQUENCY DISTRIBUTION)

Usually, the first step taken to condense the mass of quantitative data is to form a frequency distribution. Frequency distribution is a simple and effective method of organizing and presenting the data to get an overall picture of the data. Frequency distribution is an arrangement or table that groups the mass of data into non-overlapping intervals. These non-overlapping intervals are called classes. The data are then recorded in each of the classes.

Class interval is the limit within which the class limits lie. Each class interval has two limits - upper and lower. The width or length of the class interval is the difference between the upper and lower boundaries of the class. Frequency is the number of observations in each class.

2.6.1 Formation of Frequency Distribution

2.6.1.1 Ungrouped Frequency Distribution

In this method, the data are arranged in a systematic way (e.g., in ascending order). This process of arranging the observations is called an array. From the arrayed figures, the frequency distribution for each value is obtained. E.g. Weight of 10 numbers of eggs in g: 51, 58, 49, 52, 55, 61, 59, 55, 45, 48.

Formation of array

Actual data	51	58	49	52	55	61	59	55	45	48
Data in ascending order (Array form)	45	48	49	51	52	55	58	59	61	
No. of eggs in each category	1	1	1	1	1	2	1	1	1	

This representation, though appears better, does not condense the data and it is quite difficult to do if the data are huge. Hence, we have another method, i.e., grouped frequency distribution.

2.6.1.2 Grouped Frequency Distribution

Method of Tally Marks

The following are the data on the lactation period (in days) of cows in a dairy farm:

290	309	292	302	307	301	289	285
302	276	284	287	298	294	273	305
270	282	273	277	279	287	275	279
276	285	305	297	271	292	295	282
282	296	294	296	303	293	301	300

Choosing the Number of Classes

In this method, we first decide on the number of classes for the data. These classes must be non-overlapping and should contain all the observations. That is, each observation in the data must fall into exactly one class. Since there is no strict rule for the number of classes, we can decide on the number of classes by looking at the data. The range of classes should cover the entire data and the classes must be continuous. Classes should not be too large or too small. Usually, the number of classes will be between 5 and 20. Sometimes the data may be such that we should have only 3 or 4 classes.

If the number of classes is too large (>20), then each class may have only a few observations. Similarly, if the number of classes is too small, then each class may have too many observations which is also not appropriate. Then we decide on the class interval.

Choosing Class Interval

Class interval is the limit within which each class limit lies. Class intervals should be of equal width and of such size so that all the features of the data are displayed. To choose the class interval for the data, we should find the difference between maximum and minimum values in the data and we divide this difference by the number of required classes decided.

Appr. Class Interval (Width) = (Largest value – Smallest value) ÷ No. of Classes decided

Suppose we have 8 classes. The difference between the largest and smallest numbers is 39. Hence, the class interval (width) for this example is equal to (309 – 270) ÷ 8 = 39 ÷ 8 = 4.875. That is, the width of the class interval is nearer to 4.875. Then, we round off this class interval of 4.875 to the nearest whole number, i.e., 5 for convenience. If the class interval is 5, then our classes will be 270-275, 275-280, 280-285, 285-290, 290-295, 295-300, 300-305 and 305-310. i.e., The first class contains all observations from 270 up to, but not including 275.

No. of required classes can also be calculated using the formula of *Sturge's rule* or *Yule's rule*. By Sturge's rule, K = 1 + 3.322 x log N, and as per Yule's rule, K = 2.5 x $(N)^{1/4}$, where K is the number of required classes and N is the number of observations.

The following are different types of class intervals used:

a	b	c	d	e
0-10	0 and under 10	Less than 20	0-10	0-9.9
10-20	10 and under 20	20-30	10-30	10-19.9
20-30	20 and under 30	more than 30	30-70	20-29.9

- In type 'c', the first and last classes are open.
- In type 'd', there are unequal class intervals.
- Type 'b' is very similar to 'a', but it is explicitly explained here, though not necessary.
- In type 'e', class limits are exactly defined, which is also not required.
- The difficulty in 'a' is that where (in which class) to include 10, 20, etc. Generally, in such cases, the first class of 'a', defined by 0-10, will contain observations from 0 to 10, but not 10. We include 10 in 2nd class, 20 in 3rd class, and so on. Hence, the type 'a' can be said to be suitable.
- However, depending on the need and situation, an appropriate type of class interval may be chosen.

Method of Tally Marks

After forming the class interval, each class should be written one below the other. We now count and record the number or frequency of measurements belonging to each class. That is, for each item in the collected data, a stroke is marked against the class interval in which the item falls. Usually after every four such strokes in the class interval, the fifth item is indicated by striking the previous four strokes, thus, making it easy to count. These strokes are counted and this is called the formation of frequency distribution by the method of tally marks.

Classes	Tally marks	Frequency
270 – 275*	||||	4
275 - 280	卌 |	6
280 - 285	||||	4
285 - 290	卌	5
290 - 295	卌 |	6
295 - 300	卌	5
300 - 305	卌 |	6
305 - 310	||||	4
	Total	**40**

** Class contains all observations from 270 up to, but not including, 275.*

The frequency distribution is now complete. The column of tally marks is created only to facilitate the counting of measurements. It will be omitted when a frequency distribution is put in its original form, as below:

Lactation periods (in days) of cows in a farm

Lactation period (in days)	Number of cows
270 - 275	4
275 - 280	6
280 - 285	4
285 - 290	5
290 - 295	6
295 - 300	5
300 - 305	6
305 - 310	4

Array Method

An array is an orderly arrangement of the data by magnitude in ascending or descending order. Form the class interval as in the previous method. Then arrange the given data in ascending order of magnitude. From the array, we will count the number of observations belonging to each class and then we will write. This method is not easy when the number of observations is large.

2.6.2 Advantages of Presenting Data using Frequency Distribution

1. The data can be presented economically in a tabular form.
2. This form facilitates comparison of data.
3. It summarizes the collected data clearly.

2.6.3 Relative Frequency Distribution

The relative frequency is the fraction or proportion of the total number of items belonging to the class. It is obtained by dividing the frequency of each class by the total number of observations. That is, the relative frequency of a class is equal to the frequency of the class divided by the total number of observations, which is equal to the class frequency divided by the total frequency.

Classes	Tally marks	Frequency	Relative frequency
270 – 275	𝍷𝍷𝍷𝍷	4	4/40=0.100
275 - 280	𝍸𝍷	6	6/40=0.150
280 - 285	𝍷𝍷𝍷𝍷	4	4/40=0.100
285 - 290	𝍸	5	5/40=0.125
290 - 295	𝍸𝍷	6	6/40=0.150
295 - 300	𝍸	5	5/40=0.125
300 - 305	𝍸𝍷	6	6/40=0.150
305 - 310	𝍷𝍷𝍷𝍷	4	4/40=0.100
	Total	*40*	*1.000*

2.6.3.1 Percentage Frequency

Percentage frequency is calculated by multiplying the relative frequency by 100.

Classes	Tally marks	Frequency	Relative frequency	Percentage frequency (%)
270 – 275	𝍷𝍷𝍷𝍷	4	4/40=0.100	10.0
275 - 280	𝍸𝍷	6	6/40=0.150	15.0
280 - 285	𝍷𝍷𝍷𝍷	4	4/40=0.100	10.0
285 - 290	𝍸	5	5/40=0.125	12.5
290 - 295	𝍸𝍷	6	6/40=0.150	15.0
295 - 300	𝍸	5	5/40=0.125	12.5
300 - 305	𝍸𝍷	6	6/40=0.150	15.0
305 - 310	𝍷𝍷𝍷𝍷	4	4/40=0.100	10.0
	Total	*40*	*1.000*	*100.0 (%)*

2.6.3.2 Cumulative Frequency Distribution

A frequency distribution gives the number of observations lying in any class interval, whereas the cumulative frequency distribution gives the number of frequencies that lie below or above any mark. The total frequency of all classes less than the upper-class boundary of a given class is called the cumulative frequency of that class. A table showing the cumulative frequencies is called a cumulative frequency distribution. There are two types of cumulative frequency distributions:

Less than cumulative frequency distribution - It is obtained by adding successively the frequencies of all the previous classes including the class against which it is written. The cumulate is started from the lowest to the highest size.

More than cumulative frequency distribution - This is obtained by finding the cumulative total of frequencies starting from the highest to the lowest class.

The less than cumulative frequency distribution and more than cumulative frequency distribution for the frequency distribution are as below:

Class Limit	Frequency	Less than Cumulative Frequency		More than Cumulative Frequency	
		Marks	Cumulative Frequency	Marks	Cumulative Frequency
10-20	2	< 19.9	2	≥10	50
20-30	4	< 29.9	2+4=6	≥20	50-2=48
30-40	7	< 39.9	6+7=13	≥30	48-4=44
40-50	10	< 49.9	13+10=23	≥40	44-7=37
50-60	16	< 59.9	23+16=39	≥50	37-10=27
60-70	8	< 69.9	39+8=47	≥60	27-16=11
70-80	3	< 80.0	47+3=50	≥70	11-8=3
	50				

2.7 GRAPHICAL AND DIAGRAMMATIC PRESENTATION OF DATA

Data collected by the investigator are usually raw and less organized. To make them understandable, we present these data in three forms: tabular, graphic and diagrammatic. Classification and tabulation reduce the complexity of vast data, as we have seen in frequency distribution above. Still, it may not be easy to interpret even such classified and tabulated data. Hence, diagrams and graphs are drawn to present the data to make them more understandable.

2.7.1 Types of Graphs

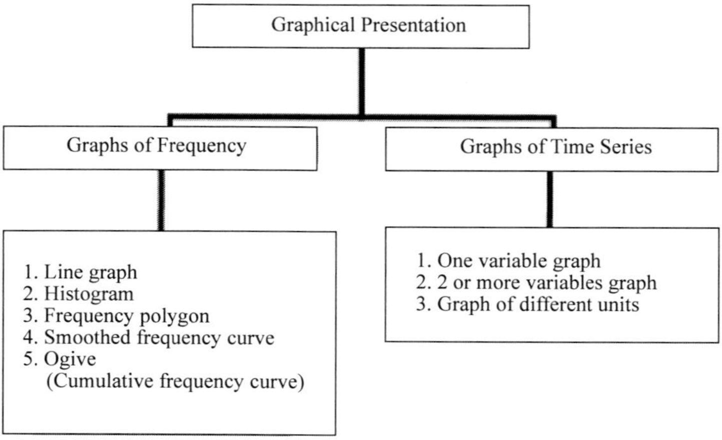

2.7.2 Types of Diagrams

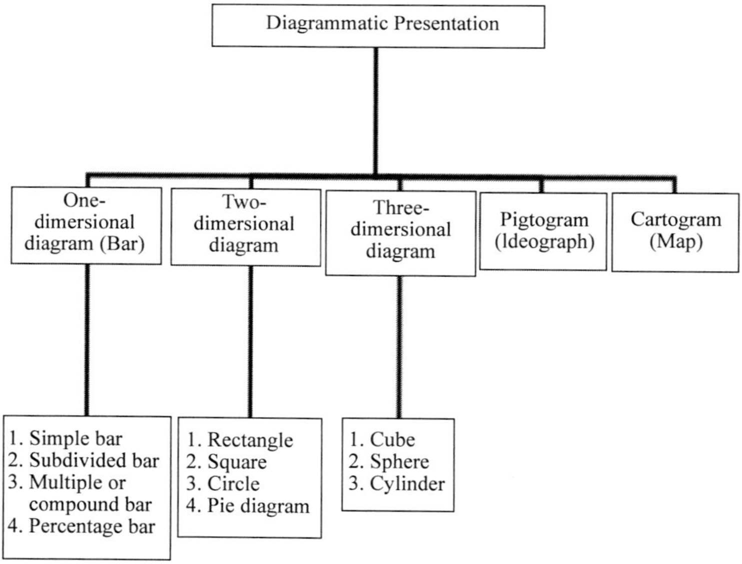

2.7.3 Advantages and Limitations of Diagrams and Graphs

Advantages

- Attract the attention of the viewers by creating a lasting impression
- Save time and space, by occupying less space than pages of numerical figures
- Facilitate the comparison of two or more sets of data more clearly

Limitations

- They are only approximate indicators.
- They fail to disclose small differences when large figures are involved.

2.7.4 Graphical Presentation of Data

A graph is a visual representation of numerical data. A graph consists of two lines: 1. A horizontal line called X axis, or Abscissa, to present the magnitudes of the independent variable, and 2. A vertical line called as Y axis, or Ordinate presents the magnitudes of the dependent variable. X and Y are perpendicular to each other. The point of intersection of X and Y is called the origin, represented by 0. Positive values of data are measured on the right side (from the origin) of the X axis and on the upper side (from the origin) of the Y axis. Similarly, negative values are measured on the left side (from the origin) of the X axis and on the lower side (from the origin) of the Y axis. The intersection of the X and Y axis divides the whole graph space into four parts called quadrants. The four quadrants are as below:

- Quadrant I: Upper right quadrant (on the north-east of the graph) where both X and Y values are positive;
- Quadrant II: Upper left quadrant (go anti-clockwise from I quadrant) where X value is negative and Y is positive;
- Quadrant III: Lower left quadrant (go anti-clockwise from II quadrant) where both X and Y values are negative; and
- Quadrant IV: Lower right quadrant (go anti-clockwise from III quadrant) where X value is positive and Y is negative.

II Quadrant (Negative X and Positive Y)	I Quadrant (Positive X and Y)
III Quadrant (Negative X and Y)	IV Quadrant (Positive X and Negative Y)

Essential steps required when drawing graphs

1. The scale for each axis should be selected in such a way that all data can be measured and marked on each axis.
2. Each axis must be labelled with the name of the variable to be measured on each axis.

2.7.4.1 Description of Types of Graphs

When the data are classified in the form of a frequency distribution, we can have the following graphical representations:

Line graph (Line diagram)

The variable is plotted on the X axis with its frequency on Y axis. This is the simplest of all the diagrammatic representations of data.

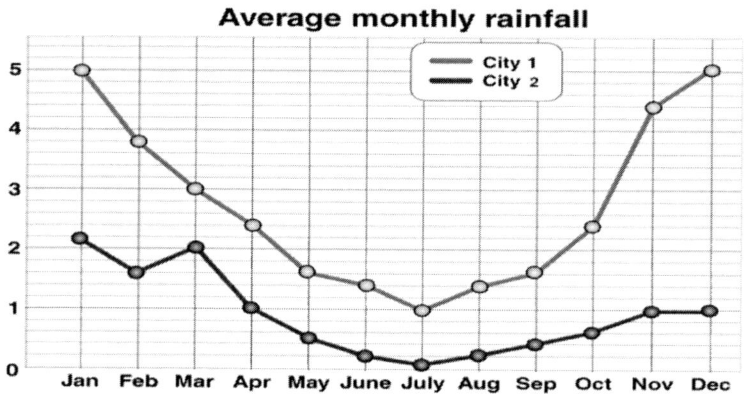

Histogram

A histogram is a graphical representation of continuous quantitative data in which the frequencies are represented as vertical bars. A histogram is constructed by marking off the class limits along the X axis and drawing a vertical rectangle, in a way that its height equals the frequency of that class, for each class interval. The vertical rectangles (called bars) in the histogram are usually drawn without gaps between the bars. The height of each bar serves as a measure of the corresponding frequency.

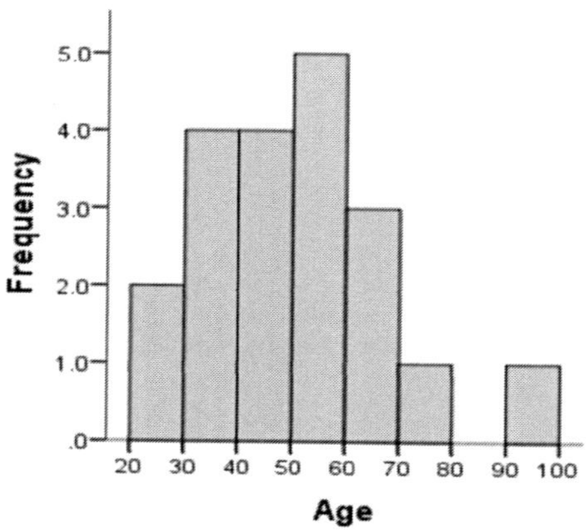

Frequency Polygon

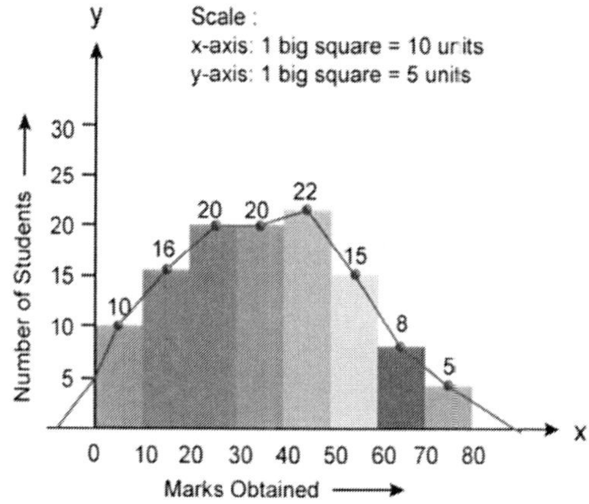

A frequency polygon is a line graph for the graphical representation of frequency distribution. The mid-point of each class interval is calculated and measured on x axis and the corresponding frequencies are plotted along y axis. Then these mid-points are joined by straight lines to give a frequency polygon. Though it is possible to connect the mid-points of the top of the bars in the histogram, the frequency polygon can be drawn directly by locating the mid-points. That is, while a histogram is a bar graph, a frequency polygon is a line graph.

Frequency Curve

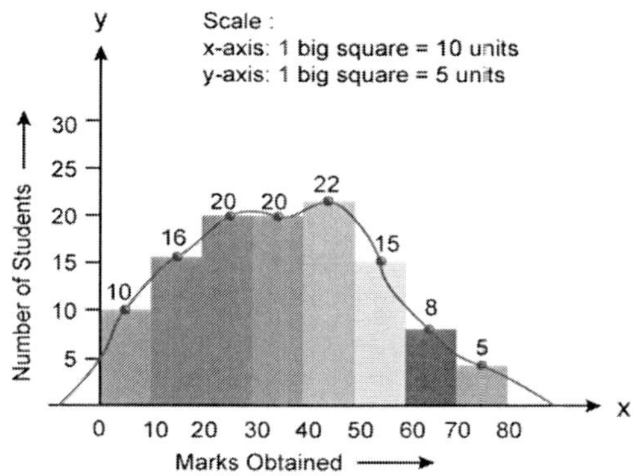

When the number of observations is large and / or the class intervals are of small widths, then the frequency curve may lose its angulations. The frequency curve is then obtained by joining the mid-points (of histogram / frequency polygon) by a freehand smoothed curve. Unlike a frequency polygon, where the points we joined by straight lines, we make use of free hand joining of those points to get a smoothed frequency curve.

Ogive (Cumulative Frequency Curve)

This curve is obtained by making use of cumulative frequency instead of the simple frequency. If we draw frequency polygons to the two cumulative distributions separately, we get two cumulative frequency polygons (less than & greater than). If we draw a frequency curve to the two cumulative distributions in the same graph, we would get a cumulative frequency curve or Ogive. The x co-ordinate of the point of intersection of less than and greater than cumulative frequency curve is the median.

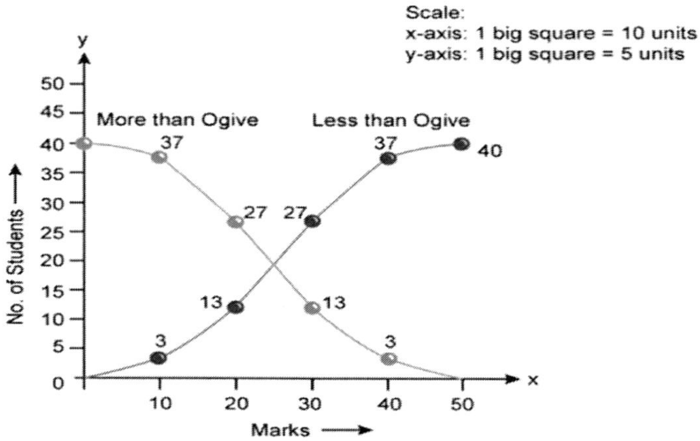

2.7.5 Diagrammatic Presentation of Data

If the data are presented by diagrams, the relation between the quantities can be easily illustrated, since a pictorial representation usually makes a clearer impression on the mind than the numbers in the tables.

Diagrams should have the following characteristics:

1. Simple to be understood.
2. Attractive and accurate.
3. Suitable heading on the top.
4. Proper scale to suit both the data and size of the paper.
5. Footnotes, if required, below the diagram to clarify important points.
6. Legend for identification of shades / colours used.

2.7.5.1 Types of Diagrams

One Dimensional Diagrams

One dimensional diagram is also called bar diagrams. It is one-dimensional, because the height of the bar is important and not the width of the bar. Following are the various types of bar diagrams:

1. **Simple Bar Diagram:** A simple bar diagram is used to represent only one variable. As one bar represents only one figure, there are as many bars as the number of figures. A simple bar diagram is drawn taking the following data:

Oxygen consumption in ml/kg/h in different months of the year in a species of rabbit

Months	Jan	Feb	Mar	Apr	May	Jun	Jul	Aug	Sep	Oct	Nov	Dec
Oxygen consumed	67	74	84	85	100	105	95	90	90	78	74	64

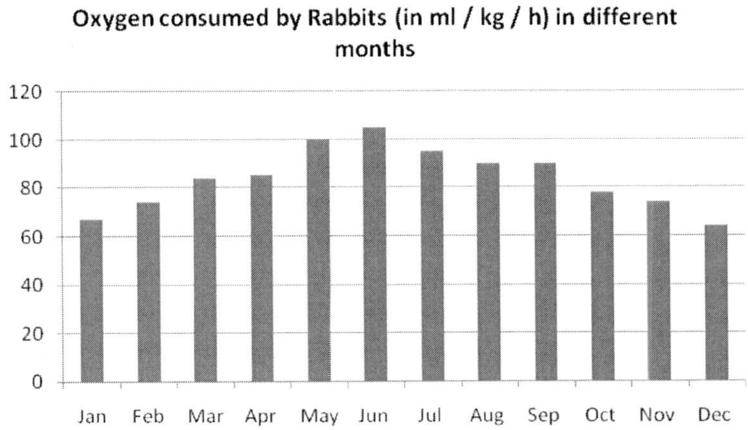

2. **Sub-divided Bar Diagram:** Here, the bars are sub-divided into different parts whose heights are proportional to the figures of different sub-divisions of items. If the animal population is subdivided into males and females, every bar representing the total population will be divided into two parts - one representing males and the other females.

Livestock Population in a Farm

Species	No. of females	No. of males	Total
Cattle	49	17	66
Buffalo	36	14	50
Sheep	20	12	32
Goat	14	8	22
Pig	13	6	19

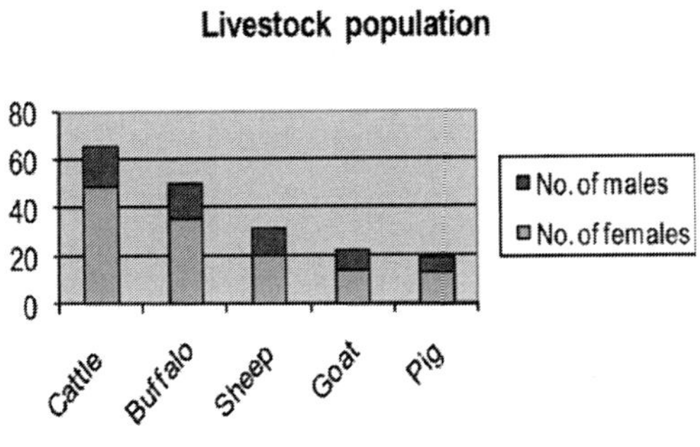

3. **Multiple or Compound Bar Diagram:** This diagram is used when we have to make a comparative study of the figures for different characters relating to different items. For example, in the above case, the bars

for two years may be compounded together. There will be one set of compound bars for each species.

Species	Comparison of Livestock Population in 2012 and 2019			
	Males		Females	
	2012	2019	2012	2019
Cattle	49	36	90	98
Buffalo	36	27	69	88
Sheep	20	18	48	56
Goat	14	15	67	79
Pig	13	8	28	41

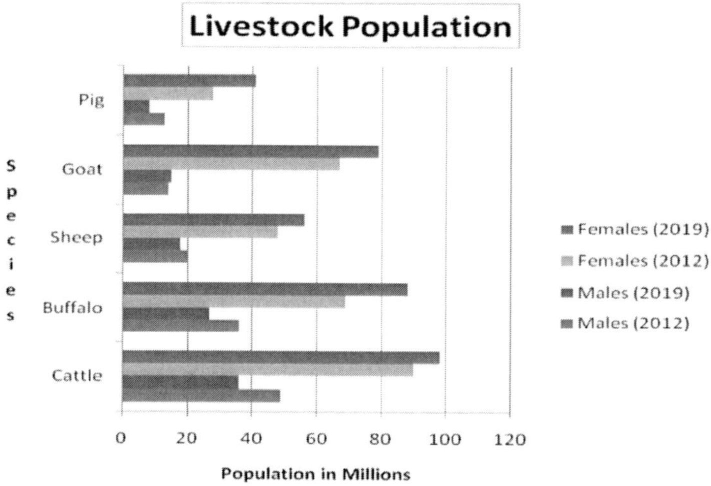

4. **Percentage Bar Diagram:** The length of the bar is kept equal to 100% and the divisions of the bar correspond to the percentage of different components.

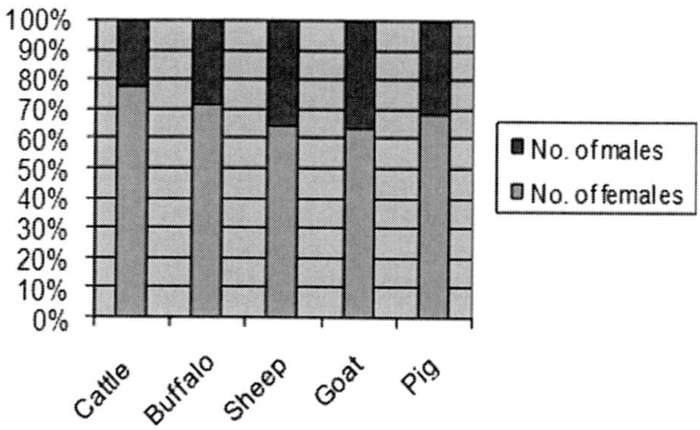

Two Dimensional Diagrams

In these diagrams, the areas, instead of lengths, are proportional to the given figures. The important diagrams of this type are:

1. **Rectangles:** When two quantities are proportional to a third quantity, one quantity is represented by length, the second is represented by the breadth and the third by the area of the rectangle.
2. **Squares:** Squares are used in place of a bar diagram when the ratio between the quantities is high. For example, if the ratio between two quantities is 25:1, the height of one bar will be 25 times the height of the other bar which is not easy to be managed in the limited space of the graph paper. In such a case, quantities are represented by squares whose areas are in the ratio 25:1, so that the sides of these squares will be in the ratio 5:1.

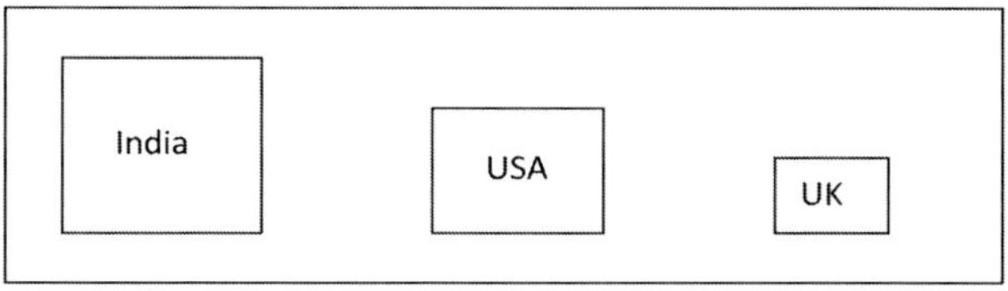

3. **Circular Diagram:** A circular diagram also serves the same purpose as a square. Here, the quantities are proportional to the areas of the circles or the squares of their radii.
4. **Pie chart:** A pie chart is a circle divided into different sectors according to the break-up of components given in percentage. The angles of sectors are proportional to the respective values of different components. As a circle represents an angle of 360^0 around the centre, 360^0 angle is divided in proportion to the percentages of different data.

Budget Outlay for the year 2023-24

Sector	Budget estimates (Million Rs)	Percentage of total	Equivalent angles
Agriculture and allied sectors	663	15.4	55.5
Cooperation	55	1.3	4.7
Irrigation and Power	2164	50.4	181.4
Industries and Mining	188	4.4	15.8
Transport and Equivalent	190	4.4	15.8
Social Services	1006	23.5	84.6
Miscellaneous	24	0.6	2.2
Total	**4290**	**100.0**	**360.0**

Percentages of budget estimates for different sectors are calculated as (663 / 4290) x 100 = 15.4; = (55 / 4290) x 100 = 1.3, etc. Angles equivalent to percentages are then calculated as (15.4 x 360) / 100 = 55.5, (1.3 x 360) / 100 = 4.7, etc. After calculating angles for other sectors also, the pie chart is drawn as below:

Budget estimates (Million Rs.)

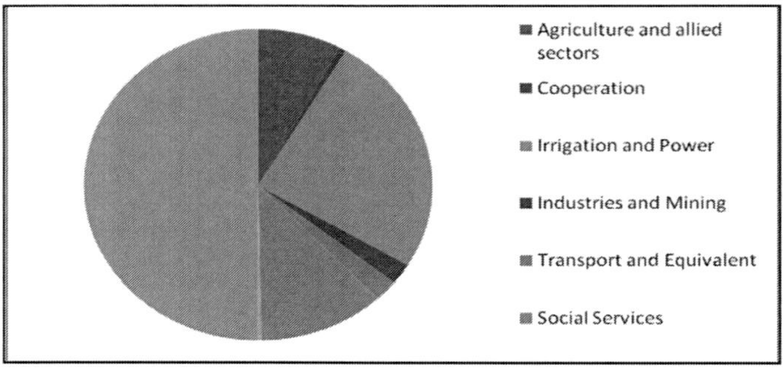

Three-Dimensional Diagrams

Cylinders, spheres, cubes, etc. are known as 3-dimensional diagrams, because 3 dimensions - length, breadth and width are used for representing figures. Unlike two-dimensional diagrams, the three diagrams have height or volume as the third dimension, which is the same as thickness or depth. Three-dimensional diagrams are used when the ratio between the highest and lowest measurements is more than 100:1. For constructing these diagrams, the cube roots of various measurements are calculated and the side of each cube is taken in proportion to the cube roots. For e.g., if the two quantities are very high (say, 125:1), the sides of the cubes will be in the ratio $(125)^{1/3}:1$, i.e., 5:1. The heights in the ratio will be in the ratio of $(125)^{1/3}:1$, i.e., 11.18:1. By convention, three dimensions are represented as spatial dimensions x, y and z, with width, height, and depth as their respective names. A cube, rectangular prism, sphere, cone, and cylinder are the basic three-dimensional figures.

Diagram	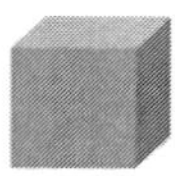	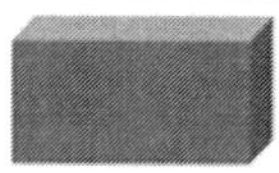	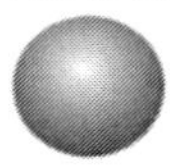	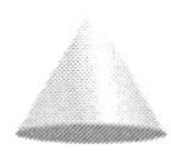	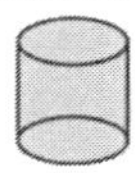
Name	Cube	Rectangular Prism or Cuboid	Sphere	Cone	Cylinder
Attributes	6 Faces, 12 Edges and 8 Vertices	6 Faces, 12 Edges and 8 Vertices	1 Curved face, 0 Edge and 0 Vertex	1 Flat face, 1 Curved face, 1 Edge and 1 Vertex	2 Flat faces, 1 Curved face, 2 Edges and 0 Vertex

Attributes of Three-Dimensional Shapes

There are three attributes of a three-dimensional figure: face, edge, and vertex.

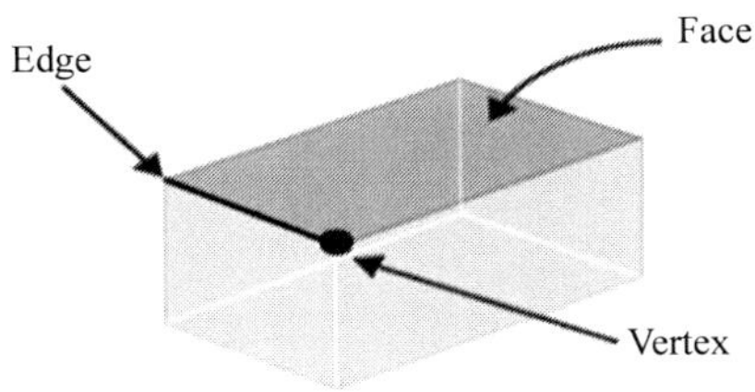

Face: Each single surface, flat or curved, of the 3D figure is called its face.

Edge: The line, where two faces of the 3D figures meet, is called its edge.

Vertex: Each corner, where three faces of 3D figures meet, is called its vertex.

Differences between a 2D Shape and a 3D Shape

2D Shape	3D Shape
A flat plane figure	A solid figure
Two dimensions - length and width	Three dimensions - length, width and height
No thickness	Thickness or depth
E.g., triangle, square, rectangle, circle	E.g., cube, cone, sphere

Pictograms

The technique of presenting data by pictures, called pictograms, has been on the rise in recent years. Pictograms are easily understood and they create a lasting impression in the mind. In pictograms, data are represented through a pictorial symbol e.g., picture of a cow or milk bottle for milk dairy, picture of a motor car for data relating to the automobile industry, etc. As pictograms are more attractive, they are used where the attention of the masses is to be drawn, such as exhibitions, fairs, etc. In a pictogram, a symbol represents a certain value and therefore there may be some difficulty in fractioning the symbol when fractions of the given value are to be represented.

Consumption of curd over the years

Year	Consumption of curd (Bottles)
2018	5,000
2019	9,000
2020	7,000
2021	8,000
2022	6,000

Consumption of curd per year (Scale: One bottle = 1000)

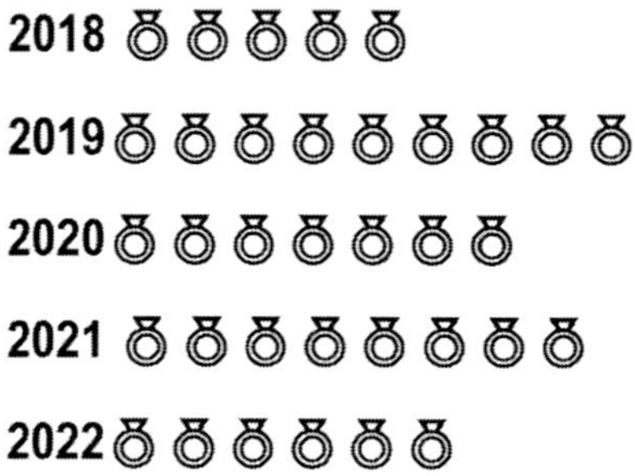

Cartograms or Maps

When numerical facts are shown in the form of maps, they are termed Cartograms. They are most suitable for geographical data. Values on a cartogram may be represented by different shades, colours, dots, lines, etc. They are used for showing rainfall, population, temperature, etc. in different parts of a region or country.

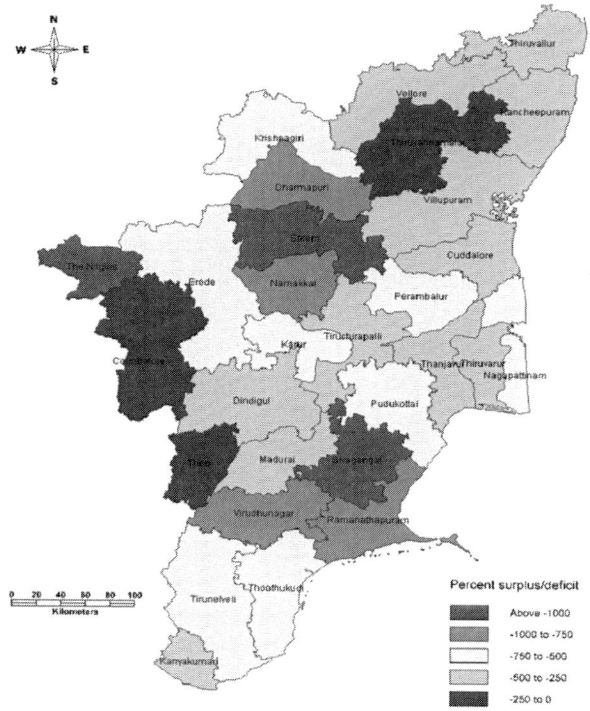

Map showing surplus and deficit districts about concentrate feed for livestock in Tamil Nadu, India

Limitations of Diagrammatic Presentation

1. Diagrams are not substitutes for tables, as minute details in data may be lost in a diagram.
2. Diagrams cannot show large data at a time, as they would become too complex.
3. Diagrams can show only approximate values. Precise differences, especially very small and very large differences between two sets of facts, are not possible in diagrams.
4. Diagrams, when not supported by tables, can misrepresent facts.
5. Diagrammatic presentation is more useful only for the layman, and not for the expert.

3

Measures of Central Tendency and Variability for Animal Health Studies

3.1 MEASURES OF CENTRAL TENDENCY (AVERAGES)

When data are presented in raw form or in the form of frequency distribution, they fail to provide a general idea of the data under study. The general idea of statistical methods is to condense the raw data into a form that can convey some meaningful characteristic(s) of the data. Though classification simplifies the data and improves the understanding of the main characteristics in the data, it is still difficult to remember. In any distribution of data, values of a variable may tend to cluster (or concentrate) around a central value. The data must be condensed into a single value. Such presentation of data is called a Central Tendency and the measures devised to consider this tendency are known as Measures of Central Tendency.

An average condenses a frequency distribution or raw data and presents it in a single representative number. It is that single value which is considered as the most representative or typical value for a set of values. Such a value usually lies somewhere near the centre of the group. That is why, an average is usually referred to as a measure of central tendency. It is located at a point around which most of the other values tend to cluster and therefore it is also termed as a measure of central location.

3.1.1 Objectives of Calculating Averages

1. To describe the distribution of data in a concise manner, i.e., to condense the mass of data into a single value to get an idea about the entire data distribution.
2. To compare two or more data distributions, i.e., when averages for two or more distributions are calculated, comparison becomes easy.
3. To compute other statistical measures, the computation of an average value is necessary and is the first step.

3.1.2 Types of Averages

The average is calculated by taking the values of all the items in the series into account. Mean is the mathematical average. The three main types of means or mathematical averages are 1. Arithmetic Mean (AM) or Mean or Average, 2. Geometric Mean (GM) and 3. Harmonic Mean (HM). Averages exhibited by their positions are called positional averages. The averages of position are 4. Median and 5. Mode.

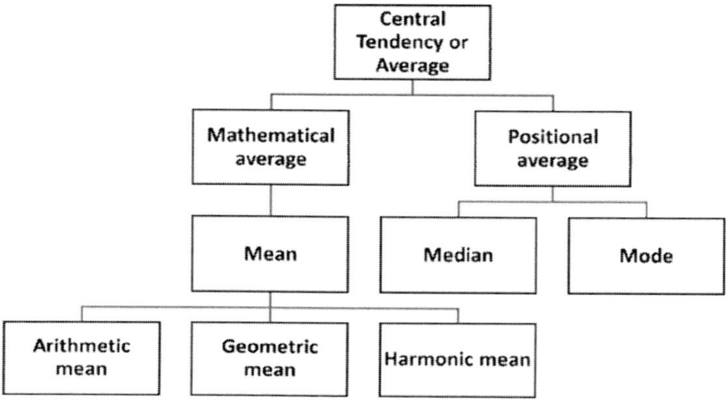

3.1.2.1 Arithmetic Mean (AM) or Mean or Average

The most popular and useful measure of central location is the arithmetic mean or simply, the mean. Commonly known as the average, it is the value obtained by dividing the sum of all the values of the given items (of a variable) by the number of items. Thus, *Mean = (Sum of values of the items / Total number of items).*

Summation Notation

Summation notation is used extensively in statistics. Consider 'n' observations $x_1, x_2, ..., x_n$, then the sum of the observations, $x_1 + x_2 + ... + x_n$ can be written using the symbol 'Σ' (Greek letter read as sigma, meaning 'sum of') as $x_1 + x_2 + \dots + x_n$. The letter i is called the index of summation. means the sum of x_i's, i taking values from 1 to n. We can write it as $x_1 + x_2 + \dots + x_n = \Sigma x$. Then, the notation $\Sigma f_i x_i = f_1 x_1 + f_2 x_2 + \dots + f_n x_n$ can be written as Σfx. It is usually denoted by.

For the 'n' no. of observations in a data series by $x_1, x_2, \dots, x_n$, the arithmetic mean or the sample mean is:

$$\bar{x} = \frac{1}{n}\sum_{i=1}^{n} x_i = \frac{1}{n}(x_1 + x_2 + \dots + x_n)$$

The population mean is expressed as:

$$\mu = \frac{1}{N}\sum_{i=1}^{N} x_i$$

$$\mu = \frac{1}{N}(x_1 + x_2 + ... + x_N)$$

where $\bar{x}$ is the sample mean, μ is the population mean, n is the number of observations in the sample and N is the number of observations in the population.

Arithmetic mean in case of frequency distribution

Let f_i be the frequency of the ith class and x_i be the mid value of the ith class, then, AM = $[f_1x_1 + f_2x_2 + \ldots + f_ix_i + \ldots + f_kx_k] / [f_1 + f_2 + \ldots + f_i + \ldots + f_k]$

$$\bar{x} = \frac{1}{N}\sum_{i=1}^{k} f_i x_i$$

$$\text{where } N = \sum_{i=1}^{k} f_i$$

Exercise

A coin is tossed 1024 times. The frequencies of heads are given below:

No. of heads	*0*	*1*	*2*	*3*	*4*	*5*	*6*	*7*	*8*	*9*	*10*
Frequency	*1*	*10*	*45*	*120*	*210*	*252*	*210*	*120*	*45*	*10*	*1*

Find the mean.

Solution

X	*0*	*1*	*2*	*3*	*4*	*5*	*6*	*7*	*8*	*9*	*10*	
f	*1*	*10*	*45*	*120*	*210*	*252*	*210*	*120*	*45*	*10*	*1*	*N = 1024*
fX	0	10	90	360	840	1260	1260	840	360	90	10	$\sum fX = 5120$

Mean $\bar{x} = \sum fX / N$

$= 5120/1024 = 5$

Short cut method

$$AM = A + \frac{1}{N}\sum_{i=1}^{k} f_i d_i C$$

$$\text{where } N = \sum_{i=1}^{k} f_i$$

A = Arbitrary Point (usually taken as the middle value of the middle-class interval)

di = (xi – A)/C

C = Class Interval

f_i = Frequency of ith class

x_i = Mid Value of ith class

Exercise

Find the arithmetic mean for the following grouped frequency distribution of birth weights of 50 adult male sheep:

Birth weight (Class)	1.8-2-0	2.0-2.2	2.2-2.4	2.4-2.6	2.6-2.8	2.8-3.0	3.0-3.2	3.2-3.4	3.4-3.6	3.6-3.8	3.8-4.0
No. of animals (Frequency i)	2	1	2	3	9	11	11	4	4	1	2

Solution

Classes	Mid Value (x_i)	f_i	f_ix_i	d_i	f_id_i
1.8 – 2.0	1.9	2	3.8	-0.20	-0.40
2.0 – 2.2	2.1	1	2.1	-0.16	-0.16
2.2 – 2.4	2.3	2	4.6	-0.12	-0.24
2.4 – 2.6	2.5	3	7.5	-0.08	-0.24
2.6 – 2.8	2.7	9	24.3	-0.04	-0.36
2.8 – 3.0	2.9	11	31.9	0.00	0.00
3.0 – 3.2	3.1	11	34.1	0.04	0.44
3.2 – 3.4	3.3	4	13.2	0.08	0.32
3.4 – 3.6	3.5	4	14.0	0.12	0.48
3.6 – 3.8	3.7	1	3.7	0.16	0.16
3.8 – 4.0	3.9	2	7.8	0.20	0.40
	Total	**50**	**147**		**0.40**

$$AM = [f_1x_1 + f_2x_2+\ldots+f_ix_i+\ldots+f_kx_k] / [f_1+f_2+\ldots+f_i+\ldots+f_k]$$
$$= 2(1.9) + 1(2.1) + 2(2.3) + 3(2.5) + 9(2.7) + 11(2.9) + 11(3.1) + 4(3.3) + 4(3.5) + 1(3.7) + 2(3.9)] / [2+1+2+3+9+11+11+4+4+1+2] = 147 / 50 = 2.94 \text{ Kg}$$

Combined mean

If $\bar{x}_1$ is the mean of the first group of n_1 items, $\bar{x}_2$ is the mean of the second group of n_2 items, then the combined mean of the two groups is $\dfrac{n_1 \bar{x}_1 + n_2 \bar{x}_2}{n_1 + n_2}$

$\bar{x}_1$ = (sum of all the observations in the first group) / n_1

$n_1\bar{x}_1$ = sum of all the observations in the first group

$\bar{x}_2$ = (sum of all the observations in the second group) / n_2

$n_2\bar{x}_2$ = sum of all the observations in the second group

$n_1\bar{x}_1+n_2\bar{x}_2$ = sum of all the observations in the two groups of size $n_1 + n_2$

Therefore $\bar{\bar{x}} = (n_1\bar{x}_1+n_2\bar{x}_2) / (n_1 + n_2)$

Extending the above result, if $\bar{x}_i$ is the mean of the ith group of n_i observations, then,

$$\bar{X} = A + \frac{\sum_{i-1}^{n} f_i d_i}{N} \times C \text{ and } \bar{X} = \frac{\sum n_i \bar{x}_i}{\sum n_i}$$

Exercise

There are two branches of a company which employ 280 and 320 persons, respectively. If the AM of the monthly salaries paid by the two companies is Rs.750 and Rs. 937.50 respectively, find the AM of the salaries of the employees of the companies as a whole.

Solution

$$\bar{X} = \frac{n_1\bar{x}_1 + n_2\bar{x}_2}{n_1 + n_2} = (280*750 + 320*937.50) / (280+320)$$

$$= (210000+300000)/600 = 510000/600 = \text{Rs.}850$$

Weighted arithmetic mean

In computing simple AM, it was assumed that all the items are of equal importance. This may not be always true. When items vary in importance, they must be assigned weight in proportion to their relative importance. Thus, a weighted mean is the mean of weighted items. In calculating weighted AM, each item is multiplied by its weight, and the products so derived are summed up. This total is divided by the total weights (and not by the number of items) to get the weighted mean.

Symbolically, if $x_1, x_2, \ldots, x_n$ are the different items with weights $w_1, w_2, \ldots, w_n$ respectively, then the weighted mean is given by

$$\bar{X}w = (W_1 X_1 + W_2 X_2 + \ldots + W_n X_n)/(W_1 + W_2 + \ldots + W_n) = (\Sigma W_i X_i)/(\Sigma W_i)$$

The AM of a grouped data is a weighted average of the class marks i.e. middle value of the class interval whose weights are the respective frequency. The weighted mean is a much better measure than the simple mean in cases when the items in a series are not equally important.

Exercise

Comment on the performance of the students of the three universities given below using simple and weighted averages:

Course	*University*					
	Chennai		*Mumbai*		*Kolkatta*	
	Pass %	*Students (in 100s)*	*Pass %*	*Students (in 100s)*	*Pass %*	*Students (in 100s)*
M.A.	*71*	*3*	*82*	*2*	*81*	*2*
M.Com.	*83*	*4*	*76*	*3*	*76*	*3.5*
B.A.	*73*	*5*	*73*	*6*	*74*	*4.5*
B.Com.	*74*	*2*	*76*	*7*	*58*	*2*
B.Sc.	*65*	*3*	*65*	*3*	*70*	*7*
M.Sc.	*66*	*3*	*60*	*7*	*73*	*2*

Solution

Course	**University**								
	Chennai			**Mumbai**			**Kolkatta**		
	Pass %	**Stu-dents (in 100s)**	**Weighted**	**Pass %**	**Stu-dents (in 100s)**	**Weighted**	**Pass %**	**Stu-dents (in 100s)**	**Weighted**
	X	**W**	**WX**	**X**	**W**	**WX**	**X**	**W**	**WX**
M.A.	71	3	213	82	2	164	81	2	162
M.Com.	83	4	332	76	3	228	76	3.5	266
B.A.	73	5	365	73	6	438	74	4.5	333
B.Com.	74	2	148	76	7	532	58	2	116
B.Sc.	65	3	195	65	3	195	70	7	490
M.Sc.	66	3	198	60	7	420	73	2	146
Σ	**432**	**20**	**1451**	**432**	**28**	**1977**	**432**	**21**	**1513**
Simple Mean	**432 / 6 = 72**			**432 / 6 = 72**			**432 / 6 = 72**		
Weighted Mean		**1451 / 20 = 72.55**			**1977 / 28 = 70.61**			**1513 / 21 = 72.05**	

From the above calculation, we know that the arithmetic mean is the same for all three universities, i.e., 72. But this is a wrong conclusion because what we should compare here is the weighted arithmetic mean. On comparing the weighted arithmetic means, we find that for Chennai University, the mean value is the highest. Hence, we can conclude that the performance of students is the best at Chennai University, among all three Universities.

Merits of Arithmetic Mean

a) **Certainty**: The arithmetic mean is rigidly defined. So, its value is always definite and certain. Mean can never be biased.

b) **Simplicity**: It is easy to calculate and simple to understand.

c) **Stability**: It is a stable measure, as it is least affected by fluctuations of sampling.

d) **Based on observations**: It is based on all the observations of a data series and therefore it is the most representative measure.

e) **Algebraic treatment**: it is capable of further algebraic treatment, as arithmetic mean is extensively used in statistical analysis.

f) **Basis of comparison**: it is the best measure for comparing two or more series of data.

g) **Balance**: Arithmetic mean balances the value on either side. The sum of the deviations of the items from the mean is equal to zero.

h) The product of the mean with the number of observations gives the total of the original data, i.e., $\Sigma x_i = n\,\bar{x}$.

Demerits of Arithmetic Mean

a) **Effect of extreme values**: Since it is calculated from all the values of the data series, it is greatly affected by extreme values (outliers). Hence, at times, it may not be a true representative value.

b) **Mean value may not appear in the series**: Mean sometimes does not appear in the data series. For e.g., the arithmetic mean of 4, 8, 15, and 21 is 12 is 12, but it is not present in the data series.

c) **Misleading conclusions**: Consider two series of data: 60, 70, and 80; 60, 30, and 120. Though the arithmetic means of both data series are 70, the mean will be misleading because the data series are different.

d) **Absurd mean values**: Sometimes the arithmetic mean may be absurd and unacceptable. E.g., we may get a mean of 2.7 children.

e) Arithmetic mean cannot be calculated for qualitative characteristics such as colours.

3.1.2.2 Geometric Mean (GM)

The geometric mean is the nth root of the product of 'n' items of a series of data. If $x_1, x_2, \ldots, x_n$ are the 'n' observations in a series, then GM is given by:

$$GM = \sqrt[n]{(x_1\, x_2 \ldots x_n)} = (x_1\, x_2 \ldots x_n)^{1/n}$$

Simplifying the above by taking logarithms on both sides,

$$\log GM = \log (x_1 x_2 \ldots x_n)^{1/n}$$

$$= 1/n (\log x_1 + \log x_2 + \ldots\ldots\ldots\ldots \log x_n)$$

$$= \frac{\sum \log x_i}{n}$$

Therefore, $GM = \text{antilog} \frac{\sum \log x_i}{n}$

Thus, the geometric mean is the antilogarithm of the arithmetic mean of the logarithmic values. The logarithm of the geometric mean is the arithmetic mean of logarithmic values.

Exercise

Calculate the geometric mean for the data - 50, 72, 54, 82, 93.

Solution

X	Log of X
50	1.6990
72	1.8573
54	1.7324
82	1.9138
93	1.9685
	∑Log X = 9.1710

Geometric mean $= \sqrt[5]{50 * 72 * 54 * 82 * 93}$

= Antilog (∑log X)N

= Antilog 9.1710/5

= Antilog 1.8342

= 68.26

In the case of a frequency distribution (grouped data), GM is given by GM = $(x_1^{f1}\, x_2^{f2} \ldots\, x_n^{fn})^{1/N}$ where N = Total frequency = Σf_i, where x_i is the midpoint of the class with frequency f_i. Simplifying by taking logarithm on both sides,

$$\log GM = 1/N \log (x_1^{f1}\, x_2^{f2} \ldots\, x_n^{fn})$$

$$= 1/N (f_1 \log x_1 + f_2 \log x_2 + \ldots + f_n \log x_n)$$

$$= \frac{\sum f_i \log x_i}{N}$$

Therefore, GM = antilog [$\sum f_i \log x_i$] / N

where xi is the mid value of the class whose frequency is f_i

Exercise

Compute the geometric mean for the following grouped data:

Marks	*0-10*	*10-20*	*20-30*	*30-40*	*40-50*
No. of students	*5*	*7*	*15*	*25*	*8*

Solution

Marks	Mid value X	Frequency f	Log X	f Log X
0-10	5	5	0.6990	3.4950
10-20	15	7	1.1761	8.2327
20-30	25	15	1.3979	20.9685
30-40	35	25	1.5441	38.6025
40-50	45	8	1.6532	13.2256
		N=60		**$\sum$f Log X = 84.5423**

Geometric mean = Antilog {($\sum$f Log X) / N}

= Antilog {(84.5243) / 60}

= Antilog 1.4087 = 25.63

Merits of Geometric Mean

a) GM, like AM, is based on all observations.

b) While AM is a bias for extremely higher values, GM is based on extremely lower values.

c) Like AM, GM is not affected much by fluctuations by sampling.

d) GM will be very useful in averaging ratios and percent rate of increase and decrease in values.

Demerits of Geometric Mean

a) Calculation of GM is highly mathematical and is not very easy to calculate.

b) GM will be zero if one or more of the values are zero.

3.1.2.3 Harmonic Mean (HM)

The harmonic mean is the reciprocal of the arithmetic mean of the given observations. It is the total number of items of a variable divided by the sum of the reciprocals of the items. If $x_1, x_2, \ldots, x_n$ are the 'n' observations, then harmonic mean (HM) is,

$$HM = n/ (1/x_1 + 1/x_2 + ... + 1/x_n) = n/ \sum 1/x_i$$

$$\frac{1}{\frac{\sum_{i=1}^{n}\frac{1}{x_i}}{n}} = \frac{1}{\text{A.M. of the reciprocals}}$$

Exercise

The monthly incomes (Rs.) of 10 families in a village are as follows:

Family	*1*	*2*	*3*	*4*	*5*	*6*	*7*	*8*	*9*	*10*
Income	*85*	*70*	*10*	*75*	*500*	*8*	*42*	*250*	*40*	*36*

Calculate the Harmonic mean.

Solution

Family	1	2	3	4	5	6	7	8	9	10	**∑1/X = 0.3469**
Income (X)	85	70	10	75	500	8	42	250	40	36	
Recip-rocal (1/X)	0.0117	0.0142	0.1	0.0133	0.002	0.125	0.0238	0.004	0.025	0.0277	

Harmonic mean = N / ∑1/X = 10/0.3469 = **Rs.28.82**

In another way, HM = 1 / AM of reciprocals = 1 / (0.3469/10) = 1 / 0.03469 = **Rs.28.82**

In the case of a frequency distribution, HM is obtained by using the formula,

$$\text{Harmonic Mean} = \frac{f_1 + f_2 + ... + f_n}{f_1/x_1 + f_2/x_2 + ... + f_n/x_n}$$

$$= N/ [\sum f_i / x_i]$$

where x_i is the mid value of the class whose frequency is f_i, and N is the total frequency.

Exercise

Find the HM for the grouped data given below:

Class	*15-25*	*25-35*	*35-45*	*45-55*	*55-65*	*65-75*
Frequency	*4*	*11*	*19*	*14*	*0*	*2*

Solution

Class	Frequency f	Midpoint X	1/X	f * 1/X
15-25	*4*	*20*	*0.0500*	*0.2000*
25-35	11	30	0.0333	0.3663
35-45	19	40	0.0250	0.4750
45-55	14	50	0.0200	0.2800
55-65	0	60	0.0166	0.0000
65-75	2	70	0.0148	0.0286
	N=50			∑(f*1/X) = 1.3499

Harmonic mean = N / ∑(f*1/X) = 50/1.3499 = 37.0398 = **37.04**

Merits of Harmonic Mean

a) HM, like AM, based on all observations.

b) As reciprocals are involved, HM gives greater weightage to smaller observations.

c) Like AM, GM is not affected much by fluctuations by sampling.

Demerits of Harmonic Mean

a) It is difficult to calculate.

b) HM cannot be calculated if any of the observation(s) is (are) zero.

3.1.2.4 Median

The median is defined as the value of the variable which has got an equal number of observations on either side, when the variables are arranged in the ascending or descending order of magnitude. In other words, if the values of a variable are arranged in ascending or descending order, the median is that value that divides the whole data into two equal parts, one having values greater than the median value and the other having values lesser than the median. That is, the median is the value of the middle observation or the mean value of two middle observations. There are two cases for which we can calculate the median.

Case (a): *When 'n' is odd:*

Arrange the observations in ascending order of magnitude and the value of $(n+1)/2^{th}$ observation is the median. E.g., Find the median of body weight of adult male sheep: 52, 58, 65, 70, 65, 55, 74, 68, and 75.

Here n = 9 (odd). Arrange the body weight in ascending order of magnitude as 52, 55, 58, 65, 65, 68, 70, 74, and 75. The Median term = $(n+1)/2^{th}$ term in the array. i.e. $(9+1) / 2^{th}$ term = 5th term in the array. Therefore, Median = 65 Kg (5th term in the array).

Case (b): *When n is even:*

Arrange the observations in ascending order of magnitude and the average value of the $(n/2)^{th}$ and $[n/(2+1)]^{th}$ terms gives the median. E.g. Find the median value of the data series: 52, 58, 65, 70, 65, 55, 74, 68, 75, and 80. Arrange data in ascending order of magnitude: 52, 55, 58, 65, 65, 68, 70, 74, 75, and 80. Here, n = 10 (even).

Hence, Median = average of $(n/2)^{th}$ and $[n/(2+1)]^{th}$ terms in the array

= average of $(10/2)^{th}$ and $[10/(2+1)]^{th}$ terms in the array

= average of 5 and 6th terms in the array

= (65 + 68)/2 = 133/2 = 66.5

In the case of frequency distribution, the median is the value of the variate, which has got an equal number of frequencies on either side (i.e., which correspond to cumulative frequency of N/2), when the variates are arranged in ascending or descending order of magnitude. The class corresponding to the cumulative frequency just greater than N/2 is called the median class.

Median = l + c (N/2–m) / f

where l = Lower limit of the median class

f = Frequency of the median class

c = Class interval

m = Cumulative frequency of the class preceding the median class

N = Total frequency

The median class is the class whose cumulative frequency just exceeds N/2.

Exercise

Find the median for the following frequency distribution of birth weights:

Classes (Birth weight)	*Frequency (fi)*	*Cumulative Frequency*
1.8 – 2.0	2	2
2.0 – 2.2	1	3
2.2 – 2.4	2	5
2.4 – 2.6	3	8
2.6 – 2.8	9	17
2.8 – 3.0	11	26
3.0 – 3.2	11	39
3.2 – 3.4	4	43
3.4 – 3.6	4	47
3.6 – 3.8	1	48
3.8 – 4.0	2	50
Total	50	

Solution

Median class = the class whose cumulative frequency just exceeds N/2

= the class whose cumulative frequency just exceeds 50/2, i.e.25

= 2.8 – 3.0 i.e., l =2.8; c = 0.2; f = 11; N/2 = 50/2 = 25; m = 17

Median = l + c (N/2–m) / f = 2.8+0.2(25–17)/11 = 2.945 Kg

Merits of Median

a) It is rigidly defined.

b) It is easy to understand and easy to calculate.

c) It is not affected by the extreme values.

d) It is the best for the qualitative data.

Demerits of Median

a) Median is relatively less stable than mean, as it is affected by fluctuations of sampling.

b) It cannot be subjected to algebraic treatment.

3.1.2.5 Mode

Mode is defined as the value of the variable, which occurs most frequently. E.g. Find the mode for the body weights: 52, 58, 65, 70, 65, 55, 74, 68, 75, and 80. Mode = 65 Kg.

If the data are ungrouped with the ungrouped frequency distribution:

Value of the variable	52	55	58	**65**	68	70	74	75	80
Frequency	1	1	1	**2**	1	1	1	1	1

Mode = 65 Kg.

For grouped frequency distribution, Mode = l + (f2 / f1 + f2) c

where l = lower limit of the model class, f1 = frequency of the class which precedes (comes after) the modal class, f2 = frequency of the class which succeeds (comes after) the modal class, c = class interval

Model Class is the class which is having the maximum frequency.

Exercise

Calculate the mode for the following frequency distribution:

Classes (birth weight)	*Frequency (fi)*
1.8 – 2.0	*2*
2.0 – 2.2	*1*
2.2 – 2.4	*2*
2.4 – 2.6	*3*

2.6 – 2.8	*9*
2.8 – 3.0	*12*
3.0 – 3.2	*10*
3.2 – 3.4	*4*
3.4 – 3.6	*4*
3.6 – 3.8	*1*
3.8 – 4.0	*2*
Total	*50*

Solution

Modal class: 2.8 – 3.0

l = 2.8; f1 = 9; f2 = 10; c = 0.2

Mode = 2.8 + (10/19) (0.2) = 2.905 Kg

Distributions with two peaks (equal or unequal in height) are called bimodal and those with more than two peaks are multimodal. In those rare distributions that are U – shaped, we refer to the low point at the middle of the distribution as an anti-mode.

Merits of Mode

- The mode is easy to calculate and understand.
- It is not affected by extreme observations and hence preferred over arithmetic mean, while dealing with extreme values.

Demerits of Mode

- Mode is not rigidly defined.
- It is affected by the fluctuations of sampling.
- It is not suitable for algebraic treatment.

3.1.3 Choice of an Average

The selection of a good average among the average measures of AM, GM, HM, Median, and Mode is not an easy task, as it is to be done with due consideration to the nature and type of data and the objective of statistical investigation. No single average can be good for all purposes, as different forms of averages have different characteristics. All the averages suffer a few limitations, despite their advantages. Thus, in selecting an average, the advantages and limitations of the averages need to be considered.

An ideal average should possess the following qualities:

1. Rigidly defined.
2. Based on all observations.

3. Be simple to understand and easy to calculate.
4. Have a minimum influence of extreme values.
5. Possesses sampling stability.
6. Be capable of further algebraic treatment.
5. Not affected by open-end classes.

The qualities essential for a good average are satisfied in varying degrees by different measures of central tendency. AM possesses the above properties more than other type of averages. Thus, AM is the most popular measure. Hence it is called the common average. Though the median and mode are more easily computed than others, they are indeterminate in many cases and are not capable of algebraic manipulations.

3.1.4 Situations where different Averages are used

- AM is applicable to all sorts of data. It should be used when the distribution is reasonably symmetrical, further statistical analysis such as computation of standard deviation is to be carried out subsequently.
- GM is used when it is desired to give more weight to small items and less weight to large items and is more useful in the case of ratios, percentages, and microorganisms.
- HM is used in averaging certain types of ratios and rates and problems involving time. It also gives more weight to small items.
- The median is to be used when the attributes of the data are not directly measurable. As it can be easily located by mere inspection, it can be calculated even when the data are incomplete. The median is used when the distribution is highly skewed and the extreme items have distorting effects on the mean.
- Mode can be used to know the most typical value or the most common item. It is also used when the quickest estimate of centrality is required.

3.1.5 Properties of Means

- AM > GM > HM or HM < GM < AM.
- When all the values are equal, AM = GM = HM.
  i. In a symmetrical distribution, mean (AM) = median = mode.
  ii. In a positively skewed distribution, mean (AM) > median > mode (short tail on the left)
  iii. In a negatively skewed distribution, mean (AM) < median < mode (short tail on right)
  iv. If a distribution is moderately asymmetrical then, mode = 3 median – 2 mean (appr.)

3.2 MEASURES OF VARIABILITY (MEASURES OF DISPERSION)

The measures of central tendency indicate only the central position of the data series. However, they may sometimes offer misleading results. E.g., Consider the following three data series.

Data series	Data	Mean
A	50, 50, 50, 50	50
B	50, 56, 48, 42, 43, 59, 52	50
C	1, 29, 120	50

All three data series have the same mean of 50. Just because the mean is the same, we cannot conclude that these data series are similar. However, the distributions in these three data series differ greatly from one another. In the first one, the values are closely packed and hence they have no variation. However, in the other two series, the data are scattered and hence show variation. The variation in data is called a scatter, spread, deviation, or dispersion. These data types with the same mean, but with varying spread indicate that an average will be meaningful only when it is provided with dispersion. The measurement of scattering of items about the average is called a measure of variation or dispersion. Variation may be more (as in series C) or less (as in series A). A measure of dispersion enables the comparison of two or more distributions about their variability or consistency and presents the deviation of individual observations around the central value in a data series.

3.2.1 Dispersion – Meaning and Measures

The measure of variation or dispersion is an important tool in biostatistical studies, as biological phenomena are more variable than physical or chemical phenomena. We need to measure dispersion 1. to determine the reliability of a central tendency calculated, 2. to serve as a basis for control of the variability, and 3. to compare two or more series of data concerning their variability.

3.2.1.1 Absolute and Relative Dispersions

When dispersion is expressed in terms of original units of series, for e.g., weight in kgs, income in rupees, etc., it is called absolute dispersion. If it is expressed in terms of a pure number, free from units of measurement, then the dispersion is relative. A relative measure of dispersion is the absolute measure of dispersion divided by an average.

3.2.1.2 Different Measures of Dispersion

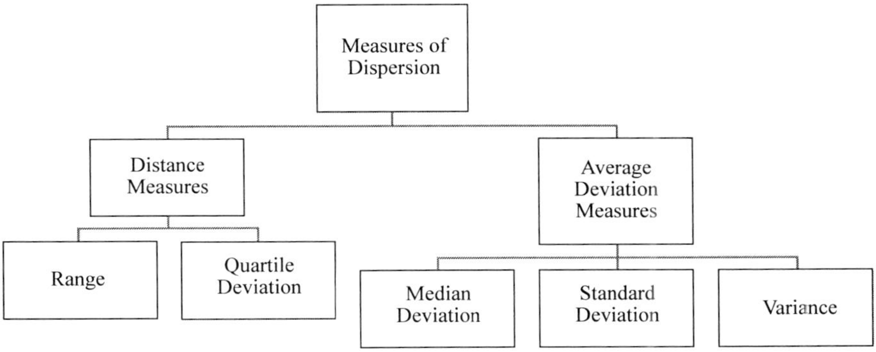

1. Range

It is the difference between the highest and lowest values in the data series. For the grouped data, the range is the difference between the lower limit of the first class and the upper limit of the last class. It is a very simple measure of dispersion. It is useful in the study of variations in money rates and rates of exchange, weather forecasts, etc. The relative measure of dispersion for range (or Co-efficient of Range) is the ratio of range.

2. Quartile Deviation (QD)

It is also known as the semi-interquartile range. It is a measure of distance, a better measure than range. It is based on quartiles (points) which divide the data into four equal parts or quarters. We define the first quartile Q_1, to be the value of the variate so that one-quarter of the observations lie below Q_1. Similarly, we define the third quartile Q_3, to be the value of the variate so that three-quarters of the observations lie below Q_3. Thus, if M (Q2) is the Median; then Q_1, M, and Q_3 divide the data distribution into four equal parts. Q_1, Q_2, and Q_3 are three quartiles that divide the data distribution into four equal parts. Each part contains 1/4th of the total observations in the distribution.

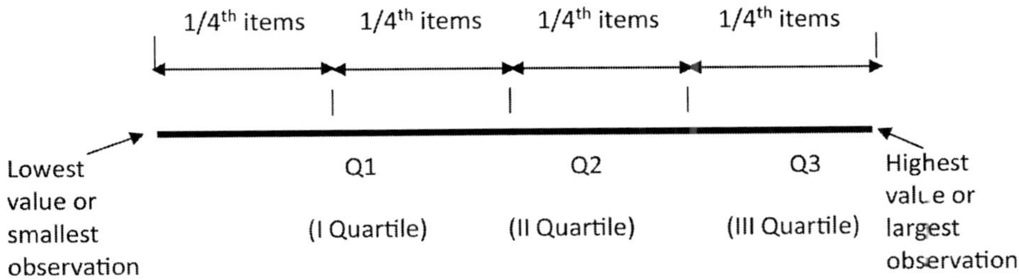

The lower or first quartile (Q_1) divides the lower half of the distribution into two equal parts, i.e., it is the value below which 25% of the observations lie and above which 75% of the observations lie. Similarly, the upper or third quartile (Q_3) divides the upper half of the distribution into two equal parts, i.e., it is the value below which 75% of the observations lie and above which 25% of the observations lie. The difference, Q_3–Q_1, is called the inter-quartile range and Quartile Deviation (QD) is given by (Q_3–Q_1)/2. QD is the distance between two values that cover the middle half of the distribution. QD is used in the case of open-end distribution. In raw data, after arranging the data in ascending order,

Q1 = Size of the [(n+1) / 4]th term

Q3 = Size of 3 [(n+1) / 4]th term

Then,

QD = (Q_3 - Q1) / 2

where Q_3 is the value of 3rd quartile or 3/4th of a range of variable or 75th percentile; and Q_1 is the value of 1st quartile or 1/4th of a range of variable or 25th percentile

In grouped data, Q_1 is the value that corresponds to the cumulative frequency of N * ¼ and Q_3 is the value that corresponds to the frequency of N * ¾. In the case of frequency distribution or grouped data,

$$Q_1 = L_1 + \frac{(N/4 - m_1)xc}{f_1}$$

where L_1 is the lower boundary of the first quartile class, m_1 is the cumulative frequency up to the first quartile class, f_1 is the frequency in the first quartile class; and c is the width of the class interval

$$Q_3 = L_3 + \frac{(3N/4 - m_3)xc}{f_3}$$

where L_3 is the lower boundary of the third quartile class, m_3 is the cumulative frequency up to third quartile class, f_3 is frequency in the third quartile class and; c is the width of the class interval

Then, QD = (Q_3 - Q_1) / 2

A relative measure of QD, also known as the Quartile Coefficient of Dispersion (QC) or Coefficient of Quartile Deviation is [(Q3-Q1)/2] / [(Q3+Q1)/2].

Important Points

- The second quartile (Q_2) is the median.
- Q_1, Q_2, Q_3 are three quartiles that divide the series into 4 equal parts.
- We can have 9 deciles to divide the entire range into 10 equal parts and they are denoted by D_1, D_2, …, D_9.

- We can have 99 percentiles to divide the entire range into 100 equal parts and they are denoted by P_1, P_2, ..., P_{99}.
- In a symmetrical distribution, $Q_3 + Q_1$ = Median / 2, and therefore, QC of dispersion is equal to 2 (Q_3 - Q_1) / Median.

3. Mean Deviation (MD)

Every value of the variable differs from the sample mean by some value which is called its deviation. This deviation (d) of an observation (X) is given by d = $X_i - \overline{X}$. Mean deviation is defined as the mean of all the deviations from the average (mean, median, or mode) of the data series. If the deviation is greater than the mean, the deviation is positive. If it is less than the mean, the deviation is negative. The deviation is calculated by adding the deviation of individual observations from their arithmetic mean without regard to their sign and dividing the sum by the number of observations. If X_1, X_2, ..., X_n are n observations, then Mean Deviation (from AM) = $1/n \sum | X_i - \overline{X} |$.

i.e., Forraw data, MD about mean $= \sum \left| \frac{x_1 - \overline{x}}{n} \right|$.

The symbol | | is read as mod, which represents modulus. The modulus refers to only the number, ignoring the + and - signs. For grouped data, the mean deviation about an average $\frac{\sum |fd|}{\sum f}$ where $\sum |fd|$ is where is the sum of the product of each frequency and deviation from the mean and is the sum of all frequencies. The relative measure of Mean Deviation is known as the mean coefficient of dispersion or coefficient of mean deviation and is obtained by dividing the MD by the average from which it is computed. Also,

Coefficient of MD about an average A = [MD about an average A] / A

Coefficient of MD about an average A (in %) = {[MD about an average A] / A} * 100

Usually, MD is calculated either from the mean or median, and mode is not used, as its value is indeterminate. Again, the median is preferred to the mean, because the mean deviation from the median is minimum.

4. Standard Deviation (SD)

Standard deviation is the positive square root of the arithmetic mean of the squares of deviations of various items from the mean of the data series. The standard deviation of the population is denoted by the Greek symbol `σ' (sigma), while the standard deviation of the sample is denoted by 's'. It is the widely used measure of dispersion, as it is an improved method over MD. SD is

$$\sqrt{\frac{\sum_{i-1}^{n}(x_i-\overline{x})^2}{n}} \text{ for raw data}$$

For grouped data,

$$\sigma = \sqrt{\frac{\sum_{i-1}^{n} fi(x_1-\overline{x})^2}{N}}$$

where x_i is the mid value of the class interval whose frequency is f_i and N is the total frequency.

Simplifying the above,

$$\sigma = \sqrt{\frac{\sum x_1^2}{n} - \left\{\frac{\sum x_1}{n}\right\}^2}$$

$$\sigma = \sqrt{\text{Mean of the squared values} - \text{Square ofthe mean for groupted data}}$$

$$\sigma = \sqrt{\frac{\sum f_i x_i^2}{N} - \left\{\frac{\sum f_i x_i}{N}\right\}^2}$$

Short-cut method (No need to calculate mean)

$$\text{Put } d_i = \frac{x_i - A,}{c}, \text{then } \sigma = c \times \sqrt{\frac{\sum f_i d_i^2}{N} - \left\{\frac{\sum f_i d_i}{N}\right\}^2}$$

Shephard's Correction

In computing the standard deviation, sometimes grouping errors may occur on account of grouping of data into different classes. For statistical adjustment of this grouping error, Shephard has suggested a correction value to be deducted from the SD of the grouped data, which is given by:

$$\frac{C^2}{12} = \frac{\text{square of width of class interval}}{12}$$

$$\text{Hence, corrected S.D.} = \sqrt{\frac{\sum f_i x_i^2}{N} - \left\{\frac{\sum f_i x_i}{N}\right\}^2 - \frac{C^2}{12}}$$

5. Variance

Variance is the square of standard deviation. It is also called mean square deviation. It is the mean of the squares of the sum of deviations from the mean value of data, divided by the number of observations. Population variance is denoted by σ^2, while sample variance is denoted by s^2.

$$\text{Variance} = \sigma^2 = \frac{1}{n}\sum(X-\bar{X})^2$$

The limitation of the mean deviation for negative values is overcome by squaring the deviations. To avoid any further errors due to the biased estimates, n – 1 degrees of freedom are used for the small number of values (<30), instead of values as such.

$$\text{Variance} = \sigma^2 = \frac{1}{n-1}\sum(X-\bar{X})^2$$

A form suitable for easy computation is = $\text{Variance} = \sigma^2 = \frac{1}{n-1}\left[\sum X^2 - (\sum X)^2\right]$

Coefficient of Variation (CV)

It is a measure of relative dispersion. It gives an idea about the extent to which variates are scattered around their central value. Therefore, two distributions having the same central values can be compared directly with the help of various measures of dispersion. When we calculate SDs for two data sets having different means, the SD alone does not give a correct idea about the extent of variability in the two data sets. Hence, a relative measure of standard deviation, known as the coefficient of variation (CV or COV), is calculated. CV is computed by dividing the mean from SD. This is also called the coefficient of standard deviation. Therefore, CV = SD / Mean. The CV is sometimes multiplied by 100 and reported as a percentage, which effectively expresses SD as a percentage of the mean. Thus, CV is the percentage variation from the mean. Higher CV indicates greater variability and less CV implies better consistency of data.

Standard Error (SE)

When more than one sample are drawn from a population, the SD for each mean may differ slightly. Theoretically, the mean of different samples drawn from the same population must be the same or very close to each other, so that the single sample is a reliable true measure of the population. However, this may not be so in actual situations, and means of different samples show variations. That is, the mean of a random sample may not be the same as the population mean. This difference between the sample mean and population mean is actually due to sampling and hence it is called sampling error or standard error of the mean. Standard error is a measure of chance or random variation and is not an error or mistake. Theoretically, the difference between means of the sample should be zero. However, in biological experiments, standard error may never be zero. The standard error (SE) is the square root of the variance of the sampling distribution, and hence given as:

$$SE = \sqrt{\sigma^2 / n} = \frac{\sigma}{\sqrt{n}}$$

where n is the size of the sample, σ^2 is the variance and σ is the SD of the sample.

SE indicates that the variation in the sample mean can be decreased by increasing the sample size (n).

Degrees of Freedom

The degrees of freedom are the number of values in a set of data, which are unrestricted, independent, and free to move or vary. For e.g., if there are 3 values A, B and C having a mean of 9, then (A+B+C) / 3 = 9. In this case, values of A and B may vary, but once they are fixed, for e.g., as A = 8 and B = 9, then the value of C has to be 10 to satisfy the mean. So, we can say that 3 numbers have 2 degrees of freedom. Hence, degrees of freedom are normally expressed as n-1 (unless specified).

Most of the statistical work in biology is carried out by taking a small sample from a large population. The inferences are then extrapolated to the whole population and generalized. However, in actuality, the statistical measures of the sample may differ from their population. The population statistics are in most cases unknown. Therefore, we have to rely only on sample statistics. It is possible to some extent to overcome this situation by using n-1 degrees of freedom rather than using the total number (n). The following table presents different degrees of freedom for various statistical tests:

Tests	***df***	**Details**
ANOVA: Mean Sum of Squares Within	N - k	n - total number of all data points; k - number of groups
ANOVA: Mean Sum of Squares Between	k - 1	
Chi-square (χ^2)	n - 1	n - sample size
Chi-square (χ^2) test for Goodness of Fit	k - 1	k - number of categories
Chi-square (χ^2) test for Independence	(r – 1) (c – 1)	r - number of rows c - number of columns
Chi-square (χ^2) test for Variance	n - 1	N - sample size
F test	n1 – 1 and n2 - 1	n1 and n2 - sizes of samples
t-test	n - 1	n - sample size
1 sample t-test, and paired t-test	n - 1	
2 (independent) sample t-test	d1 + n2 - 2	n1 and n2 - sizes of samples

Exercises

1. *The weight (in kg) of 10 goats are 16, 13, 14, 12, 17, 12, 14, 15 18 and 11. Find the range, Quartile deviation, mean deviation, standard deviation, and its relative measures of dispersion. Also, find variance and standard error.*

Solution

Arranging the data in ascending order, we get 11, 12, 12, 13, 14, 14, 15, 16, 17, 18

Range = H–L = 18-11 = 7 kg

Ratio of range = (H-L)*100 / (H+L) = (18-11) x 100 / (18+11) = (7x100)/29 = 24.14

Quartile deviation = $(Q_3-Q_1) / 2$

Q_1 = Size of ¼ (n+1)th observation = (10+1)/4 = 2.75th item = 12

Q_3 = Size of ¾ (n+1)th observation = 3(10+1)/4 = 8.25th item = 16

Quartile deviation = $(Q_3-Q_1)/2$ = (16-12)/2 = 4/2 = 2 kg

Quartile coefficient of dispersion = $(Q_3-Q_1)*100/(Q_{3+}Q_1)$ = (16-12)*100 / (16+12) = 400/28 = 14.29

Mean Deviation = 1/n ∑ |xi – Z|

xi	|xi- Z|	| xi- Z|^2
16	1.8	3.24
13	1.2	1.44
14	0.2	0.04
12	2.2	4.84
17	2.8	7.84
12	2.2	4.84
14	0.2	0.04
15	0.8	0.64
18	3.8	14.44
11	3.2	10.24
142	**18.4**	**47.60**

Z= 142/10 =14.2 kg

Mean Deviation = 1/n ∑ |xi – Z| = 1/10 * = 18.4 =1.84 kg

Mean Coefficient of Dispersion = (MD)*100/Z = (1.84*100)/14.2 = 12.96

Standard Deviation = 1/n * √ ∑ |xi – Z|^2 = 1/10 * √ 47.6 = 2.182 kg

Coefficient of Variance = SD / Z *100 = 2.182/14.2 * 100 = 15.37

Standard Error = SD / √n = 2.182/√10 = 0.69 kg

Variance = $SD^2 = (2.182)^2 = 4.76$

2. *Find out the range, quartile deviation, mean deviation, and standard deviation for the following grouped data:*

Weight in (Kgs)	No. of Goats
11-13	12
13-15	14
15-17	11
17-19	11
19-21	11
21-23	3
23-25	13

Solution

Classes – Weight in (Kg)	No. of Goats	Less than	Cumulative frequency
11-13	12	11	0
13-15	14	13	12
15-17	11	15	26
17-19	11	17	37
19-21	11	19	48
21-23	3	21	59
23-25	13	23	62
	N=75		

Range = H–L = 25-11 = 14 kg

Ratio of range = (H-L) x 100 / (H+L) = (25-11) x 100 / (25+11) = 14 x 100 / 36 = 38.89

Quartile deviation = $(Q_3\text{-}Q_1) / 2$

$Q_1 = L_1 + \frac{(N/4 - m_1)xc}{f_1}$ = 13 + (75/4 - 12) / 14 * 2 = 13+ (18.75 – 12) / 14 * 2 = 13.89

$Q_3 = L_3 + \frac{(3N/4 - m_3)xc}{f_3}$ = 19 + [(3*75)/4–48]/11*2 = 19+[(56.25–48]/11*2 = 20.50 kg

Quartile deviation = $(Q_3 - Q_1) / 2$ = (20.50 - 13.89) / 2 = 3.305 kg

Quartile coefficient of dispersion

= $(Q_3\text{-}Q_1)$ x $100/(Q_3+Q_1)$ = (20.50-13.89) x 100/(20.50+13.89)

= 661 / 34.39 = 19.22

Mean Deviation = 1/n ∑ |xi – Z|

Mid x	f	fx	|x - Z|	f |xi- Z|	|xi- Z|^2	f |xi- Z|^2
12	12	144	5.49	65.88	30.14	361.18
14	14	196	3.59	48.86	12.18	170.52
16	11	176	1.49	16.39	2.22	24.42
18	11	198	0.51	5.61	0.26	2.86
20	11	220	2.51	27.61	6.38	70.18
22	3	66	4.51	13.53	20.34	61.02
24	13	312	6.51	84.63	42.38	550.94
	75	**1312**		**262.51**		**1241.12**

Z = 1312 / 75 = 17.49

Mean Deviation = 1/n ∑ |xi – Z| = 262.51/75 = 3.5 kg

Mean Coefficient of Dispersion = MD*100/Z = 3.5*100 /17.49 = 20.01

Standard Deviation = 1/n * √ ∑f |xi- Z|^2 = √ 1241.12 /75 = 4.07 kg

Coefficient of Variance = SD/Z *100 = 4.07/17.49 * 100 = 23.27

Standard Error = SD / √N = 4.07 / √75 = 0.4699 kg

Variance = SD^2 = (4.07)^2 = 16.56

Probable error (PE)

PE $\underline{\Omega}$ 2/3 SD

Properties of Quartiles Deviation

1. QD $\underline{\Omega}$ 2/3 SD $\underline{\underline{\Omega}}$ PE
2. Mean + QD will cover 50% of the cases

Properties of Mean Deviation

1. $MD \underline{\Omega} \frac{4}{5} SD$
2. MD about median as the origin is the minimum

Interpreting Standard Deviation

Properties of Standard Deviation

1. SD is greater than MD, QD, and PE.
2. Mean square deviation will be minimum, if the deviation is taken from AM as the origin.
3. Mean + 1 SD will cover 68.27% of the items;

   Mean + 2 SD will cover 95.45% of the items;

   Mean + 3 SD will cover 99.73% of the items.

4. By adding or subtracting a constant from all the observations, SD is unaltered.
5. If $\bar{x}_1$, $\bar{x}_2$ are the means of two samples of sizes n_1, n_2 respectively with SDs σ_1, σ_2, then the combined SD (σ) is given by $(n_1 + n_2)\,\sigma^2 = n_1\,\sigma_1^{\,2} + n_2\,\sigma_2^{\,2} + n_1\,d_1^{\,2} + n_2\,d_2^{\,2}$ where $\bar{x}$ is the combined mean and $d_1 = \bar{x}_1 - \bar{x}$; $d_2 = \bar{x}_2 - \bar{x}$.

3.2.2 Merits and Demerits of Dispersion Measures

The essential requisites of a good measure of dispersion are the same as that of averages.

Dispersion measure	Merits	Demerits
Range	• Easy to calculate and simple to understand • Range given with mean gives useful information • Extensively used in statistical quality control	• Not based on the entire data set, based on extreme values, and hence not a reliable measure • Affected by sampling fluctuations • Not amenable to further mathematical treatment
Quartile Deviation	• Easy to calculate and simple to understand • Not affected by extreme items and open-ended classes	• Not based on all observations • Does not have sampling stability • Not amenable to further mathematical treatment
Mean Deviation	• Easy to calculate and understand • Based on all observations, hence is a better measure than the range	• Affected much by extreme values and open-ended classes • Does not have sampling stability • Not amenable to further mathematical treatment
Standard Deviation	• Based on all observations • Capable of algebraic treatment • Less affected by sampling • Squared deviations remove the drawbacks of ignoring signs • Helps in calculating SE	• Lengthy calculation for taking the square of deviations and then finding the square root • Affected much by extreme values and open-ended classes
Variance	• Easy to calculate • Indicates variability clearly • The most informative measure of variation	• Unit of variance not same as that of observations

3.2.3 Choice of Dispersion Measure

Among all the dispersion measures, range is unstable and its value depends on extreme items in the data. Range fails to consider central tendency of the data, while quartile deviation excludes half of the items from consideration. Mean deviation suffers from the mathematically logical defect of neglecting algebraic signs (particularly negative signs). Standard deviation (and, of course, variance) is free from all these defects to a great extent and is the most useful, reliable and most popularly used measure of dispersion.

3.2.4 Other Measures of Variability

3.2.4.1 Skewness

It has been seen that the measures of central tendency indicate the central position or central tendency of the frequency distribution and the measures of dispersion give an indication to the extent to which the items cluster around or scatter away from the central tendency. But none of these measures indicate the form or type of the distribution. Consider the following two distributions:

Class	Frequency	Class	Frequency
0-5	10	0-5	10
5-10	30	5-10	40
10-15	60	10-15	30
15-20	60	15-20	90
20-25	30	20-25	20
25-30	10	25-30	10

The above two distributions have the same mean (=15) and SD (= 6), but yet they are not identical distribution. The distribution on the left-hand side is symmetrical one, whereas the distribution on the right-hand side is asymmetrical or skewed. Skewness refers to the symmetry or departure from symmetry. Symmetry means that the number of values above the mode and below the mode is same in a data.

When a distribution departs from the symmetrical form, it is said to be asymmetrical or skewed. Evidently, in the case of symmetrical distribution, the two tails of the curve are of equal size and in asymmetrical distribution, one tail of the curve is longer than the other. A distribution is said to be skewed in the direction of the excess tail. Thus, if the right tail is longer, the distribution is positively skewed; if the left tail is longer, it is negatively skewed.

A distribution is said to be skewed if Mean, Median and Mode fall at different points, i.e. Mean ≠ Median ≠ Mode. A distribution is positively skewed, if Mean > Median > Mode. A distribution is negatively skewed, if Mean < Median > Mode. For normal (symmetrical) distribution, Mean = Median = Mode.

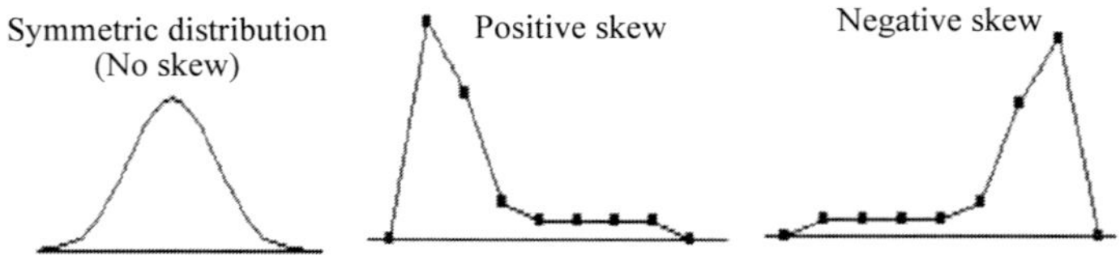

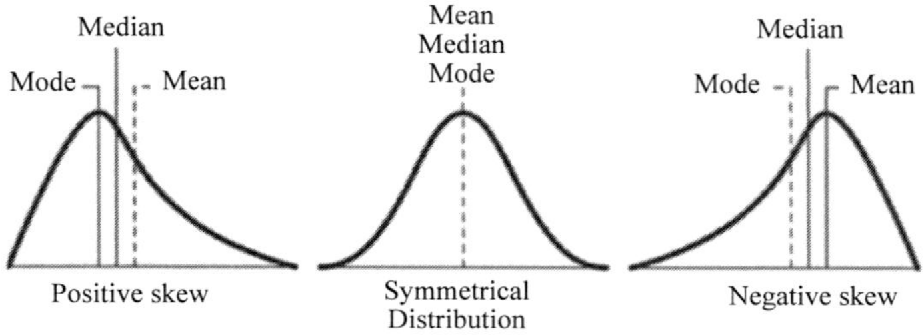

Measures of Skewness

1. **Pearsonian Measure of Skewness:** Absolute skewness is measured by mean – mode or 3 (mean - median) and the coefficient of skewness is

$$\frac{\text{mean-mode}}{\text{SD}} \text{ or } \frac{3(\text{mean-median})}{\text{SD}}$$

If mode is not well defined, then we use the second formula.

2. **Bowley's Measure of Skewness:** Absolute skewness is measured by $Q_3 - M - (M - Q_1)$. i.e. $Q_3 + Q_1 - 2M$ and the coefficient of skewness is

$$\frac{Q_3 + Q_1 - 2M}{Q_3 - Q_1}$$, where M is the median.

Exercises

1. *Calculate skewness of the following distribution:*

X	*1*	*2*	*3*	*4*	*5*	*6*	*7*
F	*5*	*7*	*3*	*1*	*4*	*6*	*9*

Solution

X	**f**	**d = X-4**	**fd**	**fd²**
1	5	-3	-15	225
2	7	-2	-14	196
3	3	-1	-3	9
4	1	0	0	0
5	4	1	4	16
6	6	2	12	144
7	9	3	27	729
	N=35		**$\sum fd = -11$**	**$\sum fd^2 = 1319$**

Mean = A + ($\sum$fd)/N = 4 – 11/35 = 4 - 0.31 = 3.69

Mode = 7

SD = Square root of ($\sum fd^2$)/N – [($\sum$fd)/N]^2

= Square root of (1319/35 – $(11/35)^2$)

= Square root of (37.69 – 0.096) = 6.13

Karl Pearson's Coefficient of Skewness = (Mean – Mode) / SD = (3.69 – 7) / 6.13 = - 0.54

2. *Compute QD and the coefficient of skewness from the following table:*

Size	*4-8*	*8-12*	*12-16*	*16-20*	*20-24*	*24-28*	*28-32*	*32-36*	*36-40*
Frequency	*6*	*10*	*18*	*30*	*15*	*12*	*10*	*6*	*2*

Solution

Size	4-8	8-12	12-16	16-20	20-24	24-28	28-32	32-36	36-40
Frequency f	6	10	18	30	15	12	10	6	2
Cumulative frequency cf	6	16	34	64	79	91	101	107	109

Median = Size of N/2th item = 109/2th item = 54.5th item which lies in the class 16-20

Median = L_1 + (N/2 – cf)/ f * i = 16 + (54.5 – 34)/30 * 4 = **18.73**

Q_1 = Size of N/4th item = Size of 109/4th item = 27.25th item which lies in the class 12-16

Q_1 = L_1 + (N/4 – cf)/ f * i = 12 + (27.25 - 16)/18 * 4 = **14.50**

Q_3 = Size of 3N/4th item = Size of 3*109/4th item = 81.75th item which lies in the class 24-28

Q_3 = L_1 + (3N/4 – cf)/ f * i = 24 + (81.75 - 79)/12 * 4 = **24.92**

QD = (Q3 – Q1)/2 = (24.92 – 14.50)/2 = 10.42/2 = **5.21**

Bowley's Coefficient of Skewness = (Q3 + Q1 – 2Median) / (Q3 – Q1)

= (24.92 + 14.50 – 2*18.73) / (24.92 - 14.50)

= (39.42 – 37.46) / 10.42 = **0.188**

3.2.4.2 Moments

Moment is a mechanical term which refers to the measure of a force with respect to its tendency to provide rotation. The strength of the tendency depends on the amount of force and the distance from the origin of the point at which the force is exerted. If a no. of forces F_1, F_2, ..., F_n at distances X_1, X_2, ..., X_n are applied, the moment of the first force about the origin is F_1X_1, the moment of the second force is F_2X_2, etc. These moments are additive so that

$\sum FX$ is the total moment about the origin. If the total moment is divided by the total force, the quotient is termed as a moment. The formula is $\sum FX/N$ where $N=\sum F$ is the total force. This formula for the moment coefficient is similar to that of arithmetic mean.

The moment about mean called the central moment is denoted by μ, thus μ_1 stands for first moment about mean, μ_2 stands for second moment about mean, etc.

$\mu_1=\sum(X-)/N$ or $\sum x/N$

μ_1 is always zero, since the sum of deviation of items from mean is zero.

$\mu_2=\sum(X-)^2/N$ or $\sum x^2/N$

$\mu_3=\sum(X-)^3/N$ or $\sum x^3/N$

Though moments can be extended to higher powers also, generally the first four moments only are calculated.

Two important constants of a distribution are calculated from μ_2, μ_3 and μ_4. They are

$= \mu_3^2 / \mu_2^3$, which measures skewness; $= \mu_4 / \mu_2^2$, which measures kurtosis.

Moments help in analyzing a frequency distribution as below:

Moment	Measure
First moment	Mean
Second moment	Variance
Third moment	Skewness
Fourth moment	Kurtosis

3.2.4.3 Kurtosis

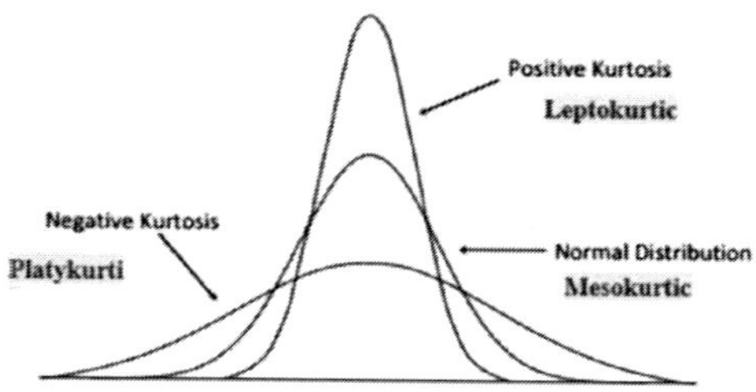

It is the measure of the peakedness. It indicates the degree of flatness or peakedness in the area relating to the mode of the frequency curve. A normal curve is symmetrical and bell-shaped. When two distributions are compared, the top of the frequency curve may be flat, narrow or peaked. This characteristic of the frequency curve is known as kurtosis or peakedness. The normal curve is known as mesokurtic. A curve more peaked than a normal curve is leptokurtic (positive kurtosis) and if it is flatter than the normal curve, it is platykurtic (negative kurtosis).

Measure of Kurtosis

It is measured by $\beta_2 - 3$ where $\beta_2 = \mu_4/\mu_2^2$ where μ_4 is the 4th moment about $\overline{x}$ which is given by $\mu_4 = \sum \frac{(x_i - \overline{x})^4}{n}$ **for raw data.**

and - $\frac{\sum f_i (x_i - \overline{x})^4}{N}$ **for grouped data.**

$\beta_2 = 3$ for a normal curve
$\beta_2 < 3$ for platykurtic curve

3.2.5 Descriptive Statistics and Graphs used according to type of data

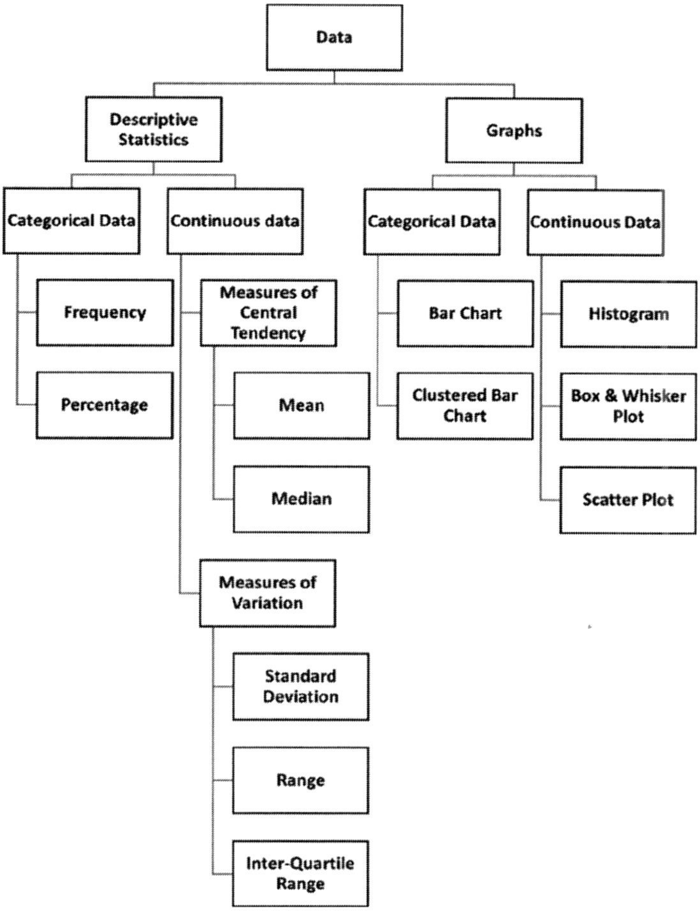

4

Sampling Methods for Animal Disease Surveys

For any statistical analysis, the required primary data are usually collected by the census or sampling methods. In the census method, the data are collected from all the individuals. E.g., If we want to study the weight of 100 cows, we have to make use of all 100 cows for data collection. That is, we collect data from the entire population or universe. However, in the sampling method, the data are collected from a small group of the population which is termed as the sample. A sample is a portion of the population selected to represent the population. E.g., we collect data only from a sample of cows, say 20 cows drawn from the population.

4.1 ADVANTAGES AND DISADVANTAGES OF CENSUS AND SAMPLING METHODS

Method	Advantages	Disadvantages
Census method	1. Data collected have a high degree of accuracy. 2. Data are representative and true. 3. Data are more reliable, as they are less biased.	1. Expensive, as it requires more time, manpower, and money. 2. Cannot be applied to all situations. E g., to analyze the blood cell count, the whole blood of an individual cannot be analyzed.
Sampling method	1. Economical, as it requires only less time, manpower, and money. 2. More suited to situations where census cannot be done.	1. Less accurate results. 2. Requires experts to plan sampling. 3. Improperly chosen samples result in poor results.

4.2 NEED FOR SAMPLING

The sampling method of data collection proves to be more appropriate in most situations, because of the following reasons:

1. Generally, populations are very large and hence it is not always possible to study every member of the population.
2. Census is expensive and time-consuming.
3. A sample can be studied more accurately and thoroughly, because of its manageable size.

4. Many times, sampling is the only way out. When the population is very large or if individuals are to be sacrificed after data collection, the census method cannot be used.

4.3 SAMPLING DESIGNS

4.3.1 Concepts in Sampling

Population: A population is the total of animals/birds about which data are to be collected. The population can be finite or infinite. A population is said to be finite if it consists of a fixed number of animals/birds so that it is possible to enumerate them. Examples of finite populations are the cows in a village or herd, the number of labourers in a farm, etc. An infinite population is a population in which it is theoretically impossible to observe all the elements, as the number of items is infinite. An example of an infinite population is the number of stars in the sky. We use the term infinite population for a population that cannot be enumerated in a reasonable time.

Sample: The sample is a part of the population that represents the characteristics of the population.

Sampling: Sampling is the process of selecting the sample to estimate the population characteristics. In other words, it is the process of obtaining data/information about the entire population by examining only a part of it.

Sampling Unit: Sampling units are the group of units of the population that can be clearly defined, identified, and observed.

Sampling Frame: A list of all the sampling units is known as the sampling frame. The sampling frame consists of a list of items from which the sample is drawn.

Sample Survey: An investigation in which data/information are collected is known as a sample survey.

Statistic: A statistic is a characteristic of the sample selected. E.g., sample mean, sample proportion, etc.

Parameter: A parameter is a characteristic of the population. E.g., population mean, population proportion, etc.

Target Population: A target population is an entire group of animals/birds about which data are collected to make some conclusions about the population.

Sampled Population: The part of the population, that we sample, is called sampled population.

Sampling indicates that a subset of the population is investigated, rather than all the individuals of the population. The investigation of a subset instead of the whole population is economical because it reduces the required time, labour, and cost. The two major reasons why a planned sample is often used in disease surveys are to describe the population characteristics (e.g., disease prevalence) and to determine the relationships between exposure to certain factors and the specified disease.

Usually, the investigator will have a sampling frame (a complete list of all the sampling units) of the target population (the population from which the data are required). The study population (the population from which the sample is drawn) should be more or less identical to the target population. The sampling fraction is the ratio of the sample size to the size of the study population.

When we study only a subset of the population, not all the data present in the total population can be collected and hence the true value of the parameter of interest in the population may not be obtained as such, and hence it needs to be estimated from the sample. The precision and accuracy of the estimate depend on the way the subset is obtained (sampling design) and on the number of units in the subset (sample size).

Sources of error in measurement may be either random or systematic. A high precision indicates a lack of random error, while a high accuracy indicates a lack of systematic error. A small sample size leads to low precision. Non-representativeness of the study population about the target population results in a lowered accuracy.

4.3.2 Purpose of Sampling

The basic purpose of sampling is to provide an estimate of the population parameter and to test the hypothesis. The advantages of sampling are:

- Sampling saves time and money.
- Sampling enables the collection of required data.
- Sampling enables better accuracy in measurement as it is conducted by trained and experienced investigators.
- Sampling remains the only way when the population is large.
- Sampling remains the only way of data collection in some situations, like in testing the pathological status of blood, etc.
- Sampling provides a valid estimation of sampling error.

4.3.3 Sample Designs

Sample designs are basically of two types *viz.*, non-probability sampling and probability sampling.

4.3.3.1 Non-Probability Sampling

Non-probability sampling is a random sampling procedure with no basis for estimating the probability. Hence, each item in the population has an equal opportunity of being included in the sample. Non-probability sampling is also known by different names such as deliberate sampling, purposive sampling, and judgment sampling. In this type of sampling, the items for the sample are selected deliberately by the researcher based on his choice. In other words, in this sampling type, the organizer of the study purposively chooses the particular units of the population to constitute a sample on the basis that the sample he/she selects from the population is representative of the population. Thus, the judgment of the organizer of the study plays an important role in the sampling. This method gives an equal probability to every sample unit of getting selected.

We define a simple random sample (or a random sample) from a finite population as a sample chosen in such a way that each of the NCn possible samples has the same probability (1/NCn) of being selected. E.g., suppose we take a finite population consisting of six elements (say a, b, c, d, e, f), i.e., N = 6 and we want to take a sample of size n = 3 from it. Then, there are 6C3 = 20 possible samples, which consist of the elements abc, abd, abe, abf, acd, ace, acf, ade, adf, aef, bcd, bce, bcf, bde, bdf, bef, cde, cdf, cef, and def. If we choose one of these samples in such a way that each has the probability of 1/20 of being chosen, we then call this a random sample.

4.3.3.2 Probability Sampling

Probability sampling is also known as non-random sampling or chance sampling. In this sampling design too, every item of the population has an equal chance of being included in the sample. It is the method in which individual units are picked up from the whole population not deliberately but through some process. Here, it is the only chance that determines whether one item or the other is selected. The results obtained from the probability or non-random sampling can be assured in terms of probability, i.e., we can measure the errors of estimation or the significance of results obtained from a random sample. This fact brings out the superiority of the probability non-random sampling design over the non-probability random sampling design.

However, in a non-random sampling method, the investigator purposively selects a sample that would yield results favourable to his point of view. However, there is a danger of bias in this technique. Because there is no assurance that every element has some specifiable chance of being included. Sampling error in this type of sampling cannot be estimated and there is always an element of bias. Hence, this sampling design is rarely adopted in large studies of importance. However, in small studies, this design may be adopted, because of the advantage of convenience, less time, and less money required for this method. However, the samples selected may not possess the characteristics, required by the investigator.

4.3.4 Features of Good Sampling

- A sample design must result in a truly representative sample.
- A sample design should ensure a smaller sampling error.
- A sample design must be commensurate with the funds available for the study.
- A sample design should ensure that the systematic bias can be controlled.
- The sample should be such that the results of the study can be applied to the population with a reasonable level of confidence.

4.3.5 Types of Sampling Methods

There are six major types of sampling methods:

1. Non-probability sampling
2. Simple random sampling
3. Systematic random sampling
4. Stratified random sampling
5. Cluster sampling
6. Multistage sampling

1. Non-Probability Sampling

Non-probability sampling methods do not rely on random techniques to decide whether or not the units are included in the sample. One example is convenience sampling, in which, the data are obtained from the units that are easily accessed by the investigator, for e.g., because the investigator knows that some farmers are known to him/her and will cooperate better. This may lead to biased data and results because farmers willing to cooperate may expect that the results of the study would reduce their problems.

2. Simple Random Sampling

In this method, the units included in the sample are selected through a random process. For example, if we want to select 50% of all units, we can flip a coin per unit and if the result is 'head', then we include that unit in the sample and if it is 'tail', we do not include it in the sample. More sophisticated methods are now available like random number tables, randomizers on pocket calculators, and random number generators in software packages to select samples randomly. When the study population is representative of the target population, random procedures will ensure that the sample is representative of the target population.

3. Systematic Random Sampling

This type of sampling implies that the units are selected at regular intervals from the sampling frame. For example, if we need to select 1% of the animals, first, we draw a random number between 1 and 100. Suppose it is 73. Then, animals 73, 173, 273, ... are selected, to end up with a 1% sample size. However, bias may occur if the sampling frame is organized systematically.

4. Stratified Random Sampling

Stratification means that the sampling frame is first divided into different strata (groups) before selection. After that, systematic or simple random sampling is performed within each group. Stratification is applied if the population is heterogeneous about the variable of interest. Then, by creating more homogeneous groups (e.g., age groups), a more robust estimate for the characteristics of interest can be obtained. A major advantage of this method is that it is possible to draw unequal percentages per stratum. This will be very useful, as the variance of the outcome will differ between strata. A disadvantage of this method is that prior information must be available to determine to which stratum each element belongs.

5. Cluster Sampling

In cluster sampling, clusters of animals (e.g., litters or herds) are randomly selected. All the animals in a cluster are then examined. These clusters may be selected by any of the above random methods. Cluster sampling may be used when not all animals can be listed in the sampling frame.

6. Multistage Sampling

This method is a more complex type of cluster sampling, with sampling also occurring at the second, third, ..., levels. It means that not all elements (animals) within a cluster are selected. This type of sampling has some practical advantages. The number of clusters (n1 primary units) and the number of elements per cluster (n2 secondary units) can be varied to obtain a higher precision of the estimate (i.e., minimize variance, if variability between clusters exists) or to reduce costs (if costs vary between sampling primary vs. secondary units).

An example of multistage sampling is that we first select n1 farms, secondly, we select n2 litters within each farm and lastly, we select n3 piglets within each selected litter from which we measure the parameters of interest. Thus, the total number of observations is n1 *n2*n3.

4.3.6 Selection Bias and Sampling Error

Naturally, survey results will have some errors. These errors can be sampling errors and non-sampling errors. The term 'error' includes systematic biases and random errors. Sampling errors and biases are necessarily brought in by the sample design. These biases and errors include 1. Selection bias, which occurs when the true selection probabilities differ from those assumed in calculating the results, and 2. Random sampling error, which arises when a random variation in the results occurs due to the elements in the sample being selected at random.

4.3.7 Non-Sampling Error

Non-sampling errors are the errors caused by problems in data collection, processing, or sample design that can impact the final survey estimates. They include:

1. Over-coverage: When data are included from outside the population
2. Under-coverage: When some members of the population are inadequately represented in the sample. It is a problem with convenience samples.
3. Measurement error: When respondents misunderstand a question or find it difficult to answer.
4. Processing error: Due to mistakes in data coding.
5. Non-response: Due to the failure to obtain complete data from all selected individuals.

4.4 SAMPLE SIZE ESTIMATIONS

One should know the sample size he has to have to collect adequate data for his study, without which his study would prove futile. Hence, sample size estimation is necessary before starting any study which will depend on the type of data to be collected and the design of the study. We cannot use the same formula for calculating the required sample size for the estimation of milk yield, for estimating disease prevalence, or for detecting whether a herd is diseased or not. We have different methods to estimate the sample size required. For e.g.:

1. To estimate a mean;
2. To estimate differences between means;
3. To estimate a proportion (e.g., disease prevalence);
4. To estimate differences between proportions;
5. To detect a disease in a population; and
6. To estimate the relationship between the exposure and the disease.

Sample size calculations are necessary before carrying out any survey or experiment. The outcomes of these calculations will guide us as to how many sample units should be included in the study. Calculations can be done by using a calculator, or software like EPISCOPE.

4.4.1 Sample size to estimate a mean

To calculate the sample size for a mean obtained from a normal distribution, we need to estimate both the mean and its standard deviation (SD). Secondly, the interval L should be defined, indicating that with a probability of x%, the true population mean will be within the interval of the sample mean ± L. This interval is therefore an indication of the precision of the estimate. Thirdly, we have to decide on x. There is no general rule for this decision, but 95 is commonly used. From x, we can determine the corresponding number (Z) of units of SD. For example, if x=95, then the significance level is 5% and $Z_{0.05}$ = 1.96, which means that 95% of all the observations will fall within the interval of mean ± 1.96*SD/√n.

Now, the confidence interval (Cl) for a mean is obtained by drawing elements from a normal distribution and can be written as:

$$CI = \overline{X} \pm \frac{Za * SD}{\sqrt{n}}$$

The ± sign is denoted as L and n is calculated as:

$$n = \frac{Z\alpha^2 * SD^2}{L^2}$$

Suppose we want to estimate the growth in calves per day. For e.g., growth is around 1000 g / day and an estimate of the SD is 50 g. How many calves should be weighed to check whether the mean growth is between 950 and 1050 g / day? A confidence level of 95% is required. To practice, determine the numbers needed like 1. SD increases by 50%, 2. the confidence level decreases to 90%, or 3. L is changed from 50 to 100. Then, the answers will be 97, 217, 68, and 25. The calculated sample size will be rounded upward.

If a large part of a population with size N is sampled, i.e., the sampling fraction (n/N) is large, the standard deviation is usually overestimated. Suppose we have all the elements of the population sampled (n=N), then the sample mean is equal to the population mean and the standard deviation will be 0. Therefore, a correction of the SD is necessary if more than 10% (thumb rule) of the population is sampled. This correction is multiplying the SD with √(1-f), where f = n/N is the sampling fraction (1 – f is called the finite population correction). If n is equal to N, then the SD becomes 0. The finite population correction can be applied directly in the above formula by dividing the calculated n by 1 + f.

$$n_a = \frac{n}{\left(1 + \frac{n}{N}\right)}$$

Suppose the number of sampled calves in the previous exercise originated from a population of 750 animals. We should calculate the adjusted sample size. Suppose the sampled calves originated from a population of 10,000 animals, then calculate the adjusted sample size, which will be 85 or 95.

4.4.2 Sample size to estimate the differences between Means

We may be interested in knowing the differences between groups of animals, for e.g., the differences in milk production between mastitic cows and healthy cows. If the milk production is a normally distributed parameter, we can perform a one-tailed test, because we know that mastitic cows will give a reduced milk yield. This will have an impact on the value of Zα: the one-sided value of $Z_{0.05}$ will be equal to the two-sided $Z_{0.10}$.

To know the sample size, we need the:

- Estimated difference between the two groups
- Standard deviation of the trait
- Level of significance, α
- Power of the test, i.e., the probability (1-β) of obtaining a significant result if the true difference is equal

The sample size formula is written as:

$$n = \frac{2 * (Z\alpha + Z\beta)^2 * SD^2}{\delta^2}$$

where Zα and Zβ are the values of the standard Normal distribution at specified levels of confidence and power, SD is the standard deviation, and δ is the estimated difference. The constant, 2, arises from the assumption that the SD is equal in both groups. The calculated sample size is the number of animals in each group.

E.g., If daily milk production in healthy cows is 25 litres and in mastitic cows, it is reduced by 10%. Thus, δ is 2.5 litres. The standard deviation of daily milk production is known to be 6 litres. Given a one-sided α of 0.05, $Z_{0.05}$ is 1.64, and a power of 80%, $Z_{0.20}$ is 0.84, we determine the sample size per group to be 71 per group.

4.4.3 Sample size to estimate a Proportion

Unlike previous calculations, when we want to investigate the presence of disease, we deal with a yes or no (binomial) situation, as each selected element is either healthy or diseased. One property of the binomial distribution is that the variance of the mean (e.g., the prevalence) is equal to p*(1 - p), when p is the proportion (i.e., p*(100 - p)), as p is the percentage. The standard deviation is the square root of p*(1 - p). Hence, the formula used to estimate a mean can be used to determine the sample size. A prominent property of the SD of a proportion is that it is symmetric around its maximum at p = 0.5 (or 50%). Hence, the sample size is maximal, when p is estimated to be 50% and this value should be used when there is no idea of the actual proportion. The finite population correction is also applicable to binomial situations. E.g., Sample sizes are given when L=0.05, Za=1.96, and infinite N at varying estimated prevalences:

Prevalence	0.10	0.20	0.30	0.40	0.50	0.60	0.70	0.80	0.90	1.00
Standard Deviation	0.30	0.40	0.46	0.49	0.50	0 49	0.46	0.40	0.30	0.00
n	139	246	323	369	385	369	323	246	139	0

Here, L is the absolute precision. Taking a lower absolute precision at low or high prevalences is often more convenient. We are not interested in whether the prevalence equals 4% ± 10%, but 4% ± 2%.

E.g.: A farmer raising 1000 calves likes to determine the prevalence of Salmonellosis in his calves. Suppose the prevalence ranges from 0 to 80%. It is sensible to put the estimated prevalence at 50%, as no information is known about the actual prevalence except that it is between 0 and 80%. By choosing 50%, we will keep the largest possible sample size for a desired value of L and Z. Also, we need to put the values on L and Z, and we choose 5% and 1.96. The ultimate result obtained is that the actual prevalence with a probability of 95% between 45 and 55%. Now, we will calculate n. We will determine whether the finite population correction is needed. If so, we determine the adjusted n. Hence, the answers are 385 and 278.

After doing the sampling, we will come to know that the prevalence is 10%, which is much lower than our initial estimate of 50%. i.e., more than enough animals have been sampled to fulfil the initial conditions (L = 0.05 and Z = 1.96) and the values of these can be recalculated (with the adjusted n equals 278). For e.g.

$$L = \frac{Za * SD}{\sqrt{n}} = \frac{1.96 * \sqrt{0.1 * 0.9}}{\sqrt{278}} = 0.035 (\text{or } 3.5\%)$$

Taking the finite population correction into account, the SD equals √(0.1 * 0.9) * √(1 – 278 / 1000) = 0.255 and, subsequently, L = 1.96 * 0.255/√278 = 0.03. The actual prevalence is, with a probability of 95% within the interval 10 ± 3.0%.

4.4.4 Sample Size to Estimate the Differences Between Proportions

Suppose we want to compare two antibiotics. Two groups of animals are infected with a pathogen and the percentages of recovery in both groups are compared. The question is how many animals should be included in each group? We use the following formula:

$$n = \left(\frac{Z\alpha + Z\beta}{p^1 - p^2} \right)^2 * (p^1 q^1 + p^2 q^2)$$

where, Zα, Zβ = values of the standard normal distribution at specified levels of confidence and power, p1, p2 = estimated proportions of recovery in groups 1 and 2, and q1, q2 = 1 - p1, 1 - p2, respectively.

A company has developed a new antibiotic against the pathogen X. No other antibiotics are available and hence no comparison can be made with the existing antibiotic treatment. However, the field data show that 70% of the infected recover from the disease. It is hoped that after the use of the antibiotic, 95% of the animals will get cured and also the duration of the disease will be reduced. Thus, p1 = 0.70 and p2 = 0.95. Choosing a one-sided (as no other antibiotic is available and using this antibiotic is better than doing nothing) confidence of 95% and a power of 80% shows that the values for Zα and Zβ are 1.64 and 0.84, respectively. Using the formula, we calculate n per group which is 26.

4.4.5 Sample Size to Estimate Equality of Proportions (Or Means)

Suppose a new antibiotic cures 95% of the sick animals. A researcher likes to prove that the new antibiotic is as effective as the existing one. We need to know how many animals should be treated in a comparative experiment. The two formulas that we have seen above can be used, but now p1 – p2 (or δ) is defined as the difference. In the case of equivalence testing, α and β are the mirror images of those used for difference testing. Thus, the typical value for the confidence level 1 - α is now 0.8, and the typical value for the power 1 - β is 0.95. In general, testing for equivalence needs a larger sample size than for testing for a difference. This is because the power is always one-sided, while the confidence level is defined either as one-sided or two-sided. The table below shows the sample sizes per treatment group to show equivalence:

Observations/treatment group for various proportions of cure in treatment groups and values for permitted difference d using a one-sided test (assuming $1 - \beta = 0.95$, $1 - \alpha = 0.8$)

	Expected proportion of cure in both groups						
d	0.30	0.40	0.50	0.60	0.70	0.80	0.90
0.05	1038	1187	1236	1187	1038	790	445
0.10	260	297	310	297	260	198	111
0.15	116	133	138	133	116	88	49
0.20	66	75	78	75	66	49	28

4.4.6 Sample size to detect a disease in a population

Suppose we are interested in the percentage of farms that are infected by a pathogen X. A farm is considered to be infected even when at least one animal is infected. Initially, the appropriate number of farms is randomly chosen and then, the status of the farm (infected or not) is determined. If the disease is present, about 50% of the animals are likely to be positive. By sampling one animal, we have a 50% probability of testing a positive farm as positive. We aim at a higher probability to classify a positive farm correctly (e.g., 95%). By selecting two animals, the probability is increased up to 75%, three animals will yield 87.5%, four animals 93.75%, and five animals 96.88%. Thus, between four and five animals should be sampled to detect positive farms with a probability of 95%, if 50% of the animals are truly diseased.

$$n = \left(1 - (1 - P)^{\frac{1}{d}}\right) * \left(N - \frac{d-1}{2}\right)$$

where n is the sample size, P is the probability of finding at least one case (= confidence level, e.g., 0.95), d is the number of (detectable) cases in the population and N is the population size.

If the test is used to evaluate the status of the animals that does not have a 100% sensitivity, d is equal to the number of diseased or infected animals multiplied by the sensitivity of the test. For e.g., we want to detect whether a flock of 1000 (= N) animals is positive for the pathogen X. If X is present, we suspect that about 50% of the animals are infected, thus d = 500. Setting P = 0.95, n = (1 - 0.0511500) * (1000 - 499/2) = 4.48 (rounded to 5). Is this number much affected by N? No, because the prevalence is higher.

The same formula can be used to determine the maximum number of positives (d) in a population given that all samples (n) are tested negative:

$$d = \left(1 - (1 - P)^{\frac{1}{n}}\right) * \left(N - \frac{n-1}{2}\right)$$

If we test 1,000 slaughtered cows as negative for *E. coli* and the total number of cows slaughtered amounted to 1 million. The maximum prevalence in the population of slaughtered cows and the maximum prevalence if the sensitivity of the test is only 85%, then, if p is set to 0.95, d equals 2990 which is about 0.3%, then 0.3/0.85 = 0.35.

4.5 ANIMAL DISEASE SURVEILLANCE

Disease surveillance is aimed at demonstrating the presence or absence of an infection and determining the distribution of infection in a population. Animal health surveillance is a tool to monitor disease trends, to facilitate the control of infection, to provide data for use in disease control, and to provide health assurances to traders. The type of surveillance depends on the objectives of the surveillance, available data sources, and outputs needed to support decision-making. We need to know the following concepts for understanding disease surveillance:

Bias: It is the tendency of an estimate to deviate from a true population parameter.

Confidence: It is the probability that the type of surveillance applied will detect the presence of infection if the population is infected, which depends on the assumed prevalence of infection.

Sensitivity: It is the proportion of the infected sampling units that are correctly identified as positive.

Specificity: It is the proportion of uninfected sampling units that are correctly identified as negative.

Surveillance system: It is the use of one or more surveillance components to generate information on the health status of animal populations.

Test: It is a procedure used to classify a unit as either positive, negative, or suspect regarding an infection.

4.5.1 Need for Animal Disease Surveillance

The main objective of disease surveillance is to detect the disease early, to prevent huge losses to the farmers, society, and the nation at large (FAO, 1999). However, many of the undeveloped, underdeveloped, and developing countries experience severe economic losses in their livestock sector, as a result of late identification of diseases. Although the words – surveillance, and monitoring - of a disease are used interchangeably, surveillance deals with observation of an animal population to see whether a disease occurs. Thus, surveillance encompasses all the activities aimed at ascertaining the health status of an animal population for early detection and control of diseases of economic importance. Monitoring, on the other hand, is a specific activity that follows, if surveillance indicates the presence of a disease in the population. Monitoring, thus, focuses specifically on the identified disease to determine the changes in the prevalence rate and direction of spread.

Besides early detection of a disease, surveillance has other roles too:

1. Surveillance monitors the spread of a disease to manage it effectively. Knowing the speed with which a disease spreads, which direction it goes, and the size of the population it affects are the key factors that help to know how much vaccine and/or prophylactic medicine are to be purchased, how many staff and where they are to be deployed, and so on.
2. Surveillance plays a key role in monitoring the progress of disease control. Surveillance is a planned activity to detect signs of the disease, which requires cooperation from all the stakeholders like management and staff of the veterinary department, private veterinarians, farmers, etc.

4.5.2 Objectives of Animal Disease Surveillance

A surveillance system will have several objectives *viz.*, to estimate the magnitude of a disease problem, determine the geographic distribution of the disease, detect the epidemics, generate a hypothesis to stimulate research, evaluate different disease control measures, and facilitate planning for control of the disease identified. These major objectives are achieved by:

1. Monitoring the trends in health, disease, and determinants of health, systematically;
2. Detecting the unusual events, epidemics, and determinants of the health of a population;
3. Evaluating the ongoing and new prevention control measures;
4. Setting priorities for the existing or new health programs;
5. Suggesting hypotheses concerning the determinants of health in the population; and
6. Informing communities to help them to take action to protect the animals and herd health.

4.5.3 Guidelines to Design an Animal Disease Surveillance System

A good surveillance system should provide quality and timely data and information on the status of animal diseases in a region to the decision-makers to enable them to develop an effective disease control programme and respond rapidly to emerging threats not only to animal health but also to public health.

FAO Animal Health (FAO, 1999) has developed the guidelines to support for designing animal disease surveillance plans. The final disease surveillance system needs to be tested, approved, and disseminated to all the actors of the system within the country. An apex national-level technical committee may review and update the system periodically to ensure its effectiveness and relevance to the country.

4.5.3.1 Contents of an Animal Disease Surveillance System

i. ***Description of the disease:*** This deals with a description of the pathogen and its epidemiology, details of the species affected, clinical signs, and method of transmission. The risk factors for the spread of the disease, at both herd and animal levels need to be identified and listed.

ii. ***Justification for surveillance:*** The purpose of the surveillance, which may be the protection of animal health, public health, protection of the economy, or prevention of issues in trade, and / or benefits for public and private partners, requires to be narrated.

iii. ***Surveillance objectives:*** Both primary and secondary objectives, including surveillance outputs and follow-up actions, need to be mentioned.

iv. ***Geographical area covered:*** The system may cover national, regional, local, and cross-border levels.

v. ***Populations monitored:*** This may include targeted species, production systems, and commodities.

vi. ***Surveillance methods and protocols:*** Surveillance methods may be active, passive, or participatory. Outbreak investigations and site-specific investigations at border posts, markets, abattoirs, etc. are done.

vii. ***Sampling strategy:*** This would entail the choice of sampling technique, selection of site, animal sampling, commodities sampling, determination of sample size, etc.

viii. ***Biosafety and public health in the field:*** These measures are required to prevent the spread of infection during surveillance and to ensure personal protection through safe carcass / waste disposal, proper disinfection, etc.

ix. ***Laboratory analysis:*** This is done at regional and national levels, on the samples collected from the field. Sample collection will involve the sampling method, pooling of samples, their preservation, required transport, and storage before sending to the laboratories.

x. ***Data collection, management, and storage:*** These would include field data collection, laboratory results, data entry and management, data analysis, and interpretation of results.

xi. ***Communication and reporting:*** This step involves reporting to the top and regional levels, sending feedback to stakeholders, communicating to the public and neighbouring countries, and publishing in scientific bulletins and journals.

xii. ***Monitoring and evaluation of the system:*** There needs to be a set of performance indicators prescribed to continuously evaluate the system itself. Besides, there may be external evaluations at specified intervals.

4.5.3.2 Design of an Animal Disease Surveillance System

a) **Population:** Surveillance should consider all animal species susceptible to infection or infestation in a region or country.

b) **Temporal Validity of Data:** The timing, duration, and frequency of surveillance should be determined taking into consideration the factors such as:

- Epidemiology (e.g. pathogenesis, vectors, transmission pathways, seasonality);
- Risk of introduction and spread;
- Husbandry practices and production systems;
- Disease prevention and control measures (e.g. vaccination, disinfection);
- Accessibility of target population; and
- Geographical and environmental factors.

c) **Epidemiology Unit:** The epidemiology unit working for the surveillance system should ensure that it meets the objectives of the system.

d) **Diagnostic Tests:** Surveillance involves the use of tests for the detection of infection or infestation. Tests used in surveillance may range from clinical observations to rapid field and detailed laboratory tests.

f) **Analytical Methods:** Surveillance data should be analyzed using appropriate methods at the appropriate level to facilitate effective decision-making. Different methods may be used for different species, pathogenic agents, production systems, and types and quantities of data.

g) **Scope of the Surveillance System:** When designing a surveillance system, due consideration should be given to the defined purposes of surveillance and how the data it generates can be used, the limitations of the data it may generate, and the availability of financial, technical, and human resources.

h) **Follow-up Action:** The design of the surveillance system should consider what actions will be taken based on the data generated.

4.5.3.3 Animal Disease Surveillance Methods

Surveillance systems vary in their primary purpose and the type of surveillance data they may provide.

1. **Disease Reporting Systems:** These systems report animal health-related events to veterinary officials. Data derived from these systems can be used with the data collected from other sources. Effective laboratory support is essential for any disease reporting system, as laboratory confirmation of suspected clinical cases is required.
2. **Surveys:** Surveys may be conducted on the entire target population (i.e., a census) or on a sample. If a survey is done on a sample, a detailed description of the sampling strategy is required to be listed.
3. **Ante-Mortem and Post-Mortem Inspections:** Inspection of animals at slaughterhouses / abattoirs will provide valuable surveillance data. The sensitivity and specificity of slaughterhouse / abattoir inspections for detecting the presence of specified diseases will be influenced by the clinical and pathological signs noticed and the training and experience of the staff.
4. **Clinical Surveillance:** Clinical observation of animals in the field is the key source of surveillance data. The sensitivity and specificity of clinical observations are highly dependent on the criteria used to define a suspected case.
5. **Interpretation of Surveillance Results:** Multiple sources of data will indicate the overall sensitivity of the surveillance system and increase confidence in the results. Past surveys may be looked back to provide a higher confidence in the current data. When assessing the results, care should be taken to identify the biases that may lead to an overestimate or an underestimate of the parameters of interest.

4.5.3.4 Role of Geographic Information System in Disease Surveillance

A Geographic Information System (GIS) is an automated and computerized system for input, storage, analysis, and output of spatial data. Many software packages are now available for visualizing geographically referenced data, of course, all being expensive. But, for an epidemiologist, it is now indispensable. The main advantage of GIS is that it is user-friendly to ascertain how a disease is distributed geographically. Also, using GIS, an animal disease can be viewed against other data like rainfall maps, vegetation maps, wind directions, rivers, etc. Ultimately, the presence of a disease can be related to other factors and can be visually appreciated.

Disease data recording in a GIS will involve georeferencing of every observation of the disease to latitude and longitude values. Each field worker will be given a list of all georeferences for the places of his area of work, which he can add to the data forms. Alternatively, someone else at the district office can fill them in, once the forms are handed over. However, using GIS is not that easy for anyone, unless he is specifically trained for that. Also, GIS software cannot be used on all computers, as GIS programs require a lot of disk space, huge operating memory, and faster processors.

4.5.3.5 Active Surveillance Vs. Passive Surveillance

A surveillance carried out routinely by the veterinary staff in their locality is called passive surveillance. Although it is routinely and infrequently done, the results of this procedure are also important, as it helps to assess the animal health situation in a locality. However, in passive surveillance, the diseases occurring in animals without access to veterinary staff will go unreported and hence, it will mostly under-report disease frequency.

However, active surveillance involves regular, frequent, and intensive efforts to identify the presence of disease in an area. When a disease is suspected to be present, active surveillance is done to confirm it. Hence, this is of greater importance in supporting the planners to control or eradicate the disease reported. Though active surveillance is expensive and time-consuming, the benefits obtained from it will offset the extra cost involved in the years to come.

5

Hypothesis Testing in Animal Health Studies

Before trying to understand Hypothesis Testing and Experimental Designs, we should be conversant with the concept of Probability Distribution.

5.1 PROBABILITY DISTRIBUTIONS

Let us look at an example to grasp the essence of a probability distribution. Let us rotate a pair of dice and observe the sum by totalling the numbers that turn upon in both the dice. Let us call this sum by a random variable X. When the first dice shows up number 1, the second dice could show 1, 2, 3, 4, 5, or 6. Likewise, when the first dice shows up number 2, the second dice could show 1, 2, 3, 4, 5, or 6. If we continue the experiment this way until all the possibilities are exhausted, the sample space will contain 36 elements. The distribution that can be observed will contain a sum = 2, 3, 4, 5, 6, 7, 8, 9, 10, 11, or 12. The starting sum will be = 2, because when both the dice show the number 1, the sum 1 + 1 = 2. Likewise, the maximum sum in the distribution will be 12, when both the dice show up a number 6. If we write the values of the random variable (sum) with associated probabilities, it is called a probability distribution.

Sample Space

(D1 D2)	(D1 D2)	(D1 D2)	(D1 D2)	(D1 D2)	(D1 D2)
(1 1)	(2 1)	(3 1)	(4 1)	(5 1)	(6 1)
(1 2)	(2 2)	(3 2)	(4 2)	(5 2)	(6 2)
(1 3)	(2 3)	(3 3)	(4 3)	(5 3)	(6 3)
(1 4)	(2 4)	(3 4)	(4 4)	(5 4)	(6 4)
(1 5)	(2 5)	(3 5)	(4 5)	(5 5)	(6 5)
(1 6)	(2 6)	(3 6)	(4 6)	(5 6)	(6 6)

Note: D1 represents Dice 1 and D2 represents Dice 2

D1 and D2 in the sample space above are used to facilitate the sum of numbers in both the dice. For example, take the case of getting eight. There are 5 possibilities [(2 6), (3 5), (5 3), (6 2)], in which the sum 8 can occur. The random variable sum can assume that there are 36 elements in the sample space. Hence, the probability of getting a sum of 8 is 5/36. Likewise, the probabilities are computed for all other values of the sums associated with this experiment. Precisely, a probability distribution is a total listing of the various values that the random variable can take along with the corresponding probability of each value.

Probability Distribution	
X = Sum	**P (X)**
2	1/36
3	2/36
4	3/36
5	4/36
6	5/36
7	6/36
8	5/36
9	4/36
10	3/36
11	2/36
12	1/36

We should note that the probability of the sample space = 1, as all the above probabilities will add up to 1.

Exercise

A bank is concerned about the waiting time of its customers before they can use the ATM for their transactions. A study of a random sample of 500 customers reveals the following probability distribution:

Waiting time in minutes	***P(X)***
0	*0.20*
1	*0.18*
2	*0.16*
3	*0.12*
4	*0.10*
5	*0.09*
6	*0.08*
7	*0.04*
8	*0.03*
Total	***1.00***

a) *What is the probability that a customer will wait more than 5 minutes?*

P (X > 5) = P (6) + P (7) + P (8) = 0.08 + 0.04 + 0.03 = 0.15

b) *What is the probability that a customer need not wait?*

P (X = 0) = 0.20

c) *What is the probability that a customer will wait less than 4 minutes?*

P (X < 4) = P (0) + P (1) + P (2) + P (3) = 0.20 + 0.18 + 0.16 + 0.12 = 0.66

Expected Value of a Random Variable is an important term, which we must know in the context of decision-making under uncertainty. The expected value of a random variable is computed by multiplying the value of the random variable by the probability of occurrence of that value and then finding the summation of these products. The probabilities are the weights that are attached to the respective values the random variable can take. In other words, the expected value of a random variable is a weighted average of all the possible outcomes of an experiment. To know how the expected value is calculated, let us use the same bank example.

X (Waiting time in minutes)	P(X)	X x P(X)
0	0.20	0.00
1	0.18	0.18
2	0.16	0.32
3	0.12	0.36
4	0.10	0.40
5	0.09	0.45
6	0.08	0.48
7	0.04	0.28
8	0.03	0.24
Total	**1.00**	**2.71**

From the table in the last row in column 3, we see the total value as 2.71. This is the expected value of X designated as E(X). Thus, the average waiting time of a customer before getting access to the ATM is 2.71 minutes.

Discrete Probability Distribution

The examples we saw above to explain the concept of a probability distribution are called discrete probability distributions. That is, the probability distribution that uses a discrete random variable is called a discrete probability distribution. The probability function P(X) associated with the discrete probability distribution is called a ***probability mass function***. A discrete random variable implies that the random variable can assume only whole numbers. For e.g., the number of aircrafts landing at an airport in an hour is an example of a discrete random variable.

Continuous Probability Distribution

The probability distribution that uses a continuous random variable is called a continuous probability distribution. The probability function P(X) associated with the continuous probability distribution is called as ***probability density function***. A continuous random variable is a variable, which takes any value within some interval of real numbers. Measurement of the height and weight of the cows is an example of a continuous random variable.

Probability of Compound Events

If p is the probability of the event, the probability that it will occur in exactly x out of n cases is $nC_x q^{n-x} p^x$.

Exercises

1. *A scientist wishes to choose three animals for his research from 8 sheep, three of which are Suffolk breed and the others are Mecheri breed. What is the probability that a randomly selected three sheep will have two Mecheri and one Suffolk?*

   Total no. of ways getting groups of 3 animals = $^8C_3$ = (8*7*6) / (1*2*3) = 56

   We can select two Mecheri out of five in $^5C_2$ ways and one Suffolk in $^3C_1$ ways.

   Hence, the total possible ways of selecting 2 Mecheri and 1 Suffolk = $^5C_2 \times {}^3C_1$ = 10 x 3 = 30. Thus, the probability of getting two Mecheri and one Suffolk is = 30 / 56 = 0.54.

2. *A scientist works with three cattle breeds to improve the efficiency of milk production. Suppose he has 10 animals, 5 of which are Jersey, 3 are Friesian, and 2 are Sindhi and he selects three animals at random. What is the probability that all the three selected are Jerseys?*

   Total no. of ways of getting 3 animals = $^{10}C_3$ = (10*9*8) / (1*2*3) = 120

   No. of ways of getting three Jerseys = $^5C_3$ = 10

   Hence, the probability of getting three Jerseys = 10 / 120 = 0.0833

3. *If we assume that male and female calves are equally likely, what is the probability that exactly three out of 10 calves born will be male calves?*

   'p' is the probability of success and 'q' is the probability of failure.

   Then, the probability of getting 'x' success in 'n' trial = $nc_x . q^{n-x} . p^x$

In the given case, n = 10, p = q = ½; x = 3

Let the event of getting a male calf be success, then we have to find probability (x = 3) is

$= {}^{10}c_3 (½)^{10-3} (½)^3 = 10c_3 (½)^{10}$

$= (10*9*8) / (1*2*3) * (½)^{10} = 120 / 1024 = 0.1171$

4. *Find the probability of a cow, having calved five times, to have i. All female calves, ii. Atleast one female calf, and iii. 2 female calves and 3 male calves.*

   Consider the event of getting the female calf as success.

   The probability of having 'x' success out of 'n' trials is $nc_x\, p^x\, g^{n-x}$; n = 5,p = q = ½

   $p(x) = 5c_x (½)^x (½)^{5-x} = 5c_x (½)^5 = 5c_x / 32$

   i. P (All are females) = P(x=5) = ${}^5c_5/32$ = 1/32 = 0.0312

   ii. P (At least one female calf) = P(x>1) = 1-P(x=0) = 1-$5c_o$/32 = 1-1/32 = 1-0.0312 = 0.9688

   iii. P (2 female calves and 3 male calves) = P(x=2) = $5C_2$/32 = 10/32 = 0.3125

5.1.1 Types of Probability Distributions

Among all the theoretical or expected frequency distributions, Binomial, Poisson, and Normal distributions are popular and extensively used. While the first two are of discrete type, the last one is of continuous type.

5.1.1.1 Binomial Distribution

Also called as Bernoulli process or distribution, Binomial distribution is a widely used probability distribution of a discrete random variable, more commonly used for quality control. Manufacturing units use binomial distribution for defective analysis. Service organizations like banks and insurance companies get ideas from customers for service quality. Binomial distribution helps to express the probability of one set of alternatives, i.e., success or failure. This distribution has the following assumptions:

- Trials are independent and random.
- The experiment is conducted under the same condition for a fixed number of 'n' trials.
- In each trial, there are only two possible outcomes, success or failure.
- The probability of success is uniform throughout n trials.
- The probability of success is denoted by 'p' which remains constant from trial to trial and the probability of failure is denoted by q = 1 - p.

In 'n' independent trials, if p is the constant probability of success in a single trial, then the variate x, i.e., the number of successes in these 'n' trials, is said to follow binomial distribution. The variate takes values from 0 to n (all integers), the probability of getting 0, 1, 2, 3, …, n successes at these n trials is q^n, $nC_1q^{n-1}p^1$, $nC_2q^{n-2}p^2$, $nC_3q^{n-3}p^3$…, $nC_xq^{n-x}p^x$, …, p^n respectively, which are the respective terms of binomial expansion $(q + p)^n$.

Suppose we have N sets of 'n' trials, the number of sets in which we will have 0, 1, 2, 3, …, n success will be given by the successive terms of binomial expansion $N (q+p)^n$. Thus, we classify the sets according to the number of successes they contain and we get a frequency distribution which is known as the binomial distribution:

No. of success	0	1	2	3	…	x	…	n
Frequency	Nq^n	$NnC_1q^{n-1}p^1$	$NnC_2q^{n-2}p^2$	$NnC_3q^{n-3}p^3$		$NnC_xq^{n-x}p^x$		Np^n

Properties of Binomial Distribution

1. It is a distribution of discontinuous or discrete variate.
2. It has two parameters (constants), n and p, where n denotes the number of independent trials and p denotes the constant probability of success in a single trial.
3. It takes values from 0 to n (all integers), i.e., 0, 1, 2, 3, …, n.
4. Its mean is np and variance is npq, where q=1-p. SD = $\sqrt{npg}$; Variance < mean.
5. The different frequencies are different terms of binomial expansion $N(q+p)^n$.
6. It is symmetrical, when p = q = ½.
7. When n is large and p is small such that np is constant, the binomial distribution tends to become a Poisson distribution.
8. When n is large and p = q = ½, ***the binomial*** distribution tends to become a normal distribution.

Binomial Probability Function

Under the conditions of a Bernoulli process, the probability of getting x successes out of n trials is the definition of a binomial distribution. The binomial probability function is given by the expression:

$$P(x) = \binom{n}{x} p^x (1-p)^{n-x}$$

where P(x) is the probability of getting x successes in n trials

$=\binom{n}{x}$ is the number of ways in which x successes can take place out of n trials

$= n! / [x! (n - x)!]$

p is the probability of success, which is the same throughout n trials; X can take values 0, 1, 2, 3, ..., n; and n! = 1.2.3.4...n (product of first n terms). For e.g., 5! = 1x2x3x4x5 = 120.

Exercise

A bank issues credit cards to customers. Based on past data, the bank has found that 60% of account holders pay their dues on time. If a sample of 7 accounts is selected at random, construct the Binomial Probability Distribution of accounts paying on time.

Solution

This problem can be structured as the Bernoulli Process, where an account holder paying on time is taken as a success, and an account holder not paying on time is taken as a failure. The random variable x represents here an account holder paying on time, which can take values 0, 1, 2, 3, 4, 5, 6, or 7. We need to prepare a table containing x and P(x) for all the values of x. Performing calculations using the Binomial probability function, we get:

$$P(x) = \binom{n}{x} p^x (1-p)^{n-x} \text{ for } x = 0,1,2,3,4,5,6,7$$

From the example, we can also answer the following questions:

1. *What is the probability of getting not more than 3 accounts paying on time?*

   We want P (x < 3). Hence, the answer is 0.2897920.

2. *What is the probability of at least 4 accounts paying on time?*

   We want P (x > 4) = P(4) + P(5) + P(6)+ P(7) = 1 – P(x < 3) = 1 – 0.2897920 = 0.710208.

3. *What is the probability of no account holder paying on time?*

   We want P (x = 0) = P(0) = 0.0016384.

Mean and Standard Deviation of Binomial Distribution

A bank issues credit cards to customers. Based on past data, it has been found that 60% of all account holders pay on time following the bill. If a sample of 7 accounts is selected at random from the current database, calculate the mean and standard deviation of the account holders paying on time.

This problem also can be structured as a Bernoulli Process where an account paying on time is taken as a success and an account holder not paying on time is taken as a failure. The random variable x represents here an account holder paying on time, which can take values 0, 1, 2, 3, 4, 5, 6, 7. Applying the formula for mean, $\mu = np$, you get mean = 7 x 0.06 = 4.2. That is, you can expect, on average, 4.2 of the accounts will pay on time. Applying the formula for standard deviation,

$\sigma = \sqrt{np(1\text{-}p)}$, we get standard deviation $= \sqrt{4.2(1\text{-}0.60)} = 1.30$.

Exercise

From a milk product company, the quality control department selects a sample of 15 items. According to the requirement, if 3 or more of the items in the sample are found to be defective, the entire production lot will be rejected and then the lot will be subjected to 100% inspection. From the past data, it is known that the probability of an item being defective is 0.04.

1. *What is the probability that the production lot will be rejected?*

   The probability of rejecting the lot = 1 – the probability of accepting the lot. We have the probability of acceptance (for n =15, x = 2, p = 0.04) as 0.9797. So, the probability of rejecting the lot is 1 – 0.9797 = 0.0203.

2. *Find the mean and SD of the binomial random variable (x = no. of defectives).*

   Mean = np = (15) * (0.04) = 0.60, Standard Deviation

   $\sigma = \sqrt{np(1-p)} = \sqrt{0.60(0.96)} = 0.76$

5.1.1.2 Poisson Distribution

Poisson distribution is another discrete distribution that is useful in quality control to reduce the number of defects in the products. The Poisson probability distribution function is worked out based on the Poisson process as below:

- The probability of getting exactly one success in a continuous interval such as length, area, time, etc. is constant.
- The probability of success in any one interval is independent of the probability of success occurring in any other interval.
- The probability of getting more than one success in an interval is 0.

Properties of Poisson Distribution

1. It has a parameter λ.
2. It is a distribution of discrete variate.

3. It takes values from 0 to α.
4. Mean is approximately equal to variance.

Probability in Poisson Distribution

$P(x) = e^{\lambda}\lambda^{x} / x!$

where P(x) = Probability of x successes given an idea of λ

λ = Average number of successes

e = 2.71828 (based on natural logarithm)

x = Successes per unit which can take values 0, 1, 2, 3, …, ∞

λ is the parameter of the Poisson distribution.

Mean of the Poisson distribution is = λ

Standard Deviation of the Poisson distribution is = $\sqrt{\lambda}$

Exercise

On average, if 6 customers arrive every two minutes at a bank during busy hours, a) what is the probability that exactly 4 customers arrive in a given minute? b) what is the probability that more than 3 customers arrive in a given minute?

Solution

λ = 3 (6 customers every two minutes implies 3 customers per minute)

a) We are required to find out P (x = 4). Substituting the value of x=4 in the formula, we can get the answer after simplifying the expression $P(x) = e^{\lambda}\lambda^{x} / x!$
b) When x = 4, the probability P (x = 4) is 0.168031.
c) We want P (x > 3) = 1 – P (x < 3) = 1 – 0.647232 = 0.352768. (P (x < 3)) is found when x = 3.

Poisson Distribution - An Approximation to Binomial Distribution

There is a general consensus among the statisticians that when n is greater than or equal to 20, and p is less than or equal to 0.05, then the Poisson approximation to the Binomial distribution is a valid assumption.

5.1.1.3 Normal Distribution

The normal distribution is the commonly used continuous distribution and inferential statistics is mainly based on the normal distribution. Binomial and Poisson distributions are the more useful distributions for discrete variables. To have a mathematical distribution suitable to deal with the quantities whose magnitudes are continuous, a continuous distribution is needed. The normal distribution is useful for the distribution of a continuous variable. Though this distribution was discovered by De Movire and later known by Laplace, Gauss was the first person who made reference to this and hence it was named after him. The frequency curve corresponding to the normal distribution is called a normal frequency curve or normal curve or Gaussian or Laplacian probability curve. In most of our analyses, the observed frequency distributions are close to the normal distribution, especially when the sample size is reasonably large.

Properties of Normal Distribution

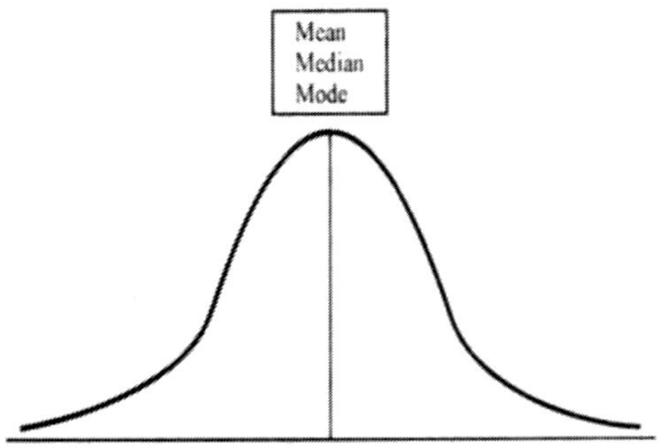

1. Normal distribution is a continuous distribution having a "Bell Shaped Distribution".
2. The variate takes values from $-\alpha$ to $+\alpha$.
3. In this distribution, mean = median = mode.
4. It is symmetrical about its mean.
5. The slope of the curve is bell-shaped, as shown in the figure. If the tails of the normal distribution extend, they would run parallel to the horizontal axis without actually touching it.
6. The normal distribution has two parameters namely mean and standard deviation (or variance).

Normal Probability Density Function

The probability density function of the normal distribution is as below:

If mean = 0; SD = 1, then the normal distribution is a standard normal distribution and its equation is

$$P(X)=\frac{1}{\sigma\sqrt{2\pi}}e^{\frac{-(x-\mu)}{2\sigma^2}}$$

where x is a continuous normal random variable with the property $-\infty < x < \infty$ (meaning that x can take all real numbers in the interval $-\infty < x < \infty$), μ is the mean of the random variable, e = 2.7183 and $\prod = 3.1416$ ($\sqrt{2\prod} = 2.5066$).

To understand the normal distribution and to apply it to practical problems, the knowledge of the probability density function is however not required. If x follows a normal distribution with mean μ and standard deviation σ, it is the practice to symbolize this expression as $x \sim N(\mu, \sigma)$. That is, it is easier to standardize the normal curve, with a mean of 0 and an SD of 1 unit.

Use of Symmetry Property of the Normal Distribution

The symmetry property of the normal distribution is important to be noted. The area under the normal curve has three distinct positions, as shown in the pictures below. The values of the area covered under each picture are close to the actual values that one can compute based on the probability density function of the normal distribution.

Case 1 - Area under the normal curve within one SD from the Mean: The total area covered within one SD from the Mean is 68%. Because of the symmetry, 68% gets divided into 34% on either side of the Mean.

Case 2 - Area under the normal curve within two SDs from the Mean: The total area covered within two SDs from the Mean is 95%. Because of the symmetry, 95% gets divided into 47.5% on either side of the Mean.

Case 3 - Area under the normal curve within three SDs from the Mean: The total area covered within three SDs from the mean is 99%. Because of the symmetry, 99% gets divided into 49.5% on either side of the Mean.

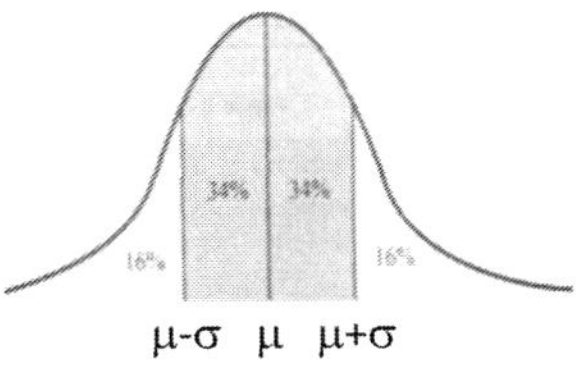

Case 1

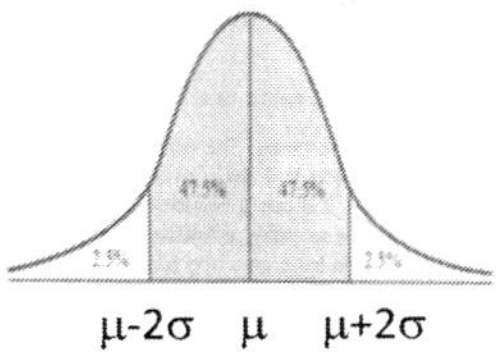

Case 2

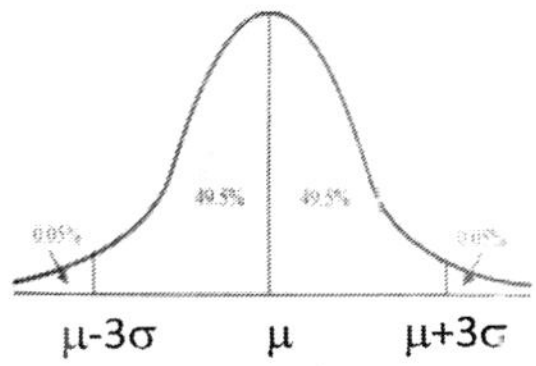

Case 3

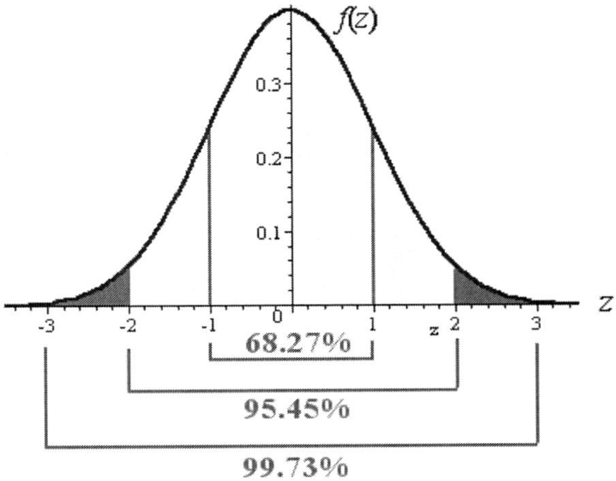

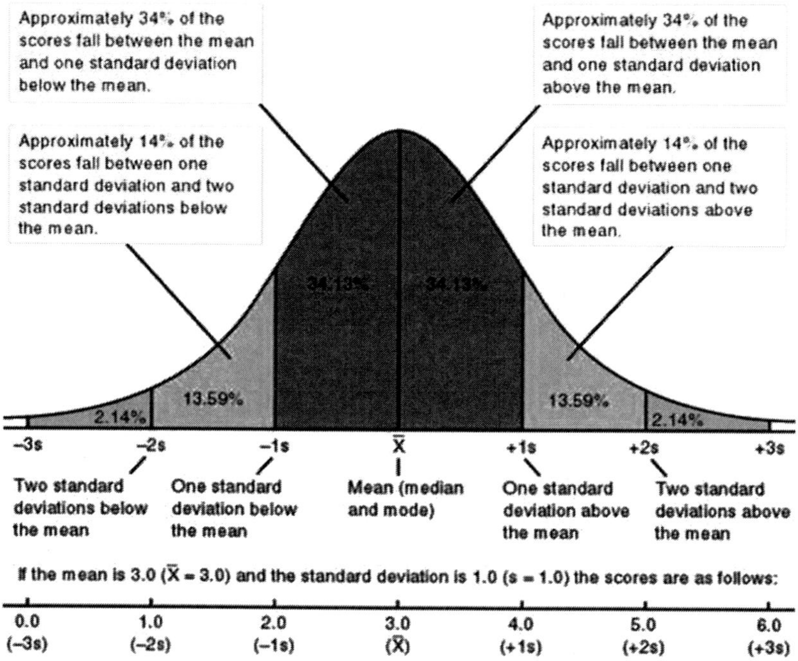

As we have seen in the measures of variation, a distribution is said to be skewed if the Mean, Median, and Mode fall at different points, i.e., Mean ≠ Median ≠ Mode. A distribution is positively skewed, if Mean > Median > Mode. A distribution is negatively skewed, if Mean < Median > Mode. For normal (symmetrical) distribution, Mean = Median = Mode.

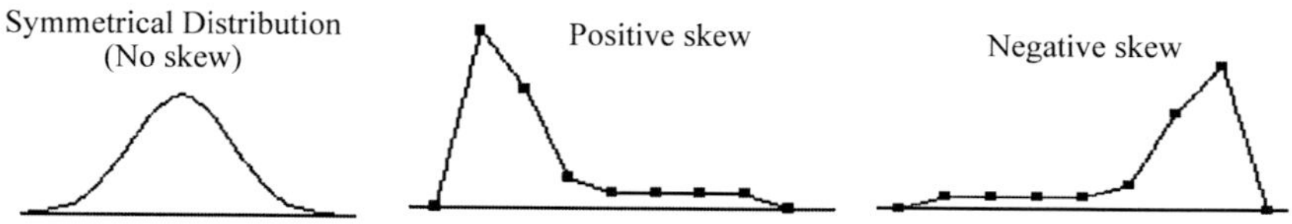

A normal (bell-shaped distribution) curve is known as a mesokurtic curve. A curve flatter than the normal curve is known as a platykurtic curve. A curve more peaked than the normal curve is known as a leptokurtic curve.

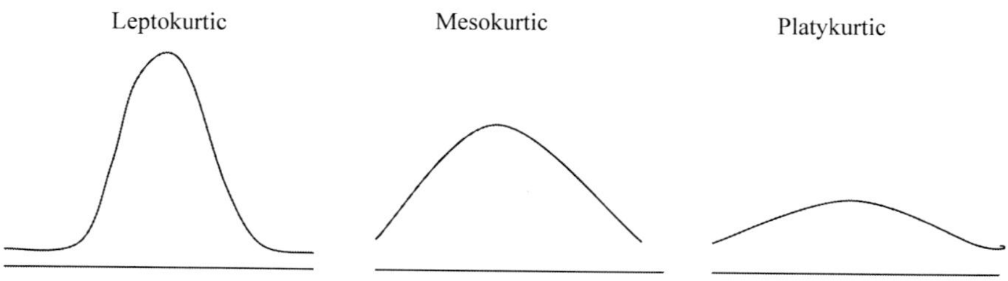

Standard Normal Distribution

For practical problems, which require the help of normal distribution for solutions, it is not possible to compute the probability in a straightforward manner because each of those normal variables may have different units of measurement. One problem may involve the unit meter, another may involve kilograms, and so on. Therefore, we need a probability distribution that can tackle any unit of measurement. Therefore, we have the Standard Normal Distribution defined as follows:

$$z = \frac{x - \mu}{\sigma}$$

z is called the standard normal variable, which is a pure number independent of the unit of measurement. The random variable z follows a normal distribution with mean = 0 and SD = 1. We first convert the original variable into z, through the transformation of scale. The probability table for z is available for computing the necessary probabilities for a given situation.

Exercise

The mean weight of a milk sachet is 0.295 kg with a standard deviation of 0.025 kg. The random variable weight of the sachet follows a normal distribution.

a) *What is the probability that the sachet weighs less than 0.280 kg?*
b) *What is the probability that the sachet weighs more than 0.350 kg?*
c) *What is the probability that the sachet weighs between 0.260 kg to 0.340 kg?*

Solution

Draw the correct diagram to the original problem. This step is crucial for getting the answer. The standard normal table displays the probability between 0 and the positive value of z. Using this table, let us answer all the parts of the above example.

Diagram for (a)

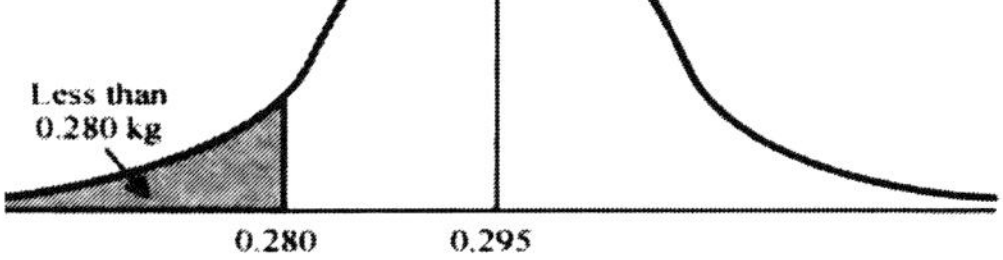

a) In the diagram above, the probability of the shaded area is required.

$z = (x-\mu)/\sigma = (0.280–0.295)/0.025 = -0.6$

In the table, this is = 0.5 - area up to z = -0.6. By the property of symmetry, this is the same as 0.5 – area from 0 to 0.6. Hence, the probability that the sachet weighs less than 0.280 kg is = 0.5 - 0.2257 = 0.2743.

Diagram for (b)

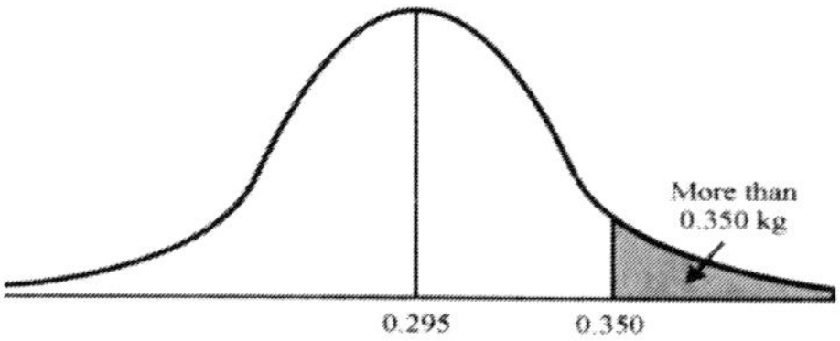

b) $z = (x-\mu)/\sigma = (0.350-0.295) / 0.025 = 2.2$

What we want is the area that is greater than 2.2. This is the same as 0.5 – area from 0 to 2.2. Hence, the probability that the sachet weighs more than 0.350 kg is = 0.5 – 0.4861 = 0.0139.

Diagram for (c)

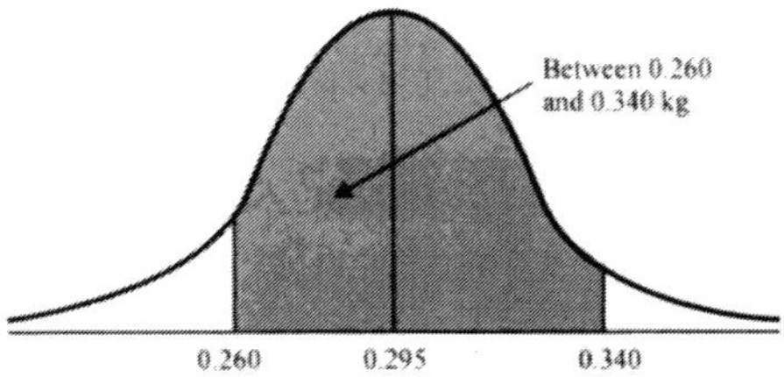

c) What we want is the area shaded above. This is the sum of the area between

$z = (x-\mu)/\sigma = (0.260-0.295) / 0.025 = -1.4$; and

$z = (x-\mu)/\sigma = (0.340-0.295) / 0.025 = 1.8$.

This is the same as –1.4 to 0 plus 0 to 1.8. But area –1.4 to 0 is the same as 0 to 1.4. Therefore, the answer is the area of 0 to 1.4 plus an area of 0 to 1.8. Hence, the probability that the sachet weighs between 0.260 kg to 0.340 kg is 0.4192 + 0.4641 = 0.8833.

Normal Approximation to Binomial Distribution

In the binomial distribution by taking n = 10, and p = 0.5, a histogram is first drawn in which the horizontal axis represents the success (x) and the vertical axis represents the probability of success P(x). A normal distribution is superimposed on the histogram. The shape of the histogram coincides with the normal curve almost perfectly. Hence, it is agreed by many practitioners that the Normal approximation for the Binomial holds true when the value of np is at least = 5.

5.2 TEST OF HYPOTHESIS AND TESTS OF SIGNIFICANCE

For all the experiments and investigations in biological sciences, only a small number of individuals, called a representative sample of the population, are studied. These samples are expected to provide estimates of the parameters of the population. In almost all the cases, two samples drawn from the same population are less likely to be similar. The process of assessing the significance of differences between two samples drawn from the same population or from two closely related populations is called as the test of significance. That is, it is a statistical procedure followed to test the significant difference between the statistic and the parameter (e.g., between the sample mean and population mean) or between two statistics (e.g., between two sample means). The test of significance helps in determining whether the observed difference between two samples is actually due to *chance* or the difference is really significant, being influenced by some factor.

The procedures followed for drawing the conclusions from the sample values are included under inferential statistics or statistical inference. In statistical inference, we deal with two aspects, *viz.*, 1. Estimation and 2. Testing of Hypothesis. Estimation helps us to estimate the population parameters based on information derived from the sample. Testing of a hypothesis is concerned with laying down a hypothesis and then testing whether the hypothesis laid down is true or not. Since the test of hypothesis helps in ascertaining whether the difference between a sample statistic and the hypothesized population parameter is significant or not, it is also called a test of significance.

5.2.1 Procedure for carrying out a Test of Significance

The procedure for the test of significance includes the following steps:

1. **Setting up a hypothesis** – This step is concerned with setting up a hypothesis about a population parameter. A hypothesis is a tentative statement about the population parameter. We collect data from the sample to know sample statistics and use this to decide how likely it is that the hypothesized population parameter is correct.
2. **Type of hypothesis** – We will have two different hypotheses in such a way that one is accepted and the other is rejected. The two hypotheses are the Null hypothesis and the True Hypothesis. The null hypothesis, denoted by H_O, will be that there is no significant difference between the statistic and parameter or between any two statistics. H_O is either accepted or rejected at some level of significance. Since many research problems aim at the establishment of statistical significance of differences, rejection of the null hypothesis thus indicates success in a project. As

against this, the alternative hypothesis is a statement contrary to the null hypothesis and is denoted by H_A.

3. **Testing of hypothesis** – There are a number of steps for testing the null hypothesis. They include setting up of H_O, computation of test statistic (SE, t-test, etc.), determining critical value (value in critical region for rejection), and making a statistical decision (to reject or accept H_O). The test statistic is some statistic that may be computed from the data of the sample. The key to the statistical inference is the sampling distribution of the relevant statistic. The general formula for a test statistic that is applied in many of the hypothesis tests is:

   Test Statistic = [relevant statistic - hypothetical parameter] / SE of the relevant statistic

   Decision rule: All the possible values that the test statistic can assume are points on the horizontal axis of the graph of the distribution of the test statistic and are divided into two groups. One group constitutes what is known as the rejection region and the other group makes up the non-rejection region. The decision rule tells us to reject the Ho if the value of the test statistic that we compute from our sample is one of the values in the rejection region and to not reject the Ho if the computed value of the test statistic is one of the values in the non-rejection region.

   Significance level: The decision as to which values go into the rejection region and which ones go into the non-rejection region is made based on the desired level of significance, designated by α. The term α (level of significance) reflects the fact that the hypothesis tests are sometimes called significance tests, and a computed value of the test statistic that falls in the rejection region is said to be significant. The level of significance specifies the area under the curve of the distribution of the test statistic that is above the values on the horizontal axis constituting the rejection region.

   The level of significance α is the probability of rejecting the true Ho. We select a small value of α in order to make the probability of rejecting a true H_O small. The more frequently encountered values of α are 0.01 and 0.05.

   Calculation of the test statistic: From the data contained in the sample, we compute a value of the test statistic and compare it with rejection and non-rejection regions that are already specified.

   Statistical decision: The statistical decision consists of rejecting or not rejecting the H_O. It is rejected if the computed value of the test statistic falls in the rejection region and it is not rejected if the computed value of the test statistic falls in the non-rejection region.

Conclusion: If H_O is rejected, we conclude that H_A is true. If H_O is not rejected, we conclude that H_O may be true.

4. **Types of errors in testing a hypothesis** – There are two types of errors possible while making a decision about H_O being correct or incorrect, *viz.*, Type I error and Type II error. When H_O is rejected when it is actually true, it is the type I error. The probability of making a type I error by rejecting H_O when it is true is α and the probability of making the correct decision of accepting H_O when it is true will be (1-α). Type II error occurs when H_O is accepted when it is actually false. It is represented by 1-β, where β is the probability of a type II error.

Hypothesis Testing - Type I and Type II Errors

Action	**Null Hypothesis**	
	True	**False**
Reject H0	Type I Error (α)	No Error
Accept H0	No Error	Type II Error (β)

5. **Fixing the level of significance** – The level of significance is the maximum probability of making a type I error and is denoted by α. It means P (i.e., probability of rejecting H_O when H_0 is true) is α and the probability of making a correct decision will be 1-α. The commonly used levels of significance are 5% (0.05) and 1% (0.01). It means that at 5% level of significance, α = 0.05 or the probability of making a type I error is 0.05. That is, there is a probability of making type I error in 5 out of 100 times. Similarly, at 1% level of significance, the error in accepting the null hypothesis is reduced, i.e., we may go wrong only in one out of 100 occasions.

5.2.2 Different Tests of Significance

A distribution will be attached to the test. The various parametric tests are:

1. Normal deviate test or large sample test or Z test
2. Students t-test or small sample test
3. Chi-square test
4. Variance–ratio test or F-test

In any test, we take any one of the following four decisions:

- Null hypothesis may be true but we reject it by our test – Type I error.
- Null hypothesis may be false but we accept it – Type II error.

- Null hypothesis is true and we accept it – Correct decision.
- Null hypothesis is false and we reject it – Correct decision.

Computation of Test of Significance

There are four types of problems for which the tests of significance are used:

1. Comparison of sample mean with population mean
2. Comparison of two sample means
3. Comparison of sample proportion with population proportion
4. Comparison of two sample proportions

5.2.3 Hypothesis Testing

Type I error says that we reject the null hypothesis when it is true. Type II error says that we accept the null hypothesis when it is false. Strictly speaking we 'don't' accept the null hypothesis. When we cannot reject the null hypothesis, it only means that the sample evidence does not warrant rejection of the null hypothesis. However, using the terminology "accept the null hypothesis" helps us to make the right decision. This little bit of dilution in terminology is permitted in the context of decision–making.

The probability of making a Type I error is called the level of significance of the test. It is designated by the Greek letter alpha (α). The probability level of this error is decided by the decision maker before the hypothesis test is performed and is based on his tolerance in terms of the risk of rejecting the true null hypothesis. The complement ($1-\alpha$) of the probability of Type I error measures the probability level of not rejecting a true null hypothesis. It is also referred to as the confidence level, which says that we are right in our assessment ($1-\alpha$)% of the time. If we set $\alpha = 0.05$ and happen to reject the null hypothesis at this level, there is a 5% probability that we have rejected the null hypothesis when in fact it is true. This also means that we are 95% confident that we have accepted the null hypothesis when it is true. The significance level desired will depend on how much risk we want to take in rejecting the null hypothesis when it is true. We can now see the connection between the confidence interval and the level of significance.

The probability of making a Type II error is symbolized by the Greek letter β. It is due to a decision to accept a false null hypothesis. The probability level of this error varies with the actual values of the population parameter being tested when H_0 is false. Thus, the level of this error is measured for different values of population parameter that make the H_0 false. The complement ($1-\beta$) of the probability of Type II error measures the probability of rejecting the false null hypothesis. It is also called the power of the test. The power of the test is the probability of rejecting the null hypothesis when, in fact, it is false. Suppose we keep $\beta = 10\%$, it means that the power of the test is 90%. That is, the probability of rejecting the null hypothesis when it is false is 90%, and only 10% of the time we commit the error of accepting the null hypothesis when it is false. It is a convention to set $\alpha = 0.05$ which responds to the confidence level of 95%.

The level of Type I error can be decreased with the increase in Type II error. Thus, for a given level of significance (i.e., the risk of Type I error), an increase in sample size will decrease the β value (i.e., the risk of Type II error). Consequently, this will increase the power of the test to detect whether the H_O is false. In other words, the level of Type II error can be reduced by considering a higher value of the level of significance as 0.05, instead of 0.01. A type I error is often considered more serious than a type II error and hence type I error should be necessarily avoided. The hypothesis test procedure should therefore be adjusted to ensure a guaranteed 'low' probability of rejecting the H_O wrongly.

5.2.4 Critical Region or Rejection Region

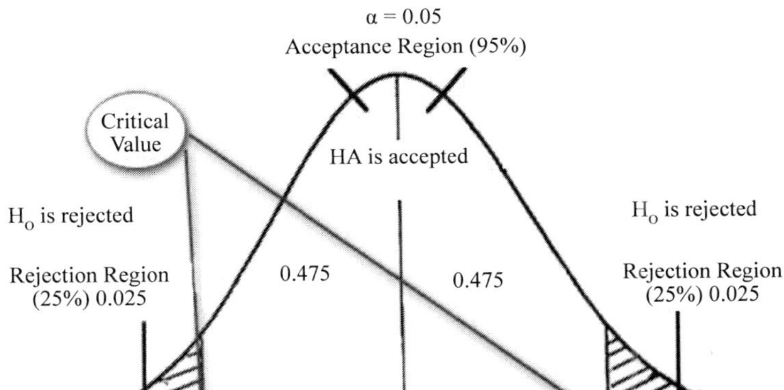

The sample space of the experiment, which corresponds to the area under the sampling distribution curve of the test statistic, is divided into two mutually exclusive regions as shown in the figure above. These regions are called the acceptance region and the critical region. If the value of the test statistic falls into the acceptance region, the H_O is accepted; otherwise, it is rejected. The rejection region consists of all the values of the test statistic that are likely to occur if H_O is true. On the other hand, these values are not likely to occur if H_O is false. The value of the test statistic that separates the region of acceptance and rejection is called the critical value.

The size of the rejection region is directly related to the level of precision to make decisions about a population parameter. Decision rules concerning the null hypothesis are:

Prob (H_O is true) ≤ α, reject H_O; Prob (H_O is true) > α, accept H_O

i.e., if the probability of H_0 being true is less than α, reject H_0; otherwise, retain H_0.

5.2.5 Calculating the Suitable Statistic

The value of the test statistic is calculated from the distribution of sample statistic:

Test statistic = (Value of sample statistic – Value of hypothesized population parameter / Standard error of sample statistic

5.2.6 Choice of Probability Distribution

The choice of a probability distribution of a sample statistic is guided by the sample size n and the value of population standard deviation σ as shown below:

Sample size n	**Population standard deviation σ**	
	Known	**Unknown**
$n > 30$	Normal distribution	Normal distribution
$n \leq 30$, the population assumed normal	Normal distribution	t - distribution

5.2.7 Reaching a Conclusion

Compare the calculated value of the test statistic with the critical value (also called the standard table value of the test statistic). The decision rules for the null hypothesis are:

$|z|_{cal} > |z|_{table}$; reject H_0

$|z|_{cal} < |z|_{table}$; accept H_0

That is, if the calculated absolute value of a test statistic is more than or equal to its critical (or table) value, then reject the H_O, otherwise accept it. The same decision rules hold for the t-distribution with the sampling distributions of means or proportions when the sample size is small.

5.2.8 Test Statistic and P value

A test statistic is a quantity calculated from sample data. Its value is used to decide whether or not the H_O should be rejected in the hypothesis test. Attached to each statistic is a Probability, or P value. It describes the chance of getting the observed effect if H_O is true. The probability value (p-value) of a statistical hypothesis test is the probability of wrongly rejecting H_O, if it is, in fact, true.

Making a Decision using the P value

According to the evidence obtained from the sample, we make a judgment about whether the data are consistent with the H_O, which leads to the decision of whether or not to reject H_O. If the observed results are not consistent with what we would expect if the H_O is true, we conclude that we have enough evidence to reject H_O. We say that the result of the test is statistically significant. If, however, the observed results are consistent with what we would expect if the H_O is true, we do not reject the H_O. We say that the result of the test is non-significant.

We should note that not rejecting the Ho is not synonymous with accepting H_A. The P value allows us to determine whether we have enough evidence to reject the H_O in favour of the H_A. If the P value is very small, then it is unlikely that we could have obtained the observed results if the H_O is true, so we reject H_A. If the P value is very large, then there is a high chance that we could have obtained the observed results if the H_O is true, so we do not reject H_A.

5.2.9 One-sided and Two-Sided Tests

Formulation of null and alternative hypotheses is the complicated part of the entire exercise of hypothesis testing. A great deal of time is required to master this part. A hypothesis can be directional or non-directional. A directional hypothesis is one in which the population parameter is structured to be greater than or equal to or less than or equal to a specified value. This is known as a one-tailed test (one-sided test). A non-directional hypothesis is one in which the population parameter is structured to be equal to a specified value. This is known as a two-tailed test (two-sided test).

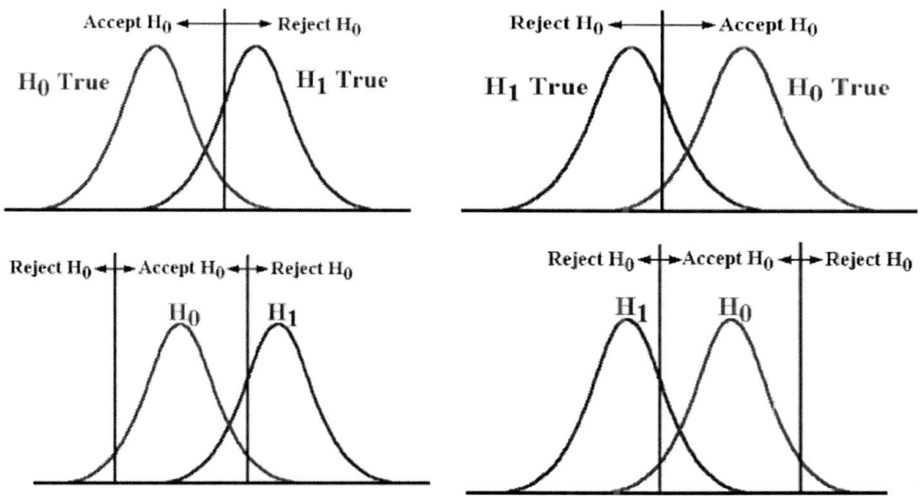

5.2.10 Hypothesis Testing - Univariate Case (One Sample)

The formulation of the null and alternative hypothesis for the univariate case can be explained.

Hypothesis Testing – Population Mean (Single Mean)

Primary Objective of the Test: To test hypotheses that compare the population mean to a specified value

Look at the illustration:

Is the average incidence of FMD in Tamil Nadu greater than 15%?

Is it a one-tailed test or a two–tailed test? It is a one–tailed test because the average incidence of FMD in Tamil Nadu is specified to be greater than 15. We will formulate the null and the alternative hypotheses for this illustration.

H_o: $\mu \leq 15$; H_A: $\mu > 15$

μ Represents the Population Mean incidence of FMD in Tamil Nadu

The null hypothesis Ho is generally the negation of the truth. The question that is raised about the population mean is, "Is the average incidence greater than 15%?". So, it is a one-sided test and the right structure is that the null hypothesis must specify the incidence of FMD in Tamil Nadu to be less than or equal to 15%. This is precisely what is given above. We will be correct in our hypothesis formulation, if we remember two things: 1) The null hypothesis is formulated to get it rejected; and, 2) We believe that the alternative hypothesis will happen. In this example, it was felt that the incidence of FMD is more than 15%. So, this is the alternative hypothesis. In other words, we must formulate the null hypothesis in such a way that its rejection automatically leads to the preferred conclusion.

If the question is rephrased as "Is the average incidence of FMD in Tamil Nadu different from 15%?", how to formulate the null and the alternative hypotheses?

H_o: $\mu = 15$ (the average incidence of FMD is equal to 15%)

H_A: $\mu \neq 15$ (the average incidence of FMD is not equal to 15%)

This formulation is undoubtedly a two-tailed test of the hypothesis, as the population mean incidence is specified to be equal to the value of 15%.

5.2.11 Hypothesis Testing – Population Proportion (One Sample)

Primary Objective of the Test: To test hypotheses that compare the population proportion to a specified value

Illustration for a Single Proportion

Is the proportion of households owning Jersey cows in Salem district less than 0.5?

It is a one-tailed test. The null and the alternative hypotheses are:

H_0: P > 0.5; H_A: P < 0.5

P represents the population proportion of households in Salem owning Jersey cows

5.2.12 Test of Hypothesis - Z Test - Large Sample Test

This test is carried out, when the sample size is > 30. When n > 30, it will follow the normal distribution.

1. **Testing the Significant Difference between Sample Mean and Population Mean**

   Step 1: H_0: No significant difference between the sample mean and population mean

   Step 2: Choice of the Test statistic (Z statistic) given by,

$$Z = \frac{\text{Sample mean} - \text{Population mean}}{\text{SE of differnce}} = \frac{\overline{x} - \mu}{SE(\overline{x} - \mu)}$$

   where $\overline{x}$ = sample mean and μ = population mean

$$Z = \frac{\overline{x} - \mu}{\frac{\sigma}{\sqrt{n}}}$$

   where σ is the SD of the population, n is the size of the sample

   When σ is not known, replace it with 's' which is the SD of the sample. Then,

$$Z = \frac{\overline{x} - \mu}{\frac{s}{\sqrt{n}}}$$

   Step 3: Conclusion (Comparison with theoretical value)

   i. |Z| < 1.96, we say that Z is not significant and Ho is accepted. We denote this by $Z = (\ )^{NS}$

   ii. |Z| > 1.96, Z is significant (at 5% level) and Ho is rejected. We denote this by $Z = (\ )^{*}$

   iii. |Z| > 2.58, Z is highly significant (at 1% level) and Ho is rejected. We denote this as $Z = (\ )^{**}$

Exercise

The mean height of a sample of 100 is 64 inches. The Standard Deviation of the distribution of the height is 3 inches. Test the statement that the mean height of the population is 67 inches.

Solution

Let us hypothesize that there is no significant difference between the sample mean and the population mean.

$$Z = \frac{\overline{x} - \mu}{\frac{s}{\sqrt{n}}}$$

Z = (64 – 67) / (3 / √100)

= -3 / (3/10) = -3/0.3 = -10

Since the difference (|Z| = 10) is more than 1.96 (at 5% level), the null hypothesis is rejected. Hence the mean height of the population cannot be 67 inches.

Exercise

A sample of size 400 was drawn and the sample mean was found to be 99. Test whether this sample could have come from a normal population with a mean of 100 and a variance of 64.

Solution

$$Z = \frac{\overline{x} - \mu}{\frac{\sigma}{\sqrt{n}}}$$

Z = 99 – 100 / (8 / √400), because SD = √variance)

= -1 / (8/20) = -2.5

|Z| = 2.5 > 1.96. Therefore, it is significant at 5% level. Hence, we conclude that the sample has not been drawn from the population with mean 100 and variance 64.

2 (a). Testing the significant difference between two sample means, when they are taken from different populations

Ho: There is no significant difference between the two sample means.

$z = \frac{\overline{x}_1 - \overline{x}_2}{SE(\overline{x}_1 - \overline{x}_2)}$ where $\overline{x}_1$, $\overline{x}_2$ are sample means with sizes n_1 and n_2, respectively

$$z = \frac{\bar{x}_1 - \bar{x}_2}{\sqrt{\frac{\sigma_1^2}{n_1} + \frac{\sigma_2^2}{n_2}}}$$ where σ_1, σ_2 are SDs of respective populations

When σ_1, σ_2 are not available S_1, S_2 are used.

$$z = \frac{\bar{x}_1 - \bar{x}_2}{\sqrt{\frac{s_1^2}{n_1} + \frac{s_2^2}{n_2}}}$$

Exercise

An examination was conducted for 50 students at College A and for 60 students at College B. At College A, the mean mark was 75 with a SD of 9. At B, the mean was 79 with an SD of 7. Is there a significant difference between the performance of students at A and that of B?

Solution

H_O: There is no difference in the marks obtained by the students of Colleges A and B.

$$z = \frac{\bar{x}_1 - \bar{x}_2}{\sqrt{\frac{\sigma_1^2}{n_1} + \frac{\sigma_2^2}{n_2}}}$$

Z = (75 – 79) / sqrt {(9^2/50) + (7^2/60)}

= -4 / sqrt {(81/50) + (49/60)} = -4 / sqrt (1.62 + 0.817)

= -4 (1.56) = - 2.56 > 1.96

Since the difference between the two colleges is significant at 5% level, we reject H_O. However, 2.56 < 2.58 and hence we accept the Ho at 1% level.

2. **(b). Testing the significant difference between two sample means, when they are taken from the same population**

   Ho: There is no significant difference between the two-sample means

$$Z = \frac{x_1 - x_2}{\sigma\sqrt{\frac{1}{n_1} + \frac{1}{n_2}}}$$

$$Z = \frac{\bar{x}_1 - \bar{x}_2}{\sqrt{\frac{s_1^2}{n_2} + \frac{s_2^2}{n_1}}}$$

where σ (SD of Population) is not known

$$\text{replace}\,\sigma^2 = \frac{n_1 s_1^{\,2} + n_2 s_2^{\,2}}{n_1 + n_2}$$

Exercise

A test on two groups of students gave the following results:

Group	*Mean mark*	*SD*	*N*
Boys	*70*	*20*	*250*
Girls	*75*	*15*	*150*

Is there a significant in the mean scores obtained by boys and girls?

Solution

Ho – There is no significant difference in the mean scores obtained by boys and girls.

$$Z = \frac{\overline{x}_1 - \overline{x}_2}{\sqrt{\frac{S_1^{\,2}}{n_2} + \frac{S_2^{\,2}}{n_1}}}$$

$$\begin{aligned} Z &= (75\text{-}70) / \text{sqrt}\ \{(20^2/250) + (15^2/150)\} \\ &= 5 / \text{sqrt}\ (1.5 + 1.6) \\ &= 5 / 1.761 = 2.84 \end{aligned}$$

Since the difference (2.84) is more than 2.58 at 1% level, Ho is rejected. Hence, we conclude that there seems to be a significant difference in the mean marks obtained by boys and girls.

3. **Testing the significant difference between sample and population proportions (Test for proportion of successes)**

   If n is the number of trials, p is the proportion of success out of n trials, and P is the expected proportion of success, then p follows the normal distribution when n is large. Hence, Ho: There is no significant difference between p and P.

   $$\text{Teststatistic}\ Z = \frac{p - P}{SE(p - P)} = \frac{p - P}{\sqrt{\frac{pq}{n}}} \quad \text{where } q = 1 - p$$

Exercise

A wholesaler of apples claims that only 4% of the apples supplied by him are defective. A random sample of 600 apples contained 36 defective apples. Test the claim of the wholesaler.

Solution

The wholesaler claims that only 4% of his apples are defective. Hence, the 95% confidence limit is mean + 1.96 SE.

SE = sqrt (pq/n) = sqrt {(0.96*0.04)/600} = 0.008

95% confidence limits = mean + 1.96 SE.

= 0.96 + 1.96 (0.008)

= 0.96 + 0.0157

= 0.9443 to 0.9757

That is, out of 600 apples, the good apples may be between 0.9443*600 = 566.58 or 557 to 0.9757*600 = 585.42 or 585. Hence, the number of defectives (out of 600) is expected to lie between 15 and 33. Since the actual number is 36, his claim that only 4% (i.e., 24 out of 600) is defective cannot be accepted.

4. **Testing the significant difference between two proportions**

   Ho: There is no significant difference between the two proportions

   Let p_1, p_2 be observed proportions of success out of n_1, n_2 trails, respectively.

$$z = \frac{p_1 - p_2}{SE(p_1 - p_2)}$$

$$= \frac{p_1 - p_2}{\sqrt{\frac{p_1 q_1}{n_1} + \frac{p_2 q_2}{n_2}}} \text{ where } q_1 = 1\ p_1\ q_2 = 1\ p_2$$

(or)

$$\frac{p_1 - p_2}{\sqrt{PQ\left(\frac{1}{n_1} + \frac{1}{n_2}\right)}} \text{ where } P = \frac{n_1 p_1 + n_2 p_2}{n_1 + n_2} \text{ and } Q = 1 - P$$

Exercise

In a random sample of 1000 persons from town A, 400 are found to be consumers of wheat. In a sample of 800 from town B, 400 are found to be consumers of wheat. Is there a significant difference between these towns as far as the proportion of wheat consumers is concerned?

Solution

Ho – There is no significant difference between towns A and B with regard to the proportion of wheat consumers.

Z = p_1p_2 / sqrt [PQ /(1/n_1 + 1/n_2)]

n_1 = 1000, p_1 = 400/1000 = 0.4

n_2 = 800, p_2 = 400/800 = 0.5

p = [(1000*0.4) + (800*0.5)] / (1000+800) = 800/1800 = 4/9

q = 1 – 4/9 = 5/9

Z = (0.4 – 0.5) / sqrt {4/9*5/9 (1/1000 + 1/800)

= -0.1 / sqrt (20/81 * 9/4000)

= -4.17

|Z| = 4.17 is greater than 2.58 at 1% level. Therefore, there is a significant difference between town A and town B, so far as the proportion of wheat consumers is concerned.

5.2.13 Test of Hypothesis - t Test - Small Sample Test

When the sample size is large and variates are normally distributed, the normal test is employed to test the significance of differences. With small samples and when the degrees of freedom less than 30, the variates are not normally distributed. Hence, we make use of the t-distribution and t-test of significance. Tables are available relating to t at different probability levels for various degrees of freedom.

1. **Testing the significant difference of sample mean from the population mean**

   Step 1: Ho: There is no significant difference between the sample mean and population mean

   Step 2: Test statistic is given by

$$t = \frac{\text{difference in the mean of the sample and population}}{\text{S.E of difference}}$$

$$t = \frac{\overline{x} - \mu}{SE(\overline{x} - \mu)} = \frac{\overline{x} - \mu}{\frac{S}{\sqrt{n-1}}} \text{ with d.f} = (n-1)$$

   $\overline{x}$ = mean of the sample of size 'n' with SD 's' and df = n-1

   μ = population mean

   Step 3: Conclusion

   i. If |t| < table value of t for (n-1) df at 5% level, t is non-significant, and H_o is accepted. We denote this as t = ( )$^{N.S.}$

   ii. If |t| > table value of t for (n-1) df at 5% level, t is significant and Ho is rejected. We denote this as t = ( )*.

   iii. If |t| > table value of t for (n-1) df at 1% level, t is highly significant and H_o is rejected. We denote this as t = ( )**

Exercise

A sample of 20 items has mean 42 units and SD 5 units. Test the Ho that it is a random sample from a normal population with a mean of 45 units.

Solution

Ho - μ=45 and H_A - $\mu \neq 45$

N = 20 (small sample), $\bar{x}$ = 42 and s = 5

$$= \frac{\bar{x} - \mu}{\frac{s}{\sqrt{n-1}}} = (42 - 45) / (5 / \sqrt{(20-1)})$$

$|t| = 3/5\sqrt{19} = 2.62$

Table t for df = 19 at 5% level is 2.09. $|t| > t_{0.05}$. That is, the difference between the sample mean and the population mean is significant. Hence, the sample could not have come from the population.

2. **Testing the significant difference between two sample means when the sizes are less than 30 and they are dependent (Paired t-test)**

   Two samples are dependent when they have some common factor linking the observations in the two samples.

   Step 1: H_O: There is no significant difference between the two-sample means.

   Step 2: Test statistic is given by $t = \frac{\bar{d} - 0}{SE of \bar{d}} = \frac{\bar{d}}{\frac{s}{\sqrt{n-1}}}$ with d.f = (n – 1)

   $\bar{d}$ = Difference in the observation of the two samples; s = SD of $\bar{d}$

   Conclusion: As in the previous test

Exercise

The memory capacity of 9 students was tested before and after a course for a month. State whether the course was effective or not from the data below (in the same units).

Before: 10, 15, 9, 3, 7, 12, 16, 17, 4

After: 12, 17, 8, 5, 6, 11, 18, 20, 3

Solution

Here, we adopt paired test as we are concerned with the same set of students and the data are correlated. H_O – the course was effective. $\mu_1 = \mu_2$; H1 - $\mu_1 \neq \mu_2$

Before the course	After the course	Difference d	d^2
10	12	2	4
15	17	2	4
9	8	-1	1
3	5	2	4
7	6	-1	1
12	11	-1	1
16	18	2	4
17	20	3	9
4	3	-1	1
		$\sum d = 7$	**$\sum d^2 = 29$**

$\bar{d} = 7/9 = 0.7778$

$s^2 = \sum d^2/n - \bar{d}^2 = 29/9 - 0.7778^2 = 3.222 - 0.605 = 2.617$, hence $s = 1.6177$

$t = \bar{d} / [s/\sqrt{(n-1)}] = 0.7778/(1.6177/\sqrt{8}) = 1.360$

At df 8 and at 5% level, table value of t is 2.31. That is $|t| < t_{0.05}$.

We accept the Ho. Hence, the course was effective in improving the performance.

3. **Testing the significant difference between two samples, when they are independent (Non-paired or Un-paired t-test)**

   By independence of the two samples, we mean that there is no relationship between individuals contributing to the sample. Thus, the sample drawn from different populations or different parts of the same population will be independent.

   Step 1: H_o: There is no significant difference between the sample means.

   Step 2: Test statistics t is given by

$$\text{i.e. } t = \frac{\text{difference in the mean of the sample}}{\text{S.E of difference}}$$

$$= \frac{\bar{x}_1 - \bar{x}_2}{\sqrt{s^2\left(\frac{1}{n_1} + \frac{1}{n_2}\right)}} \quad \text{With d.f} = n_1 + n_2 \quad \text{where } s^2 = \frac{(n_1 - 1)s_1^2 + (n_2 - 1)s_2^2}{n_1 + n_2 - 2}$$

   $\bar{x}_1, \bar{x}_2$ are the means of the two samples with SD s_1, s_2 of sizes n_1, n_2 respectively

   Conclusion: as in the previous test (with respect to d.f.)

Exercise

Following are the data on first lactation yield of Sindhi and Sahiwal. Test whether there is any significant difference between these two breeds.

Sindhi	*66*	*47*	*54*	*64*	*56*	*66*	*51*	*28*	*55*	*56*	*29*
Sahiwal	*68*	*53*	*53*	*72*	*54*	*63*	*41*	*33*			

4. **Test of significance of an observed correlation coefficient**

Let 'r' be the sample correlation coefficient and 'ρ' be the population correlation coefficient.

Ho: There is no significant difference between correlation coefficients of the sample and population.

$$t = \frac{r - \rho}{SE(r - \rho)} = \frac{r}{\sqrt{1 - r^2}}\sqrt{n - 2}$$

Conclusion: as in the previous test.

If t is not significant, then we conclude that r is not significant, i.e., there is no correlation between the variables studied. If t is significant, then there is a significant correlation. Then, we denote this as r = ( ).* If t is highly significant, then we say that r is highly significant and r = ( )**. In both cases, both variables studied are related.

Exercise

A random sample of 27 pairs of observations from a normal population gave a correlation coefficient of 0.40. Is this value significant of correlation in the population?

Solution

Ho – Variables have r = 0.

$t = \{0.40 / \text{sqrt}(1\text{-}0.4^2)\} * \text{sqrt}(27\text{-}2)$

$= \{0.4 / \text{sqrt}(0.84)\} * \text{sqrt}(25)$

$= (0.4 / 0.92) * 5 = 2.17$

It is greater than 2.05 at $t_{0.05}$. Hence the H_O is rejected.

5.2.14 Test of Hypothesis - χ^2 Test (Chi-Square Test of Significance)

This test is used to test the observed frequencies for their fit with expected or theoretical frequencies or to test whether two factors of classification of a set of individuals presented in the form of a two-way table are independent or not.

χ^2 test of goodness of fit

This test is performed to test whether the deviation of observed frequencies in a given data from the expected frequencies is due to real causes or due to chance. This test is used to decide whether the given data has a good fit with one of the known forms of distributions, *viz.*, Normal, Binomial, or Poisson. The test statistic for goodness of fit is given by:

$$\chi^2 = \sum \frac{(O-E)^2}{E}$$

where O - observed frequency and E - Expected frequency; df = No. of classes-1

In this case, Ho: The fit is good or there is no significant difference between observed and expected frequency.

Conclusion

1. If calculated χ^2 is less than table χ^2 for the respective df at 5% level, χ^2 is not significant which is denoted by $\chi^2 = (\ )^{N.S}$, i.e., Ho is accepted. The fit is good.
2. If calculated χ^2 is greater than table χ^2 for the respective df at 5% level, χ^2 is significant and is denoted by $\chi^2 = (\ )^*$. H_o is rejected. The fit is not good.
3. If calculated χ^2 is greater than table χ^2 for the respective df at 1% level, χ^2 is highly significant and is denoted by $\chi^2 = (\ )^{**}$. H_o is rejected.

Exercise

A tobacco company claims that there is no relationship between smoking and lung diseases. To investigate this claim, a random sample of 300 males in the age group of 40-50 was tested and the results are given below:

Details	*Lung disease*	*No lung disease*	*Total*
Smokers	*75*	*105*	*180*
Non-smokers	*25*	*95*	*120*
Total	*100*	*200*	*300*

Can we conclude that smoking and lung diseases are independent?

Solution

H_O – Smoking and lung diseases are not associated. Calculating expected frequencies,

Observed frequencies	Attribute B1	Attribute B2	THUS	Expected frequencies	Attribute B1	Attribute B2
Attribute A1	a	b		Attribute A1	(a+b)(a+c)/N	(a+b)(b+d)/N
Attribute A2	c	d		Attribute A2	(a+c)(c+d)/N	(b+d)(c+d)/N

That is, the expected frequency in each cell is = Product of column total and row total / Whole total. Hence, the table of expected frequencies is:

(100*180)/300 = 60	120	180
40	80	120
100	200	300

When applying χ^2 test,

O	E	O-E	$(O-E)^2$	$(O-E)^2/E$
75	60	15	225	3.750
25	40	-15	225	5.625
105	120	-15	225	1.875
95	80	15	225	2.813
				$\sum(O-E)^2/E$ = 14.063

df = (r-1)(c-1) = (2-1) (2-1) = 1

The table value of χ^2 for 1 df at 5% level of significance is 3.841. The calculated value of χ^2 14.063 is more than the tabular value. Hence the hypothesis may be rejected. Thus, we conclude that smoking and lung diseases are not independent and they are associated attributes.

Chi-square test of independence

This is performed when the data are presented in the form of a contingency table. A table, giving the simultaneous classification of the body of data in two different ways, is called a contingency table. If there are r rows and c columns, the table is said to be an r x c contingency table. χ^2 test is applied to test whether the factors classified are independent or not, i.e., the 2 factors are associated or not. In the contingency table, both factors may be qualitative or one qualitative and the other quantitative or both quantitative. The degrees of freedom for r x c contingency table is (r-1) (c-1).

Application of χ^2 statistics in a 2 x 2 χ^2 contingency table

Level – I	Level – II		Total
Level I	a	b	a + b
Level II	c	d	c + d
Total	a+c	b+d	a+b+c+d=n

Step 1: H_O: The factors are independent

Step 2: χ^2 is given by

$$\chi^2 = \frac{(ad - bc)^2 xn}{(a+b)(c+d)(a+c)(b+d)} \text{ with df} = (2\text{-}1)\ (2\text{-}1) = 1$$

Conclusion: as in the case of χ^2 test of goodness of fit (with the respective d.f). The above formula is applicable when all a, b, c, and d are greater than 5. If one or more is / are less than 5, Yate's correction of continuity is to be applied which is as below:

$$\chi^2 = \frac{(|ad - bc| - n/2)^2 xn}{(a+b)(c+d)(a+c)(b+d)}$$

In a (r x c) contingency table, the expected value (E) in the ith row and j^{th} column is

Calculated by $\frac{R_i X C_j}{N}$

where Ri = Sum of all the values in the ith row

Cj = Sum of all the values in the jth column

N = Grand total i.e., the sum of all the values in the given contingency table

Then $\chi^2 = \sum \frac{(O-E)^2}{E}$

Conclusion: as in the previous test (with the respective df)

5.2.15 Test of Hypothesis - F Test or Variance-Ratio Test

This is the test to compare the variance of 2 samples.

i. H_O: There is no significant difference between the variances of two samples

ii. The F Statistics is given by

$$F = \frac{\text{Estimated variance of first sample}}{\text{Estimated variance of second sample}} = \frac{S_1^2}{S_1^2} \text{ with d.f - } (n_1 - 1).\ (n_2 - 1)$$

S_1^2 and S_2^2 are the variances of the sample of sizes n_1 and n_2 respectively. F has 2 df, one for higher variance and another for smaller variance.

NB: We have to put the greatest variance (S_1^2, S_2^2) in the numerator.

Conclusion

i. If cal |F| < tab F for df = $(n_1-1), (n_2-1)$ at 5% level, F is not significant. H_o is accepted.

ii. If cal |F| > tab F for df = $(n_1-1), (n_2-1)$ at 5% level, F is significant, F = ( )*. Ho is rejected

iii. If cal |F| > tab F for df = $(n_1-1), (n_2-1)$ at 1% level, F is highly significant. F = ( )**. Ho is rejected.

Exercise

Two independent samples of sizes 9 and 7 from a normal population had the following values of variables:

Sample I (X_1)	*18*	*13*	*12*	*15*	*12*	*14*	*16*	*14*	*15*
Sample II (X_2)	*16*	*19*	*13*	*16*	*18*	*13*	*15*		

Do the estimates of the population variance differ significantly at 5% level?

Solution

										Total
Sample I (X_1)	*18*	*13*	*12*	*15*	*12*	*14*	*16*	*14*	*15*	***129***
X_1^2	*324*	*169*	*144*	*225*	*144*	*196*	*256*	*196*	*225*	***1879***
Sample II (X_2)	*16*	*19*	*13*	*16*	*18*	*13*	*15*			***110***
X_2^2	*256*	*361*	*169*	*256*	*324*	*169*	*225*			***1760***

n1 = 9, n2 = 7

$\overline{X}_1 = \sum X_1/n_1 = 129/9 = 14.3333$

$\overline{X}_2 = \sum X_2/n_2 = 110/7 = 15.7143$

$s_1^2 = \sum X_1^2/n_1 - (\overline{X}_1)^2 = 1879/9 - 14.3333^2 = 208.7777 - 205.4435 = 3.3342$

$s_2^2 = \sum X_2^2/n_2 - (\overline{X}_2)^2 = 1760/7 - 15.7143^2 = 251.4286 - 246.9392 = 4.4894$

$S_1^2 = n_1 / (n_1-1) * s_1^2 = 9/8 * 3.3342 = 3.7510$

$S_2^2 = n_2 / (n_2-1) * s_2^2 = 7/6 * 4.4894 = 5.2376$

$S_2^2 > S_1^2$

$F = S_2^2 / S_1^2 = 5.2376 / 3.7510 = 1.3963$

$F_{0.05}$ at (6,8) df is 3.58

That is, Calculated F < Tabular value ($F_{0.05}$). Therefore, H_O is accepted. The difference is not significant.

Let us now summarize different averages with their null hypotheses, distributions and usage in the following table:

Test for	Null Hypothesis (H0)	Distribution	Used when
Population mean (μ)	$\mu = \mu_0$	Z	Normal distribution or n > 30; σ known
		t_{n-1}	n < 30 and / or σ unknown
Population proportion (p)	$p = p_0$	Z	n, n(1-) $\geq$ 10
Difference of two means (μ_1 - μ_2)	$\mu_1 - \mu_2 = 0$	Z	Both normal distributions, or n_1, n_2 $\geq$ 30; σ_1, σ_2 known
		t distribution with df = smaller of $n_1 - 1$ and n_2 - 1	n_1, n_2 < 30; σ_1, σ_2 unknown
Mean difference μ_d (paired data)	$\mu_d = 0$	t_{n-1}	n < 30 pairs of data and or σ_d unknown
Difference of two proportions ($p_1 - p_2$)	$p_1 - p_2 = 0$	Z	n, n(1-) $\geq$ 10 for each group

5.3 NON-PARAMETRIC TESTS

Non-parametric tests are the methods of statistical analysis that do not require a distribution to meet the required assumptions to be analyzed, especially if the data are not normally distributed. Due to this reason, they are referred to as distribution-free tests. Non-parametric tests serve as alternatives to parametric tests such as t-test or ANOVA which can be employed only if the underlying data satisfy certain criteria and assumptions. They are used when there are skewed data, and they comprise techniques that do not depend on data about any particular distribution. The word non-parametric does not mean that these models do not have any parameters. The fact is that the characteristics and number of parameters are flexible and not predefined. Therefore, these models are called distribution-free models.

5.3.1 Parametric Tests Vs. Non-Parametric Tests

Under probability distributions and hypothesis testing, we studied that there are several assumptions attached to each probability distribution. Parametric tests are used when the information about the population parameters is completely known, whereas non-parametric tests are used when there is no or little information available about the population parameters. In simple words, a parametric test assumes that the data are normally distributed. However, non-parametric tests make no assumptions about the distribution of the data.

We know that the parameters are the characteristics of the population that cannot be changed. For e.g., a dairy farmer calculates the average daily milk yield per animal produced by his milch animals by dividing the total daily milk yield by the number of milch animals in his farm. That is, the farmer considers all his milch animals while calculating the total yield. Assuming that measuring of milk yield is done accurately, we cannot change the total yield produced by the animals. Therefore, average yield is called a parameter of the population, as it cannot be changed. If the average (mean) of the data more accurately represents the centre point of the distribution, and the sample size is large enough, we can use a parametric test. Whereas, if the median of the data more accurately represents the centre point of the distribution, and the sample size is large, we can use non-parametric distribution.

5.3.2 Reasons to Use Nonparametric Tests

Let us consider an example: 1). A sample of 20 sick cows undergoes a treatment. The improvements found after treatment are observed – maybe no improvement, slightly improved, much improved, and completely cured. Unfortunately, these observations are not scalable, because these observations are based on the experience of the veterinarian and are not calculated. In such a case, parametric tests are not valid, as no parametric tests exist for such nominal data.

There can be some others like 2). The limit of detection is the lowest quantity of a substance that can be detected, but not necessarily quantified. For e.g., COVID 19 viral load in the blood, which may either be beyond the limit of detection or it can have a higher value, and 3). In a factory, considering the average salary of employees, the CEO's salary will be very high and lies at an abnormal distance from the income of others, which can be called an outlier. Non-parametric tests are applied in these situations, where a). data do not follow any probability distribution, b). data constitute ordinal values or ranks, c). there are outliers in data and d). data has a limit of detection. However, it is important to note that if there exists a parametric test for a problem, then using a non-parametric test will yield only inaccurate results.

To achieve the correct results from the statistical analysis, we should know the situations in which the application of non-parametric tests is appropriate. The main reasons to use the non-parametric tests are the following:

a) ***Underlying data not meeting the assumptions about the population sample:*** Generally, the application of parametric tests requires various assumptions to be satisfied. For e.g., Suppose the data follow a normal distribution and the population variance is homogeneous. However, some data samples may show skewed distributions. Skewness in data makes the parametric tests less powerful, because the mean is no longer the best measure of central tendency, as it is strongly affected by extreme values. At the same time, non-parametric tests work well with skewed distributions and distributions that are better represented by the median.

b) ***Too small sample size:*** If a sample size is reasonably large, an appropriate parametric test can be used. However, if a sample size is too small, it is possible that we may not be able to validate the distribution of data. Thus, the application of non-parametric tests is the only suitable option.

c) ***Ordinal or nominal data:*** Unlike parametric tests that can work only with continuous data, non-parametric tests can be applied to other data types such as ordinal or nominal data. For such types of variables, the non-parametric tests are the only appropriate solution.

5.3.3 Types of Non-parametric Tests

The parametric tests and their non-parametric test alternatives are:

Parametric tests	Non-parametric alternatives
One-sample Z-test, One sample t-test	Sign test
One sample Z-test, One sample t-test	Wilcoxon Signed Rank test
Two-way ANOVA	Friedman test
One-way ANOVA	Kruskal-Wallis test
Independent samples t-test	Mann-Whitney test
Correlation Coefficient	Spearman Rank Correlation

When we say that the non-parametric tests are alternative methods to parametric tests, it does not mean that they are the substitutes to the parametric tests. In other words, if the data meet the required assumptions for performing the parametric tests, only the relevant parametric test must be used. In addition, even if the data do not meet the necessary assumptions, but the sample size of the data is large enough, we can still apply the parametric tests, instead of the nonparametric tests.

5.3.4 Approach (Hypothesis testing) to (in) a Non-Parametric Test

To conduct non-parametric tests, we follow a five-step approach as below:

i. ***Set up hypotheses and select the level of significance α.*** Similar to parametric testing, the research hypothesis can be one or two-sided (one or two-tailed).

ii. ***Select the appropriate test statistic.*** The test statistic is a single number that summarizes the sample information. In non-parametric tests, the observed data are converted into ranks and then, ranks are summarized into a test statistic.

iii. ***Set up a decision rule.*** The decision rule is a statement that tells under what circumstances we should reject the null hypothesis. In some nonparametric tests, we reject H_0 if the test statistic is large, while in others we reject H_0 if the test statistic is small.

iv. ***Compute the test statistic.*** We compute the test statistic by summarizing the ranks into the test statistic identified in Step 2.

v. ***Conclusion.*** The conclusion is made by comparing the test statistic to the decision rule. It is either to reject the null hypothesis or not to reject the null hypothesis.

5.3.5 Types of Non-Parametric Tests

Non-parametric tests are completely based on the ranks, which are assigned to the ordered data. They are summarized below with their uses, null hypothesis, test statistic, and the decision rule:

5.3.5.1 Kruskal Wallis Test

Kruskal Wallis Test is used to compare the continuous outcomes in greater than two independent samples. This test is extremely useful when we deal with more than two independent groups and it compares the median among k populations. This test is an alternative to one-way ANOVA, when the data violate the assumptions of normal distribution and when the sample size is too small. This test can be used both for continuous and ordinal-level dependent variables.

The null hypothesis, H_O is that the K Population medians are equal. The test statistic is that if N is the total sample size, k is the number of comparison groups, Rj is the sum of the ranks in the jth group and nj is the sample size in the jth group, then the test statistic, H is given by:

$$H = \left[\frac{12}{n(n+1)} \sum_{j=1}^{k} \left(\frac{Rj^2}{nj}\right)\right] - 3(n+1)$$

Where k = number of comparison groups, n = total sample size, nj = sample size in j^{th} group and Rj = sum of the ranks in j^{th} group

The decision rule is that reject $H_{O,}$ if $H \geq$ critical value.

Example

Patients suffering from a disease were divided into 3 groups and 3 different types of treatment were given to them. A blood parameter (in some unit) of the patients after following a 3-day course of treatment is given below:

Treatment 1	Treatment 2	Treatment 3
4.9	6.7	7.8
4.6	7.2	8.5
5.7	8.3	6.7
4.9	7.6	6.8
5.2		7.2
5.0		

The sample size is different for the 3 treatments, which can be analyzed using Kruskal-Wallis test. Sample sizes for treatments 1, 2, and 3 are n1 = 6, n2 = 4 and n3 = 5. That is, total sample size n = n1 + n2 + n3 = 6 + 4 + 5 = 20.

The hypotheses here are: H_O – Three population medians are the same and H_A – Three population medians are different. Let us select 5% level of significance. Now, let us order these samples from the smallest to the largest and then assign ranks to the clubbed sample, as below:

Treatments			Ranks in Treatment		
1	**2**	**3**	**1**	**2**	**3**
4.6			1		
4.8			2		
4.9			3		
5.0			4		
5.2			5		
6.7	6.7	6.7	6	6	6
		6.8	9		
	7.2	7.2		10.5	10.5
	7.6			12	
		7.8			13
	8.3			14	
		8.5			15

We know that the sum of ranks will always be equal to n(n+1)/2. Here, the sum of ranks = 78. i.e., n (n+1) / 2 = (15*16) / 2 = 120. Now, we have to check if there is a difference between 3 population medians. We will now summarize the sample information in a test statistic based on ranks. We calculate the test statistic, H, using the formula given above, which is equal to 3.2632.

We now determine the critical value of H using the table of critical values and the test criteria are given by rejecting $H_{0,}$ if $H \geq$ critical value and accepting $H_{0,}$ if $H <$ critical value. H is 3.2632 and the critical value is 0.19562. Therefore, we reject H_O and conclude that there is no significant evidence to conclude that the three treatment medians are the same.

5.3.5.2 Mann Whitney U Test

Mann Whitney U Test is known as Mann Whitney Wilcoxon test or Wilcoxon rank sum test. It is an alternative form to the independent sample t-test. This test is used to compare the continuous outcomes in the two independent samples. The null hypothesis (H_O) in this test is that the two populations are equal. The sums of ranks in group 1 and group 2 are denoted as R_1 and R_2, respectively. The test statistic is U. The decision rule is that we reject H_O, if the test statistic, U, is less than or equal to the critical value from the table.

Example

A company produces a new weedicide to kill weeds in paddy fields and observes the results on a group of 5 plots after a week. Another group of 5 plots is applied with the old weedicide. The company then records the number of plots with weeds after the week:

Plots with weeds in plots	*After using old weedicide*	*7*	*8*	*4*	*9*	*8*
	After using new weedicide	*3*	*4*	*2*	*1*	*1*

We know from the table that the number of plots with weeds after applying the new weedicide has decreased. We are interested in knowing whether the two groups of plots applied with two different weedicides present the same number of plots with weeds or not. The hypothesis can be H_O: The two groups of plots report the same number of weed cases; and H_A: The two groups of plots report different numbers of weed cases. Let us select 5% level of significance for the test.

For Mann Whitney U test, the test statistic is denoted by U which is the minimum of U1 and U2.

$$U1 = n1n2 + \frac{n1(n1+1)}{2} - R1$$

$$U2 = n1n2 + \frac{n2(n2+1)}{2} - R2$$

where R1 is the sum of the ranks of group 1, R2 is the sum of the ranks of group 2, n1 is the size of group 1 and n2 is the size of group 2.

We now compute the ranks by combining the two groups. Ranks are an important component of non-parametric tests and therefore learning how to assign ranks to a sample is vital.

1. *We combine the two samples and arrange them in ascending order. We use OW for the old weedicide and ND for the new weedicide.*

Weedicide	NW	NW	NW	NW	NW	OW	OW	OW	OW	OW
Sample	1	1	2	3	4	4	7	8	8	9

The lowest value here is assigned the rank 1 and the second lowest value is assigned the rank 2 and so on.

Weedicide	NW	NW	NW	NW	NW	OW	OW	OW	OW	OW
Sample	1	1	2	3	4	4	7	8	8	9
Rank	1	2	3	4	5	6	7	8	9	10

The numbers 1, 4, and 8 appear more than once in the combined sample. So, the ranks assigned are wrong. Look at the position of number 1 in the sample after sorting the data. The number 1 is appearing at 1st and 2nd position. In such a case, we take the mean of 1 and 2 and assign the mean to the number 1. We follow the same steps for numbers 4 and 8. We assign the mean rank when there are ties in a sample to make sure that the sum of ranks in each sample of size n is the same.

Weedicide	NW	NW	NW	NW	NW	OW	OW	OW	OW	OW
Sample	1	1	2	3	4	4	7	8	8	9
Rank	1.5	1.5	3	4	5.5	5.5	7	8.5	8.5	10

Therefore, the sum of ranks will always be equal to n (n + 1) / 2.

2. *The next step is to compute the sum of ranks for group 1 and group 2.* R1 = 15.5; R2 = 39.5
3. *Using the formula, compute values.* U1 = 24.5; U2 = 0.5; Now, U = min (U1, U2) = 0.5

   For the Mann Whitney U test, the value of U lies in the range (0, n1*n2) where 0 indicates that the two groups are completely different from each other and n1*n2 indicates some relation between the two groups. Also, U1 + U2 (24.5 + 0.5) is always equal to n1*n2 (5*5). The value of U is 0.5 here which is close to 0.

   We then determine a critical value (denoted by ρ), using the table for critical values, which is a point derived from the level of significance of the test and is used to reject or accept the H_O. In Mann Whitney U test, the test criteria are: Reject H_O: U < Critical value; Accept H_O: U > Critical value. Here, ρ = 2. Since U < critical value, we reject H_O and conclude that there is no significant evidence that the two groups of plots report the same number of weeded plots.

5.3.5.3 Wilcoxon Signed-Rank Test

Wilcoxon Signed-Rank test is used to compare the continuous outcomes in two matched samples or the paired samples. This test can be used in place of a paired t-test whenever the sample violates the assumptions of a normal distribution. The null hypothesis, H_O, in this test, is that the median difference is zero. The test statistic, W, is defined as the smaller of W+ or W-, where W+ and W- are the sums of the positive and the negative ranks of different scores. The decision rule is that we reject H_0, if the test statistic, W, is less than or equal to the critical value from the table.

Example

A dairy farmer wants to test the efficacy of a new feed regimen for improving the milk yield of his animals and hence he records the milk yields of his 6 animals before starting the new feed. The milk yields of his 6 cows are as below:

Dairy cow	*1*	*2*	*3*	*4*	*5*	*6*
Milk yield in litres before new feed	*8*	*5*	*4*	*4*	*6*	*7*

After that, he starts feeding his cows with new feed and checks the milk yield after 10 days. The milk yields 10 days after the new feed regimen are:

Dairy cow	*1*	*2*	*3*	*4*	*5*	*6*
Milk yield in litres after new feed	*10*	*8*	*3*	*7*	*5*	*10*

Let us check whether the milk yields of the cows have improved after 10 days of the new feed regimen:

Dairy cow	**Milk yield**		**Yield difference (Before new feed – After new feed)**
	Before new feed	**After new feed**	
1	8	10	2
2	5	8	3
3	4	3	-1
4	4	7	3
5	6	5	-1
6	7	10	3

In the table, there are some cases where the cows have yielded more than that yielded by them before and in some cases, they yielded less. This could be due to some random effect. We will analyze if the difference in yield is systematic or is due to chance, using this test. We assign ranks to the absolute value of differences. This can be done after arranging the data in ascending order.

Difference	**Ranks**
-1	1.5
-1	1.5
2	3
3	5
3	5
3	5

In Wilcoxon Signed-Rank test, we need signed ranks which are obtained by assigning the signs associated with the differences to the ranks, as shown below:

Difference	Ranks	Signed ranks
-1	1.5	-1.5
-1	1.5	-1.5
2	3	3
3	5	5
3	5	5
3	5	5

Now, the hypotheses are H_O: The median difference is zero, and H_A: The median difference is positive. The hypothesis can be one-sided or two-sided, but let us consider the one-sided hypothesis at 5% level of significance. Therefore, $\alpha = 0.05$. The test statistic for this test is W, which is the smaller of W1 and W2, where W1 is the sum of positive ranks and W2 is the sum of negative ranks. Here, W1 = 18 and W2 = 3. Hence, W = min (W1, W2) = 3.

If W1 is similar to W2, we accept H_O. Otherwise, if the difference reflects a greater improvement in the yields, then, we reject H_O. The critical value of W can be looked for in the table. The criteria to accept or reject H_O are: Reject H_O, if W < Critical value, Accept H_O, if W > Critical value. Here, W is greater than the critical value of 2. Hence, we accept H_O and conclude that there is no significant difference between the milk yields before and after new feed regimen.

5.3.5.4 Sign Test

A sign test is used to compare the continuous outcomes in paired samples or two matched samples. This test is similar to Wilcoxon Signed-Rank test and this can also be used in place of a paired t-test if the data violate the assumptions of normality. The H_O here is that the median difference is zero. The test statistic is the smaller of the number of positive sign or negative sign. The decision rule is that we reject H_O, if the smaller of number of the +ve or the –ve signs is less than or equal to the critical value from the table. We use the same example that we used in the Wilcoxon Signed-Rank test, assuming that it does not follow the normal distribution, to explain sign test.

Dairy cow	Milk yield		Yield difference (Before new feed – After new feed)	Sign
	Before new feed	After new feed		
1	8	10	2	+
2	5	8	3	+
3	4	3	-1	-
4	4	7	3	+
5	6	5	-1	-
6	7	10	3	+

In Sign test, we do not consider magnitude, thereby ignoring the ranks. The hypothesis is the same as before and hence, the hypotheses are H_O: The median difference is zero and H_A: The median difference is positive. Here, if we see a similar number of positive and negative differences, then the H_O is true. Otherwise, if we see more of positive signs, then the H_O is false. The test statistic is smaller of the number of positive and negative signs. Now, we determine the critical value and the criteria is to Reject H_O, if the smaller number of + and – signs is less than or equal to the critical value and Accept H_O, if the smaller number of + and – signs is greater than the critical value. Here, the smaller number of + and – signs = 2 which is less than the critical value of 6 (table value). Therefore, we reject H_O and conclude that there is no significant evidence to state that the median difference is zero.

5.3.5.5 Spearman Rank Correlation

The Spearman Rank Correlation test is used when we want to find a correlation between two sets of data. Suppose a farmer goes to a market to buy 60 kg of NPK fertilizer of a particular brand for his paddy farm. Another farmer buys the same quantity of the same brand of fertilizer from another market at a higher price. Now, the question here is whether the market influences the price of the fertilizer. If the market influences the price, then we can say that there is a link between the market and the price of the fertilizer. In such occasions, we use Spearman rank correlation to establish if there is a correlation between two datasets. Spearman rank correlation method can be to check the direction and strength of correlation.

The hypothesis in this test will be: H_O – There is no relation between the price and the market and H_A - There is a relation between the price and the market. Spearman rank correlation method can be used to check the direction and strength of correlation. It is a non-parametric alternative to the Pearson correlation coefficient and is denoted by ρ. The value of ρ lies in the range of -1 to 1), where -1 represents a negative correlation between the ranks, 0 represents no correlation between the ranks and 1 represents a positive correlation between the ranks. After assigning ranks to the sample, we use the following formula to calculate the Spearman rank correlation coefficient:

$$\rho = 1 - \frac{6\sum d_i^2}{n(n^2 - 1)}$$

where ρ is the Spearman rank correlation coefficient, di is the difference between the two ranks of each observation, and n is the number of observations

Example

The following table presents the marks given by two judges for 12 students who participated in an essay writing competition:

Judge 1	*60*	*34*	*40*	*50*	*45*	*41*	*22*	*43*	*42*	*66*	*64*	*46*
Judge 2	*75*	*32*	*34*	*40*	*45*	*33*	*12*	*30*	*36*	*72*	*41*	*57*

Use Spearman Rank Correlation method to find out is there a relationship between the marks given by the judges.

The H_O here will be that there is no relationship between the marks awarded by the judges and the H_A is that there is a relationship between the marks awarded. Let us have a 5% level of significance for this test. Calculate the ranks and d which is the difference between the ranks and n which is the sample size, which is 12:

Judge 1	60	34	40	50	45	41	22	43	42	66	64	46
Judge 2	75	32	34	40	45	33	12	30	36	72	41	57
Ranks (Judge 1) - Rx	3	11	10	4	6	9	12	7	8	1	2	5
Ranks (Judge 2) - Ry	1	10	8	6	4	9	12	11	7	2	5	3
d = (Rx – Ry)	2	1	2	-2	2	0	0	-4	1	-1	-3	2
d^2	4	1	4	4	4	0	0	16	1	1	9	4
$\sum d^2$	48											

Now, we use the formula to calculate the Spearman rank correlation coefficient.

$$\rho = 1 - \frac{6\sum d_i^2}{n(n^2 - 1)}$$

P = 1 – [(6 * 48) / (12 (12^2 – 1)] = 1 – [288 / 1716] = 1- 0.1678 = 0.8322

Hence, the Spearman rank correlation coefficient ρ is 0.83. We look at this coefficient for the direction and the strength of the association between the ranks. While the value indicates the strength of the correlation between the ranks, the sign of it implies the direction of the association. The coefficient will be between -1 and +1, where -1 indicates a perfect negative correlation and +1 a perfect positive correlation. Hence, from the result of +0.83, we can infer that there is a positive relationship between the ranks obtained with the two judges. Also, since the value is higher than 0.7, we can infer that there is a very strong relationship between the ranks given by the judges.

We reject H_0, if the calculated ρ (sign not considered) value is greater than the tabular critical value and accept H_0, if ρ value is less than the tabular critical value. The critical value for this example, where there are 12 pairs of data (n=12), is 0.504. As the value of ρ is greater than the critical value, we can say with 95% certainty that the results have not occurred by chance and the results are highly significant. Hence, we reject the H_0.

To summarise, non-parametric tests are more powerful when the assumptions for parametric tests are violated and can be used for all data types such as nominal, ordinal, and interval, and also when data has outliers. If any of the parametric tests is valid for a problem then using a non-parametric test will give highly inaccurate results. Mann Whitney U test is used for testing the difference between two independent groups with ordinal or continuous dependent variable. Wilcoxon signed-rank test is used for testing the difference between two related variables which takes into account the magnitude and direction of difference; however, the Sign test ignores the magnitude and only considers the direction of the difference. Kruskal-Wallis test compares the outcome among more than 2 independent groups by making use of the medians. The Spearman Rank Correlation technique is used to check if there exists a relationship between the two data sets and it also talks about the type of relationship.

5.3.6 Advantages of Non-Parametric Tests

i. We achieve better statistical power, especially when assumptions for parametric tests are violated.

ii. There are only fewer assumptions (i.e., assumption of normality is not required) than parametric tests.

iii. Even small sample sizes are acceptable.

iv. They can be used for all data types, including nominal variables, interval variables, or data that have outliers or that have been measured imprecisely.

5.3.7 Disadvantages of Non-Parametric Tests

i. They are less powerful than parametric tests, especially when the assumptions are not violated.

ii. If there exists any parametric test for a set of data, then using a non-parametric test could lead to a terrible error.

iii. These tests are more labour-intensive to calculate by hand and hence, the use of computers is required for calculations.

iv. Critical value tables for many tests are not available. Hence, the values are compared to the tables for parametric tests (like the z-table or t-table).

6

Design of Experiments For Animal Health Studies

A scientific experiment is a planned research to obtain new facts or to confirm or refute the results of previous experiments. Research is usually conducted in a controlled environment to study the effect of one or more variables on observations. The objective of research may be to answer a question, verify a hypothesis, or estimate the effect of an independent variable on a dependent variable. After stating the research problem, we need to outline the methodology (or materials and methods) of the research, which includes developing an experimental design.

Scientific experiments are conducted to study the causal relationships between independent variable(s) and dependent variable(s). The researcher manipulates one or more independent variables and measures their effect on one or more dependent variables. Designing an experiment is planning an experiment. It is a complete sequence of steps taken before experimenting to ensure that appropriate data are obtained to perform a data analysis to get valid inferences about the problem. It must be seen that the data collected are relevant to the problem investigated. E.g., studying the effect of breed, age, feed, etc. on milk output. Here, the objects like breed, age, feed, etc. are called treatments. That is, any specific experimental conditions (like the addition of feed additives, new feed formula, etc.) applied to the experimental units are called treatments. The basic objects on which the experiment is done are called experimental units (E.g., a bird, an insect, an animal). However, the responses in all the experimental units receiving the same treatments may not be similar, due to the inherent differences in the experimental units, called experimental error, caused by extraneous factors.

The observed difference between the effects of the two treatments is the sum of the true difference and the contribution due to experimental error. If the error is small, we can obtain a better estimate of the true difference. If the error is large, we get a poor estimate of the true difference. Hence, experimental error is the basis for deciding whether the observed difference in response due to treatments is real or is just due to chance. Hence, for proper interpretation of the results, we should have a correct estimate of the experimental error.

6.1 CONCEPTS

Treatment: What we apply on the subject of investigation is called treatment. e.g. application of feed to animals, application of fertilizer to fodder crops, etc.

Experimental unit and experimental material: The individual or group of individuals that is subjected to a treatment is called the experimental unit and the collection of such units is the experimental material.

Response: Response is the outcome of an experiment. i.e., it is the effect of treatment in the experimental units.

Experimental error: It refers to the variation within the treatment group due to uncontrollable causes. It also describes the failure of two identically treated experimental units to yield identical results.

Factor: A factor is a discrete variable used to classify experimental units. For example, gender is a factor with two levels - male and female and diet is a factor with three levels - low, medium, and high protein. The levels within each factor can be discrete, such as drug A and drug B, or may be quantitative like 0, 10, 20, and 30 mg/kg.

Fixed effects factors: Fixed effects factors are variables that can be controlled by the investigator. These include gender, dose, diet, and any treatment that can be administered to the animals. Most experiments are designed to study the fixed effects.

Random effects factors: Random effects factors are variables that cannot be controlled by the investigator. They include inter-individual differences, time effects, and environmental effects. The aim of some experimental designs, such as randomized blocks, is to partition these effects out, so that they do not obscure the fixed effects.

6.2 PRINCIPLES OF EXPERIMENTAL DESIGNS

Replication

If a farmer gives his sick cow a medicine and if the cow gets cured after 2 days, it cannot be called an experiment, as there is only one treatment. Any experiment must have at least two treatments, one of which may be a control involving no treatment. Suppose that the farmer has two sick cows and he gives his medicine to one of them. If the cow that received the medicine gets cured in 3 days or so and the other untreated cow takes a month to recover. This can be called an experiment. But this is unreplicated. Next, if the farmer has six cows showing similar symptoms and he gives the medicine to three of them which recover in 3 to 5 days, while the other three cows which were untreated take 30 to 40 days to recover, then the medicine given has to be considered seriously. This experiment is now a replicated experiment. Animals sometimes recover from illness on their own and so we need controls (animals not treated) and replication to evaluate whether the medicine given is the cause of early recovery.

Replication means the number of experimental units receiving a particular treatment. If an experiment has equal replication for all the treatments studied, then the design is called an Equi-replicated design. If a design has an unequal replication for different treatments, then it is known as a design with unequal replication. Replication provides an estimate of experimental error and helps us to obtain a more precise estimate of the mean effect of any factor. By increasing the sample size, the precision of the experiment can be increased. The more the replication, the better the precision will be.

Randomization

From the six ailing cows, if we choose three cows that are least affected to receive the medicine, then the 'experiment' is not properly designed. Because the question of which cows are to be treated should have been determined at random. If the animals chosen are blind (or masked) to the identity of the treatment they receive, then such a study is called a *placebo*, which is a name the scientists use for inactive treatments given to animals. Placebo means a practice of concealing the information about which patient is receiving which treatment from both patients and doctors who record the results of the trial. Patients are randomly allocated to a medicine or medicines and a placebo (that is a tablet, cream, or solution looking exactly like the real medicine but lacking the active ingredient).

Randomization is a process for eliminating personal bias. By randomly assigning treatments to the experimental units, we avoid personal bias. It is aimed at giving equal chances to all the experimental units to be subjected to different treatments. Randomization may be achieved by the use of a random number table or by drawing lots. There are different randomization procedures for different designs. By avoiding personal bias, this process makes the test valid.

Local Control

It refers to the blocking and grouping of the experimental units in the experiment. It refers to the logical way of grouping the experimental units to ensure more uniformity within the same group and greater variability between groups. Local control makes the experimental design more efficient and the test procedure more powerful. Local control imposes some restrictions on the random allocation of treatments to account for the known initial differences in the experimental materials. The most common form of local control is blocking. A block refers to a subset of items under investigation in an experiment. The variability within a block is expected to be less. The general purpose of dividing the materials into blocks is to isolate the sources of heterogeneity. The items within a block are believed to be more or less homogenous. Another kind of local control, often used in survey work, is stratification.

For example, one might be interested in mastitis in dairy cows and the correlation between various husbandry and hygienic practices and the incidence of the disease. For this purpose, we may classify farms according to the size of the farm. We then draw similar proportions (at random) from each size class to ensure that we take samples in all small, medium, and large herds, to give a clear picture of mastitis in the region.

Benefits of Randomization, Replication, and Local Control

Almost all the experiments involve the above three basic principles, *viz.*, randomization, replication, and local control. These principles are complementary to each other to increase the accuracy of the experiment and to provide a valid test of significance. A bird, a cow, or a collection of animals may be an experimental unit, also referred to as a plot. A collection of plots is a block. Observations made on experimental units vary considerably, partly produced by manipulation of certain variables, called treatments. E.g., levels of feed additives in feed trials can be called a treatment.

Besides variations due to known sources, variations may also occur due to the unknown sources of the environment and genetic variations in the experimental materials which are unavoidable in any experiment. These variations are called experimental errors, produced by factors beyond the control of the experimenter. These errors may be systematic or random. Error arising due to an equipment like a defective weighing machine is an example of systematic error. Random errors usually result from the experimenter›s inability to take the measurement exactly in the same way. Any number of repeated measurements would not overcome the systematic error, whereas random errors can be avoided with repeated measurements. The basic principles *viz.*, randomization, replication, and local control are devices to avoid systematic error and to control random error.

To conclude, we can say that randomization is assigning treatments or factors to be tested to the experimental units according to probability to eliminate systematic error. Through randomization, every experimental unit will have the same chance of receiving any treatment. Replication is the repetition of an experiment under identical conditions. Replication, along with randomization, provides a basis for estimating the error variance. Without randomization, no amount of replication can produce a true estimate of error. A greater number of replications is likely yield to greater precision. The number of replications depends on factors like homogeneity of experimental material, number of treatments, degree of precision required, etc. Local control means control of all factors except the ones about which we are investigating. Local control, like replication, reduces the variation due to extraneous factors and increases the precision of an experiment. If an experimental field is heterogeneous (e.g., soil fertility), then the field can be divided into blocks, so that the plots within each block are more homogeneous. This homogeneity of experiment units ensures an unbiased comparison of treatment means. In short, while randomization is a method of eliminating a systematic error (i.e., bias), thereby leaving only the random error component of variation, the other two *viz.*, replication and local control keep this random error as low as possible. All three hence are essential for making a valid estimate of error variance and to provide a valid test of significance.

6.3 ANALYSIS OF VARIANCE (ANOVA)

Once we get the experimental results, they have to be analyzed and interpreted. We should see whether all treatments have the same effect. i.e., to test the null hypothesis (H_O): $\mu_1 = \mu_2 = \mu_3 = \ldots = \mu_t$ (all means are equal), against the alternative hypothesis (H_A): $\mu_1 \neq \mu_2 \neq \mu_3 \neq \ldots \neq \mu_t$ (at least one mean differs from others). Student's t-test and ANOVA examine whether group means differ from one another. Student's t-test compares two groups, while ANOVA does for more than two groups. ANOVA is a systematic algebraic procedure and statistical method for decomposing overall variation in responses in an experiment into different components. It is used to determine whether there are any statistically significant differences between the means of three or more independent (unrelated) groups. The essence of ANOVA is that the total amount of variation in a set of data is broken down into 1. the amount that can be attributed to chance and 2. the amount that can be attributed to specified causes.

Each component is attributed to an identifiable cause or source of variation. Suppose that we have a factor T with t levels (t treatments), with equal replication r and their responses Y. The results can be tabulated as below:

Replications	Treatments						
	1	2	...	i	...	t	
1	Y_{11}	Y_{21}	...	Y_{i1}	...	Y_{t1}	
2	Y_{12}	Y_{22}	...	Y_{i2}	...	Y_{t2}	
...	...	...	...	...	...	...	
j	Y_{1j}	Y_{2j}	...	Y_{ij}	...	Y_{tj}	
...	...	...	...	...	...	...	
r	Y_{1r}	Y_{2r}	...	Y_{ir}	...	Y_{tr}	
Total	$Y_{1.}$	$Y_{2.}$	...	$Y_{i.}$	...	$Y_{t.}$	**Y.. = Grand total**
Mean	y_1	y_2	...	y_i	...	y_t	

For example,

Replications	Treatments				
	1	2	3	4	
1	Y_{11}	Y_{21}	Y_{31}	Y_{41}	
2	Y_{12}	Y_{22}	Y_{32}	Y_{42}	
3	Y_{13}	Y_{23}	Y_{33}	Y_{43}	
4	Y_{14}	Y_{24}	Y_{34}	Y_{44}	
Total	$Y_{1.}$	$Y_{2.}$	$Y_{3.}$	$Y_{4.}$	**Y.. = Grand total**
Mean	y_1	y_2	y_3	y_4	

The response of the jth individual unit in the ith treatment can be represented by the equation:

$$Yij = yi + eij$$
$$= i^{th} \text{ treatment mean} + \text{random deviation}$$
$$= \mu + (yi - \mu) + (Yij - yi)$$
$$Yij - \mu = (yi - \mu) + (Yij - yi)$$

That is, the variation of an individual response from the overall mean is the sum of two components. One is the variation in the means of the treatments yi from the overall mean μ. The other is the variation within each of the treatments and hence it is the error term. The significance of the difference $(yi - \mu)$ is based on the magnitude of the components $(yi - \mu)$ compared with $(Yij - yi)$. The statistical test of the significance involves the use of the following identity:

$$\sum\sum (Yij - \mu)^2 = \sum\sum [(yi - \mu) + (Yij - yi)]^2$$
$$= \sum\sum (yi - \mu)^2 + \sum\sum (Yij - yi)^2 + 2\sum\sum (yi - \mu)(Yij - yi)$$
$$= \sum\sum (yi - \mu)^2 + \sum\sum (Yij - yi)^2$$

The last term will vanish, because $\sum$ (Yij – yi) = 0. Thus, we have the total sum of squares = treatment sum of squares + error sum of squares. That is, SS (Y) = SS (T) + SS (E). Total variation can thus be partitioned into two components: variation between treatments and variation within treatments. Before the magnitude of two components can be compared, they must be divided by the number of degrees of freedom. For the component "between treatments", the degrees of freedom is t – 1 and that for the "within treatments" is (tr – t) = t(r-1). The quantity SS(T) / t-1 is known as the treatment mean square, MS (T). The quantity SS(E) / n-t is known as the error mean square, MS (E). The ratio between the two estimates F = MS (T) / MS (E) follows the F distribution with t-1 and n-t degrees of freedom. The significance of the F can then be determined by using Tables of F.

6.4 STEPS IN THE DESIGN OF EXPERIMENTS

- Set objectives;
- Select variables;
- Select an experimental design;
- Execute the design;
- Check that the data are consistent with the experimental assumptions;
- Analyze the data and interpret the results; and
- Present the results.

6.5 CRITERIA FOR MAKING BLOCKS

Characters that influence the response value before the commencement of the experiment are considered as the criteria for making blocks. E.g., in milk yield studies, the breed can be considered as a criterion for making blocks, and in weight gain studies, the initial weight is a criterion for making blocks. In a Completely Randomised Design (CRD), there is no local control applied, while in a Randomized Block Design (RBD), local control is applied in one direction with one criterion, and in Latin Square Design (LSD) in two directions with two criteria.

Besides the three principles of experimental designs, *viz.*, randomization, replication, and control, there are also auxiliary variables that could be considered while experimenting. Some characters are not altered by the treatments applied, but may have an influence on the characters under study. They are called Auxiliary variables which can be utilized to improve the precision of the estimate and the efficiency of designs. They are chosen in a way that the collection of data about them does not involve any cost or labour.

6.6 MAJOR EXPERIMENTAL DESIGNS

- ***Completely Randomised Design (CRD):*** CRD has one or more fixed effect factor(s), often called treatment(s). Subjects are assigned to treatments randomly, regardless of the characteristics of the experimental material(s). This is the most commonly used and simple design. It tolerates unequal numbers in each group.
- ***Randomised Block Design (RBD):*** Also known as within subject, crossover, or matched subjects design, RBD has one random effect variable that is of *no interest* and one or more fixed effect factors (treatments) that *are* of interest. This design is used to 1). Increase the power by better control of variation, 2). Provide a convenient way of breaking up the experiment into smaller and more convenient parts, and 3). Take account of some natural structures of the experimental material, such as litter differences.
- ***Latin Square Design (LSD):*** This design has two random effect variables (designated as rows and columns) and one or more fixed effects. This design is used to further increase the power in special situations, taking into account the two sources of random effects.
- ***Factorial Design:*** This has two or more fixed effect factors. Strictly they are the arrangements of the treatments rather than designs, so it is possible to have a factorial treatment structure in a CRD, RBD, or LSD.
- ***Split Plot Design:*** This is an RBD with a factorial treatment structure, in which a main effect is confounded with the blocks. It may be possible to design such an experiment, because they make good use of the experimental subjects. For example, a within-animal experiment is a type of RBD. But, suppose half of the available animals are males and the other half are females. The gender differences can be assessed using whole set of animals, while the treatment differences can be assessed within the animals.
- ***Repeated Measures Design (RMD):*** RMD is a design in which each experimental unit is measured several times without different treatments being applied. Some authors use the term RMD for crossover experiments, in which a subject receives different treatments over a period of time.

6.7 COMPLETELY RANDOMIZED DESIGN (CRD) OR ANALYSIS OF VARIANCE (ANOVA)

Completely Randomized Design (CRD), the simplest of all experimental designs, is also called a one-way Analysis of Variance (One-way ANOVA). In a CRD, treatments are allocated to experimental units in a completely random manner, so that each experimental unit has the same chance of receiving any one treatment. That is, it imposes no restrictions on the allocation of treatments to the experimental units. Further, any number of experimental units and treatments can be utilized in this design. The experimental units are allotted to different treatments randomly. The difference among the experimental units receiving the same treatment is considered as experimental error. Hence, CRD is appropriate only for experiments with homogeneous experimental units, such as laboratory experiments, where environmental effects are easy to control. For field experiments, where there is generally large variation among experimental plots, CRD is rarely used. Analysis of data in this design is simple, even if some values are missing.

After having randomized the experimental units over different treatments, initial recordings (if any) of the experimental units are noted against each experimental unit. For e.g., in a weight gain study, initial weights may be recorded. Then, the experimental units are subjected to respective treatments and after the experimental period, the response values are observed.

6.7.1 Procedure for a CRD

Ho: There is no significant difference between the treatments.

Step 1

a) Determine the total number of experimental plots (n) as the product of number of treatments (t) and number of replications (r); that is, n = rt; That is, if there are 4 treatments (for e.g., A, B, C and D), each replicated 5 times, then n = 4 x 5 = 20.

b) In case, the number of replications is not the same for all treatments, then the total number of experimental plots is obtained as the sum of the replications for each treatment. i.e.,

$$n = \sum_{i=1}^{t} ri$$

where r_i is the number of times the ith treatment is replicated

Step 2: Assign a number to each experimental plot; may be from 1 to n.

Step 3: Assign the treatments to experimental plots randomly, maybe by using a random number table

Step 4: Form the CRD layout with 4 treatments (A, B, C, and D), each replicated 5 times in 20 plots, the layout will appear as below:

Plot number Treatment	1 D	2 A	3 B	4 B	5 B	6 D	7 D	8 A	9 C	10 A
Plot number Treatment	11 C	12 C	13 A	14 A	15 B	16 C	17 D	18 B	19 C	20 D

Step 5

a) Calculation of Treatment Total $T_1, T_2, \ldots, T_t$

b) Calculation of Grand Total (GT) = $T_1 + T_2 + \ldots + T_t$

c) Calculation of Correction Factor (CF) = $(GT)^2 / N$

Step 6: Calculation of Sum of Squares

1. Total Sum of Squares (TSS) = $y_{11}^2 + y_{12}^2 + \ldots + y_{ntt}^2 - CF$
2. Treatment Sum of Squares (TrSS) = $[T_1^2 / n_1] + [T_2^2 / n_2] + \ldots + [T_t^2 / n_t] - CF$
3. Error sum of squares (ESS) = TSS – T_rSS

Step 7: Formation of Analysis of Variance Table

ANOVA Table

Source of variation	**Degrees of freedom (df)**	**Sum of Squares (SS)**	**Mean Squares (MS) = SS/df**	**F**
Treatments	(t-1)	T_r SS	T_rSS = T_rMS / (t-1)	T_rMS / EMS
Error	(N-t)	ESS	EMS = ESS / (N-t)	
Total	(N-1)	TSS		

Error df = Total df – Treatment df = (N-1) – (t-1) = N-1–t+1 = N–t

Step 8: Interpretation

i. If cal F < tab F for (t-1), (N-1) df at 5% level, F is not significant. H_0 is accepted. All the treatments are alike.

ii. If cal F > tab F for (t-1), (N-1) df at 5% level, F is significant. F = ( )*. Ho is rejected.

iii. If cal F > tab F for (t-1), (N-1) df at 1% level, F is highly significant. F = ( )**. Ho is rejected.

If F is significant or highly significant, the Critical Difference (CD) between treatment means is to be worked out. CD between any two treatment means is defined as the least significant difference between any two treatment means, to be exceeded by the difference between two treatment means to declare them as significantly different.

CD between any two treatment means at 5% level	=	SE of the difference between the treatment means x table value of t for error df at 5% level.
CD between any two treatment means at 1% level	=	SE of the difference between the treatment means x table value of t for error df at 1% level.

Critical difference between Tr_1 and Tr_2 at 5% (1%) $=\sqrt{E.M.S.[1/n_1+1/n_2]}*t$ error df at 5% (1%)

Critical difference betweenTr_1 and Tr_3 at 5% (1%) $=\sqrt{E.M.S\left(\frac{1}{n_1}+\frac{1}{n_3}\right)}$ *t error df at 5% (1%)

Step 9: After this, write treatment means $\overline{Tr}_1\ \overline{Tr}_2 \ldots \overline{Tr}_n$. Bar chart representation can be made to show the significant differences among the treatments.

Note: If we have equal number of replications, i.e, $n_1 = n_2 = \ldots n_t = n$, then, we have in step 2 Treatment sum of squares $=\frac{T_1^2+T_2^2+\ldots+T_r^2}{n}-CF$

CD between any two treatment means at 5% or 1% level = $\sqrt{\frac{2EMS}{n}}$ * table t for error df at 5% or 1% level

Exercise

Data from a laboratory experiment are as below, in which the observations were made on the growth of different isolates on a medium:

Isolates	*Growth (mm diameter) of the colony of X isolates on Y medium after 14 hours of incubation*		
	Replication	***Replication***	***Replication***
1	*29.0*	*28.0*	*29.0*
2	*33.5*	*31.5*	*29.0*
3	*26.5*	*30.0*	
4	*48.5*	*46.5*	*49.0*
5	*34.5*	*31.0*	

Find out whether the above treatment differences are significant.

Solution

For the above problem, we can use One-way ANOVA to find whether the treatment differences are significant. First, we calculate Treatment Totals (Ti), Treatment Mean, Grand Total (G), and Grand Mean:

Isolates	Replication	Replication	Replication	Treatment Total (Ti)	Treatment Mean
1	29.0	28.0	29.0	86.0	28.67
2	33.5	31.5	29.0	94.0	31.33
3	26.5	30.0		56.5	28.25
4	48.5	46.5	49.0	144.0	48.00
5	34.5	31.0		65.5	32.72
Grand Total (G)				**446.0**	
Grand Mean					**34.1**

Next, with the above treatment totals (T_i) and grand total (G), compute the correction factor (CF) and various sums of squares (SS).

Correction Factor (CF) = $G^2 / n = 446^2 / 13 = 15301.23$

Total Sum of Squares (TSS) = $29^2 + 28^2 + \dots + 31_t^2 - CF = 789.27$

Treatment Sum of Squares (TrSS) = $[86^2 / 3] + [94^2 / 3] + \dots + [65.5^2 / 2] - CF = 762.69$

Error sum of squares (ESS) = TSS – T_rSS = 789.27 – 762.69 = 26.58

Now, let us enter all the values of sums of squares in ANOVA table and compute mean squares and F value. Tabular F value is found with treatment df = t - 1 = 4 and error df = n – t = 8 at 5% level of significance.

ANOVA Table

Source of variation	Degree of freedom	Sum of squares	Mean square	Computed F	Tabular F 5%
Treatment	(t-1) = 4	762.69	762.69 / 4 = 190.67	TrMS / EMS = 190.67 / 3.32 = 57.43*	3.84
Error	(N-t) = 8	26.58	26.58 / 8 = 3.32		
Total	(N-1) = 12	789.27			

* Significant at 5% level

We compare the computed F value (57.43) with the tabular F value (3.84). Since the computed F value is larger than the tabular F value at 5% level of significance, we conclude that the variation due to treatments is significant and such a result is generally indicated by placing an asterisk on the computed F value. If the computed F value is smaller than or equal to the tabular F value at 5% level of significance, then we say that the variation due to treatments is said to be non-significant and such result is indicated by placing 'NS' on the computed F value or by leaving the F value without any marking.

A non-significant F in ANOVA indicates the failure of the experiment to detect any differences among treatments. It does not prove that all treatments are the same. Because, the failure to detect treatment differences based on a non-significant F test could be the result of either a very small or no difference among the treatments or due to a large experimental error, or both. Thus, whenever the F test is non-significant, the researcher should examine the size of the experimental error and the numerical differences among the treatment means. If both values are large, the trial may be repeated and efforts may be made to reduce the experimental error so that the differences among treatments, if any, can be detected.

On the other hand, if both values are small, the differences among treatments are probably too small to be of any value, and thus no additional trials are needed. In the above example, the computed F value of 57.43 is larger than the tabular F value of 3.84 at the 5% level of significance. Hence, the treatment differences are said to be significant. In other words, chances are less than 5 in 100 that all the observed differences among the five treatment means could be due to chance. Such a significant F test verifies the existence of some differences among the treatments tested, but does not specify the particular pair (or pairs) of treatments that differ significantly.

6.8 RANDOMIZED BLOCK DESIGN (RBD) – TWO-WAY ANOVA

For a CRD, the experimental materials should be homogenous. However, in reality, the experimental materials are not homogenous, particularly in biological research. Hence, the principle of local control is adopted and experimental materials are grouped into homogenous sub-groups, called blocks. Since each block will consist of the entire set of treatments, a block is equivalent to a replication. Hence, the terms block and replication are used synonymously in RBD.

In RBD, we use the principle of local control to reduce the variability due to experimental error. First, we arrange the experimental units into homogeneous blocks in such a way that within the blocks, the experimental units are homogeneous, and between the blocks, there is variability. Blocking has to be done based on any observable character, which is likely to have an influence over the factor under study. E.g. in the study of effects on weight gain in chicks, the chicks may be grouped according to strains. If we conduct an RBD in 't' number of treatments, we need `rt' number of experimental units, where r is the number of blocks (replications). RBD is an equi-replicated design.

6.8.1 Blocking Technique

The purpose of blocking is to reduce the experimental error by eliminating the contribution of known sources of variation among experimental units. It is done by grouping the experimental units into blocks in such a way that the variability within each block is minimized and the variability among blocks is maximized. For e.g., in animal experiments, breed, age, litter or weight may form blocks. Suppose the experimental material is divided into 'r' blocks (replications). Let there be 't' treatments. Each block is divided into 't' units and treatments are allocated within a block randomly. Since only variation within a block becomes part of experimental error, blocking is most effective. E.g., studying different breeds of pigs, in a feed trial. Variability between pigs will be greater than expected, because of variability between breeds. In such a trial, breeds need to be defined as blocks, and pigs within each breed are fed different feeds.

6.8.2 Randomization

Having formed the number of blocks, experimental units will be allotted independently to different treatments for each block randomly and the response values are tabulated as below:

Treatment	Replication				Total
	Tr_1	Tr_2	…	Tr_t	
1	y_{11}	y_{12}	…	y_{1t}	B_1
2	y_{21}	y_{22}	…	y_{2t}	B_2
…	…	…	…	…	…
b	y_{b1}	y_{b2}	…	y_{bt}	B_t
Total	T_1	T_2	…	T_t	GT

6.8.3 Stepwise Procedure for RBD

Ho: Treatment means do not differ significantly.

Step 1:

a) Calculation of treatment total, i.e. $T_1, T_2, \ldots, T_t$

b) Calculation of block total, i.e. $B_1, B_{2,} \ldots, B_t$

c) Calculation of grand total (GT) = $[T_1 + T_2 + \ldots + T_t] = [B_1 + B_2 + \ldots + B_t]$
= Sum of the treatment totals = Sum of the block totals

d) Calculation of correction factor (C.F) $= \frac{(G.T)^2}{hvt} N = bt$

Step 2: Calculation of sum of squares

a) Total sum of squares (T.S.S.) $= \sum\sum y_{ij}^2 - CF$. i.e sum of square of all the b t values – CF

b) Treatment Sum of Square (TrSS) $= \frac{T_1^2 + T_2^2 + \ldots + T_r^2}{h} - C.F$

c) Block sum of Squares (BSS) $= \frac{B_1^2 + B_2^2 + \ldots\ldots\ldots + B_b^2}{+} - C.F$

d) Error sum of Squares (ESS) = TSS - (TrSS + BSS)

Step 3: Formation of ANOVA table

There are three sources of variability in an RBD: treatment, replication (or block) and experimental error, which is one more than that for a CRD, because of the addition of replication, which corresponds to the variability among blocks. Total variance is thus divided into three sources of variation, *viz.*, between replications, between treatments and error. Hence, ANOVA for data from a RBD is given by:

$Y_{ij} = \mu + t_i + b_j + e_{ij}$

where, μ = the overall mean

t_i = i^{th} treatment effect

b_j = j^{th} replication (block) effect; and

e_{ij} = error term

Hence, the required sums of squares are

$CF = (GT)^2 / bt$

Total sum of squares (TSS) = ΣY_{ij}^2 - CF

Block (Replication) sum of squares (BSS) = $(1/t) \Sigma b_j^2$ – CF

Treatment sum of squares (TrSS) = $(1/r) \Sigma T_i^2$ – CF

Error sum of squares = Total sum of squares – Block sum of squares – Treatment sum of squares

ANOVA Table

Source of variation	**Degrees of freedom**	**Sum of squares**	**Mean squares**	**F**
Treatment	(t-1)	T_rSS	$T_rMS = T_rSS$ / (t-1)	T_rMS / EMS
Block (Replication)	(b-1)	BSS	BMS = BSS / (b-1)	BSS / ESS
Error	(b-1) (t-1)	ESS	EMS = ESS / (b-1)(t-1)	
Total	N-1	TSS		

Step 4: Interpretation

i. If calculated F < table value of F for (t-1), (b-1) (t-1) df at 5% level, F is not significant. H_0 is accepted. Hence, we can say that all the treatments are alike.

ii. If calculated F > tab F for (t-1), (b-1) (t-1) df at 5% level, F is significant. F = ( )*. Ho is rejected.

iii. If calculated F> tab F for (t-1), (b-1) (t-1) df at 1% level, F is highly significant. F = ( )**. Ho is rejected.

If we find a significant difference between treatments by F test, then, we have to use critical difference (CD) for comparing treatments. Hence, in the last two cases, we have to calculate the critical difference between any two treatment means at 5% (or 1%) level.

$$= \sqrt{\frac{2EMS}{b}} \text{ x table value of `t' for error d.f. at 5\% (1\%) level}$$

Such differences can also be tested by Duncan's Multiple Range Test (DMRT). Finally, bar chart representation may be done to show the significance between treatments.

6.8.4 Advantages of RBD

a) It is more efficient than CRD.

b) RBD is a simple design with one local control for efficient utilization of the available experimental units. RBD eliminates the assignable source of variation among the experimental units by grouping the more homogeneous units together.

c) This reduces the experimental error, which results in increased precision of the experiment due to reduction in experimental error, and hence, the test of significance becomes more efficient.

d) There is better flexibility and hence any number of treatments and any number of replications may be included. However, each treatment should have the same number of replications.

Because of these advantages, RBD is widely used in biological research.

6.8.5 Disadvantages of RBD

a) RBD is not suitable for a large number of treatments.

b) When data from some experimental units are missing, then RBD will not be useful, for which we need to use the Missing plot technique. If the missing observations are more, this design is less convenient than CRD.

c) Each block is a replication by itself and the number of replications is equal to the number of blocks. This is the restriction in RBD.

Exercise

An experiment was conducted to study the performance of different varieties of fodder sorghum under rain-fed conditions and the green matter yields of sorghum in kg per plot are given below:

Green matter yield of sorghum, kg/plot				
Variety	***Replication***			
	I	***II***	***III***	***IV***
1	*22.9*	*25.9*	*39.1*	*33.9*
2	*29.5*	*30.4*	*35.3*	*29.6*
3	*28.8*	*24.4*	*32.1*	*28.6*
4	*47.0*	*40.9*	*42.8*	*32.1*
5	*28.9*	*20.4*	*21.1*	*31.8*

Find out whether the varietal yields are significantly different.

Solution

Let us first find the treatment (variety) totals, block (replication) totals and treatment (variety) means:

Green matter yield of sorghum, kg/plot						
Variety	**Replication**				**Total**	**Mean**
	I	**II**	**III**	**IV**		
1	22.9	25.9	39.1	33.9	121.8	30.4
2	29.5	30.4	35.3	29.6	124.8	31.2
3	28.8	24.4	32.1	28.6	113.9	28.5
4	47.0	40.9	42.8	32.1	162.8	40.7
5	28.9	20.4	21.1	31.8	102.2	25.6
Total	**157.1**	**142.0**	**170.4**	**156.0**	**625.5**	**31.3**

Then, we will find the Correction Factor and Sums of Squares:

CF = $(625.5)^2 / 20$ = 19562.5125

TSS = $[(22.9)^2 + (29.5)^2 + \ldots + (31.8)^2]$ – CF = 952.4375

RSS (BSS) = $1/4\ [(157.1)^2 + \ldots + (156.0)^2$ – CF = 80.8015

TrSS (VSS) = $1/5\ [(121.8)^2 + \ldots + (102.2)^2$ – CF = 520.53

ESS = TSS – BSS – TrSS = 351.106

Source of Variation	**Degree of Freedom (df)**	**Sum of Squares (SS)**	**Mean Square (MS)**	**Computed F**
Treatment / Variety	4	520.5300	130.1325	**4.448***
Replication / Block	3	80.8015	26.9338	<1
Error	12	351.1060	29.2588	
Total	19	952.4375		

* Significant at 5% level

SE (d) = Square root of (2 x EMS / r) = Square root of (2 x 29.2588 / 4) = 3.8248

CD = t x SE (d) = 2.179 X 3.8248 = 8.33

If the difference between the two treatment means is less than the CD, then they do not differ significantly. If it is greater than the CD, then they differ significantly. The treatment mean of only variety 4 differs from the treatment means of other varieties by more than CD (8.33), this variety can be said to produce significantly higher green matter than all other varieties.

6.9 LATIN SQUARE DESIGN (LSD) – THREE-WAY ANOVA

RBD is an improvement over CRD, as it provides error control measures. In some experiments, there may be two sources of variation. Hence, two-directional blocking is necessary to reduce experimental error considerably. By providing such an opportunity to reduce experimental error, Latin Square Design (LSD) is an improvement over RBD. In LSD, rows represent levels of one factor and columns that of another factor. E.g., the age of animals may form rows and the weight of animals may form columns.

6.9.1 Layout of LSD

When the experimental material is divided into rows and columns, treatments are allocated in such a way that each treatment occurs only once in a row and once in a column. In LSD, the numbers of rows and columns are equal and hence, the arrangement will form a square. Each row and each column are a complete block or replication in LSD. In LSD, treatments are denoted by alphabets A, B, C, etc.:

Square 1					**Square 2**				
A	B	C	D	E	A	B	C	D	E
B	A	E	C	D	B	A	D	E	C
C	D	A	E	B	C	E	A	B	D
D	E	B	A	C	D	C	E	A	B
E	C	D	B	A	E	D	B	C	A

These squares are called standard squares. In a standard square, the first row and first column are ordered alphabetically. Two standard squares are called conjugate squares when rows of one square are columns of another square. Hence, the squares 1 and 2 are conjugate. A standard square is called self-conjugate if its arrangement remains same when its rows and columns are interchanged. Now, look at the square 3 below, which is a self-conjugate square:

Square 3				
A	B	C	D	E
B	C	D	E	A
C	D	E	A	B
D	E	A	B	C
E	A	B	C	D

The layout of LSD starts with dividing the experimental materials into a number of rows and columns depending on the number of treatments. The columns of the square are rearranged randomly using random number tables. Then, keeping the first row of the rearranged square as such, the remaining rows are randomised. Treatments are then allocated to the final arrangement. For a 5 X 5 Latin square, there are 56 possible standard squares.

The first step is to select a random number between 1 to 56 (both inclusive) using a random number table. If the selected random number is 50 or below, see whether it is odd or even. If it is odd, the standard square with that number is taken as such. If it is even, then the conjugate of the standard square with that number is written. If the number is between 51 and 56, then the corresponding standard square is selected. Suppose the selected random number is 48, then the standard square corresponding to this number is:

A	B	C	D	E
B	E	A	C	D
C	D	B	E	A
D	C	E	A	B
E	A	D	B	C

The conjugate of this square is:

A	B	C	D	E
B	E	D	C	A
C	A	B	E	D
D	C	E	A	B
E	D	A	B	C

In the second step, the columns of the square are randomised. For this, a set of 5 single-digit numbers from 1 to 5 are selected. For e.g., the random numbers may be 5, 1, 3, 2, and 4. They represent the column numbers and their random order. i.e., the original column 5 will be column 1 in the rearrangement and column 1 will be column 2. This randomization will result in:

E	A	C	B	D
A	B	D	E	C
D	C	B	A	E
B	D	E	C	A
C	E	A	D	B

The next step is randomizing the rows of the square got in the 2nd step, keeping the first row as such. For this, select a set of 4 single-digit random numbers from 2 to 5, which may be 4, 2, 5, and 3. i.e., row 4 should be placed after row 1, row 2 next, and so on. Thus, we now have the square below, which is the final layout of 5 X 5 LSD, to which treatments are allocated.

E	A	C	B	D
B	D	E	C	A
A	B	D	E	C
C	E	A	D	B
D	C	B	A	E

6.9.2 Analysis and Interpretation of LSD Results

ANOVA Model for LSD

$Y_{ijk} = \mu + r_i + c_j + t_k + e_{ijk}$

where, μ = the overall mean

r_i = i^{th} row effect

c_j = c^{th} column effect

t_k = k^{th} treatment effect; and

e_{ijk} = error term

The results of LSD will be in the form of two-way tables according to rows and columns. Results have to be arranged according to treatments also. Let Ri be i^{th} row total, Cj be j^{th} column total, Tk be k^{th} treatment total and GT be Grand total. Different sums of squares for t X t LSD are:

$CF = (GT)^2 / t^2$

Total SS = $\Sigma\, Y_{ijk}^2$ - CF

Row SS = $(1/t)\, \Sigma\, R_j^2$ – CF

Column SS = $(1/t)\, \Sigma\, C_j^2$ – CF

Treatment SS = $(1/t)\, \Sigma\, T_k^2$ – CF

Error SS = Total SS - Row SS – Column SS – Treatment SS

These results can be summarised in the ANOVA table:

ANOVA Table for t x t LSD

Source of variation	**Degree of freedom (df)**	**Sum of Squares (SS)**	**Mean Square**	**Computed F**
Rows	t – 1	RSS	RMS	RMS / EMS
Columns	t – 1	CSS	CMS	CMS / EMS
Treatments	t - 1	TSS	TMS	**TMS / EMS**
Error	(t – 1) (t - 2)	ESS	EMS	
Total	t^2 - 1	Total SS		

If F is not significant, we can conclude that the treatments do not differ significantly among themselves. If F is significant, the significance of any treatment can be tested by CD value in the same way as done in RBD.

CD = t x SE (d)

where t = table value of t for a specified level of significance and error df

9SE (d) = Square root of (2 x EMS / r), where r is the number of rows

Exercise

In a trial on paddy to test the yielding ability of five varieties (A, B, C, D and E), an experiment was laid out in a 5x5 LSD. The results are:

Grain yield of paddy, kg / plot				
D 39.0	*A* 24.1	*E* 26.1	*B* 37.0	*C* 42.2
E 21.2	*B* 38.1	*A* 24.0	*C* 39.3	*D* 33.1
C 35.6	*E* 33.5	*B* 38.1	*D* 40.8	*A* 24.2
A 30.8	*C* 31.1	*D* 46.7	*E* 28.7	*B* 44.9
B 44.3	*D* 29.6	*C* 41.1	*A* 26.3	*E* 24.4

Find out whether the varietal differences are significantly different.

Solution

Let us first calculate the correction factor and Sums of Squares, for which we need to find the row and column totals in the table:

Grain yield of paddy, kg/plot						
						Total
	D 39.0	A 24.1	E 26.1	B 37.0	C 42.2	168.4
	E 21.2	B 38.1	A 24.0	C 39.3	D 33.1	155.7
	C 35.6	E 33.5	B 38.1	D 40.8	A 24.2	172.2
	A 30.8	C 31.1	D 46.7	E 28.7	B 44.9	182.2
	B 44.3	D 29.6	C 41.1	A 26.3	E 24.4	165.7
Total	170.9	156.4	176.0	172.1	168.8	844.2

$CF = (844.2)^2 / 25 = 28506.95$

Total SS $= [(39.0)^2 + (24.1)^2 + \ldots + (24.4)^2] - CF = 1385.91$

Row SS $= [1/5\ (168.4)^2 + (155.7)^2 + \ldots + (165.7)^2] - CF = 74.49$

Column SS $= [1/5\ (170.9)^2 + (156.4)^2 + \ldots + (168.8)^2]$ - $CF = 44.17$

We shall then rearrange the table of results treatment-wise and find the variety total, to find the Variety SS and Error SS:

	A	B	C	D	E
	24.1	37.0	42.2	39.0	26.1
	24.0	38.1	39.3	33.1	21.2
	24.2	38.1	35.6	40.8	33.5
	30.8	44.9	31.1	46.7	28.7
	26.3	44.3	41.1	29.6	24.4
Total	129.4	202.4	189.3	189.2	133.9

Variety SS $= [1/5(129.4)^2 + (202.4)^2 + \ldots + (133.9)^2]$ - $CF = 947.14$

Error SS = TSS – RSS – CSS – VSS = 1385.91 - 74.49 - 44.17 - 947.14 = 320.11

ANOVA Table for the above LSD

Source of variation	**Degree of freedom**	**Sum of Squares**	**Mean Square**	**Computed F**
Rows	4	74.49	18.62	< 1
Columns	4	44.17	11.04	< 1
Treatments (Varieties)	4	947.14	236.78	**8.87****
Error	12	320.09	26.66	
Total	24	1385.91		

The table value of t for α = 0.05 (5% level) and 12 df is 2.179. Hence, we can say that the treatments differ significantly. Hence, let us find the critical difference:

SE (d) = square root of [2 (26.66) / 5] = 3.263 and CD = t x SE (d) = 2.179 X 3.263 = 7.11

6.9.3 Advantage of LSD

- Because of double grouping, the experimental error is small in LSD, compared to CRD and RBD and thus LSD is more efficient than CRD and RBD.

6.9.4 Disadvantages of LSD

- With the increase in size of the square (increase in no. of rows / columns), the experimental error is likely to increase. Hence, LSD is normally not used for more than 12 treatments.
- In 2 X 2 Latin square, the error df is 0, and hence, error variance cannot be estimated. Also, in 3 X 3 and 4 x 4 Latin squares, the error df are too few and hence, the estimate of error variance will not be precise. Hence, LSD is not suitable for less than 5 treatments. Hence, despite its potential, LSD is not used widely.

6.10 MISSING PLOT TECHNIQUE

A missing data situation occurs whenever an observation is not available for an experimental unit. Missing data may be due to improper application of treatments, erroneous observations, destruction of experimental units due to natural calamities like fire, damage due to wildlife, etc. It is important to examine the reasons for these missing data. Destruction of experimental material should not be the result of treatment effect. If a plot has no surviving chicks because it has been eaten by rodents, etc., or taken away by thieves, it is not treatment-related, and hence, missing data should be appropriately declared. On the other hand, if a control plot in a vaccine trial is damaged by the disease, destruction of that control plot is required.

Thus, the plot data should be accepted as valid (i.e., zero yield if all chicks in the plot are destroyed, or the actual low value if some chicks survive), instead of treating it as missing data. The occurrence of missing data results in two major difficulties – 1. loss of data and 2. non-applicability of standard ANOVA. That is, when an experiment has one or more missing observations, then the standard procedure of ANOVA can no longer be applied. One alternative design in such cases is the missing data formula technique.

In the missing data formula technique, an estimate of a missing observation is calculated through an appropriate formula. This estimate is used to replace the missing data and the resulting new data set is then subjected to standard ANOVA. This estimate of missing data does not supply any additional information, as data once lost is not retrievable through any amount of statistical manipulation.

This procedure allows us to compute ANOVA in the usual manner (i.e., as if the data are complete), without resorting to more complex procedures needed for incomplete data sets. A single missing value in a RBD is estimated as:

$$y = \frac{rBo + tTo - Go}{(r-1)}(t-1)$$

where y = Estimate of missing data

t = No. of treatments, r = No. of replications

B_0 and T_0 = Total of observed values of replication and treatment, respectively, that contain missing data

G_0 = Grand total of all observed values

Missing datum (data) is then replaced by the computed value of y and the usual computational procedure of analysis of variance is applied to the new (augmented) dataset with some modifications.

Example of Data with One Missing Observation

Treatment	Replication			Treatment total (T)
	Replication I	Replication II	Replication III	
1	30.85	38.01	35.1	103.96
2	30.24	28.43	35.93	94.6
3	30.94	31.64	34.95	97.53
4	29.89	29.12	36.75	95.76
5	21.52	24.07	20.76	66.35
6	25.38	M	32.19	(57.57=T_0)
7	22.89	19.66	26.92	69.47
8	29.44	24.95	37.99	92.38
Replication total (R)	**221.15**	**(195.88=B_0)**	**260.59**	
Grand total (G)				**(677.62=G_0)**

6.10.1 Computation of ANOVA and Comparisons of Treatment Means

Step 1: Estimate the missing values and values of totals.

$$y = \frac{3(195.88) + 8(57.7) - 677.62}{(3-1)(8-1)} = 26.47$$

Step 2: Replace the missing data with its estimated value computed in Step 1 and carry out the ANOVA of the augmented data set based on standard procedure.

Missing data replaced by value estimated

Treatment	Replication			Treatment total (T)
	Replication I	Replication II	Replication III	
1	30.85	38.01	35.1	103.96
2	30.24	28.43	35.93	94.6
3	30.94	31.64	34.95	97.53
4	29.89	29.12	36.75	95.76
5	21.52	24.07	20.76	66.35
6	25.38	**26.47**[a]	32.19	**84.04**
7	22.89	19.66	26.92	69.47
8	29.44	24.95	37.99	92.38
Replication total (R)	**221.15**	**222.35**	**260.59**	
Grand total (G)	[a] **Estimate of missing data from missing data formula technique**			**704.09**

Step 3: Make modifications to the ANOVA obtained in Step 2 and subtract 1 from both the total and error df.

In the example, total df of 23 becomes 22 and error df of 14 becomes 13. Now, let us compute the correction factor for bias (B) as,

$$B = \frac{[Bo-(t-1)y]^2}{t(t-1)} = \frac{[195.88-(8-1)(26.47)]^2}{8(8-1)} = 2.00$$

Subtract the computed B value of 2.00 from treatment SS (SST) and total SS (SSTO), computed in Step 2 from augmented data are 680.12 and 432.09, respectively. We obtain Adjusted SST = 432.09 - 2.00 = 430.09 and Adjusted SSTO = 680.12 - 2.00 = 678.12.

Resulting ANOVA with missing values estimated

Source of variation	**Degree of freedom**	**Sum of Squares**	**Mean Square**	**Computed F**	**Tabular F (5 %)**
Replication	2	125.80	62.90	6.69	
Treatment	7	430.09	61.44	**6.53***	2.83
Error	13	122.23	9.40		
Total	22	678.12			

* Significant at 5% level of significance

6.11 REPEATED MEASURES DESIGN (RMD)

Repeated measures design is a research design that involves multiple measures of the same variable taken on the same or matched subjects either under different conditions or over two or more time periods. For instance, repeated measurements are collected in a longitudinal study in which changes over time are assessed. For e.g., in animal clinical research, we may select dairy animals suffering from mastitis and test them for their response to different drugs. Every animal included in the study is given the medicines to cure mastitis. After giving the medicines, the chosen sick animals are evaluated.

Types of Repeated Measures Designs

1. **Ordinary repeated measures** – An ordinary repeated measures design is where sick animals are assigned a single treatment and the results are measured over time (e.g., at 1, 2, and 3rd day).
2. **A crossover design** - A crossover design is where patients are assigned all the treatments and the results are measured over time.

The term repeated measures design is often interchanged with the term within-subjects design, known as a crossover study. The primary strength of the repeated measures design is that it makes the experiment more efficient and helps to keep the variability low, resulting in higher validity of the results. This design has some disadvantages too. The biggest drawbacks are known as order effects, and they are caused by exposing the subjects to multiple treatments. Because, order effects may be related to the order that treatments are given, but not due to the treatment itself.

6.12 FACTORIAL EXPERIMENTS

We have seen experiments in which the effects of a single treatment (or a factor) were estimated and compared, keeping other factor(s) constant. However, in reality, the response of biological phenomena to a factor often differs due to other factor(s) too. For e.g., milk yields may differ under different feeding patterns, housing patterns, breed, etc. Hence, we should know what happens with a combination of factors. When several factors are investigated together in a single experiment, such an experiment is called a factorial experiment.

Terminologies

Factor – Factor refers to a set of related treatments. E.g., different combinations of feed to milch cows. Here, feed, irrespective of combinations, is a factor.

Levels of a factor – Different components making up a factor are known as the levels of that factor. The levels of a factor may be quantitative (quantity of feed) or qualitative (breed of cow). These levels are usually indicated by codes such as 0, 1, 2, 3, etc.

6.12.1 Types of Factorial Experiments

A factorial experiment is named based on the number of factors and the levels of each factor. E.g., if there are 4 factors, each at 2 levels, then the experiment is known as 2x2x2x2 or 2^4 factorial experiment. If there are 2 factors, each with 3 levels, then the experiment is known as a 3x3 = 3^2 factorial experiment. i.e., if there are n factors each with p levels, then the experiment is known as a p^n factorial experiment. So, for differing numbers of levels, the arrangement is described by their products. E.g., an experiment with 3 factors, first at 2 levels, second at 3 levels, and third at 4 levels, is designated as a 2x3x4 factorial experiment; if all factors have the same levels, the experiment is called a symmetrical factorial experiment, otherwise, it is called as a mixed factorial experiment.

The factors and the numerical measures of their effects are usually represented by the capital letters of the English alphabets, while the treatment combinations are represented by small letters. For e.g., an experiment in which,

- 2 breeds of cows (b0 and b1) are tried.
- 2 dates of insemination (d0 – June and d1 – July), and
- 2 levels of feeds (f0 = 40 kg/ha and f1 = 80 kg/ha)

Hence, there will be 8 treatment combinations, *viz.*, f0d0b0, f1d0b0, f0d1b0, f1d1b0, f0d0b1, f1d0b1, f0d1b1, and f1d1b1. These treatment combinations are written as (1), f, d, fd, b, fb, db, and fdb. Symbol (1) indicates the combination of the first or basal level of all the factors. In other combinations, the first level of a factor is signified by the absence of a corresponding letter. Corresponding capital letters G, F, D, B, FD, FB, DB, and FDB denote numerical measures of the mean response of respective treatment combinations. Treatment combinations are written in a specified order, called standard order.

6.12.2 Simple and Main Effects

The effects of a factor are usually termed as simple effect or main effect. The simple effect is the difference between its responses for a fixed level of other factors. The mean of the simple effects of a factor is called as main effect. e.g. of 2x2 factorial experiment:

Yield of milk, kg/animal			
Breed	**Date of insemination**		**Response (= d1 – d0)**
	d0	**d1**	
b0	28	36	8
b1	34	44	10
Response (= v1 – v0)	6	8	

d1 has increased the yield by 8 kg / animal in breed b0 and by 10 kg / animal in b1. These responses are known as simple effects of the date of insemination d1. Similarly, the simple effect of b1 at do is 6 kg / animal and at d1, it is 8 kg / animal. The main effect of the date of insemination is (8+10) / 2 = 9 kg / animal and the main effect of the breed is (6+8) / 2 = 7 kg / animal.

Interaction

In the example, the simple effects of dates of insemination at b0 and b1 are not the same. Similarly, the simple effects of breeds at d0 and d1 are not the same. Effect of one factor changes, as the level of the other factor changes. This means that the factors are not independent. Dependence of factors in their responses is known as interaction. Interaction is measured as the mean of the differences between simple effects of factors.

In the e.g., interaction between breeds and dates of insemination is (8-6) / 2 = 1 kg / animal. If the mean is 0, it is indicative of the absence of interaction. Interaction can be positive or negative. Interaction between the two factors is known as two-factor interaction or first-order interaction. Interaction between n factors is known as n factor interaction or $(n-1)^{th}$ order interaction. Interaction between factors is denoted by the product of factors. If factors are A, B, and C, the three-factor interaction is ABC. With n factors, there will be n/1 = n main effects, n/2 two-factor interactions, n/3 three-factor interactions, and so on.

Computation of Main Effects and Interactions

Main effects and interactions can be computed by different methods. They are 1. Fisher's Algebraic Method, 2. Algebraic Method, 3. Yate's Algorithm Method and 4. Modular Arithmetic Method.

6.12.3 Layout of Factorial Experiments

When a factorial experiment is chosen, we would know the total number of treatment combinations to be tested. For the number of treatments, any basic design like CRD, RBD, or LSD may be adopted. For e.g., for a 3^2 factorial experiment, there will be 9 treatment combinations. We can arrange the 9 treatments in RBD or in 9x9 LSD. Depending on the basic design, randomization is to be carried out. Thus, we can have a factorial CRD, a factorial RBD, or a factorial LSD.

6.12.4 Analysis and Interpretation of Factorial Experiments

Analysis of results of factorial experiments is the same as that for the basic design. However, treatment df and treatment SS will be split up according to the components. Suppose we have a factorial RBD with 3 factors A, B, and C, having p, q, and s levels, respectively, we will have pqs treatment combinations. Analysis of variance model for this experiment is:

$$Y_{ijkl} = \mu + r_i + a_j + b_k + ab_{jk} + c_l + ac_{jl} + bc_{kl} + abc_{jkl} + e_{ijkl}$$

The terms ab, ac, bc, and abc represent the interaction effects. This can be generalized for any number of factors. Sums of squares can be computed using the effect total. For e.g., in the case of 2^n experiment with r replications, SS (X) = [(effect total of X)^2] / [2n * R], where X represents the main effect or interaction. The degree of freedom associated with a factor is equal to its level minus one. For interactions, the degrees of freedom will be the product of the df of the individual factors of that interaction. For three factors A, B, and C with p, q, and s levels, respectively, the degrees of freedom will be as follows:

Factorial effect	Degrees of freedom
A	p-1
B	q-1
C	s-1
AB	(p-1) (q-1)
AC	(p-1) (s-1)
BC	(q-1) (s-1)
ABC	(p-1) (q-1) (s-1)

ANOVA table can be completed with these results. Once ANOVA is completed, computation of critical difference and other steps can be done, as with single factor experiments. General formula for SE(d) is:

SE(d) for X = square root of [2EMS / r.D]

where X = main factors or interactions

D = product of levels of left out factors in X

r = no. of replications

E.g., Consider a factorial RBD with factors A, B, and C with levels p, q, and s, respectively;

- SE (d) for A = √2EMS / rqs
- SE (d) for B = √2EMS / rps

- SE (d) for C = √2EMS / rpq
- SE (d) for AB = √2EMS / rs
- SE (d) for AC = √2EMS / rq
- SE (d) for BC = √2EMS / rp
- SE (d) for ABC = √2EMS / r

Exercise

An experiment was conducted in RBD on paddy crop with 3 factors each at 2 levels. The factors were 1. Paddy variety – v0: ADT 31 and v1: IR 20; 2. Plant protection – p0: old practice and p1: new practice and 3. Irrigation – w0: local schedule and w1: new schedule. The order of treatment combination is vpw, represented by the levels of factors. Results are given in the following table:

Paddy Yield (kg/plot) from a 2^3 Factorial Experiment arranged in Randomised Blocks

Replication I	*100*	*001*	*111*	*101*	*110*	*000*	*011*	*010*
	108.2	*128.9*	*116.8*	*112.4*	*115.8*	*122.8*	*119.8*	*114.6*
Replication II	*110*	*111*	*011*	*001*	*101*	*010*	*000*	*100*
	108.6	*125.3*	*122.8*	*129.1*	*123.8*	*113.3*	*127.8*	*117.6*
Replication III	*000*	*010*	*001*	*011*	*100*	*111*	*110*	*101*
	126.0	*119.5*	*134.6*	*120.4*	*107.1*	*116.5*	*124.0*	*115.8*

Statistical analysis is carried out in 2 stages. In the first stage, analysis is done as in the case of RBD with 8 treatments. In the second stage, treatment SS is split into components. The first stage starts with the rearrangement of data as below:

Treatment combinations	**Replication**			**Total**
	I	**II**	**III**	
000: (1)	122.8	127.8	126.0	**376.6**
100: v	108.2	117.6	107.1	**332.9**
010: p	114.6	113.3	119.5	**347.4**
110: q	115.8	108.6	124.0	**348.4**
001: w	128.9	129.1	134.6	**392.6**
101: vw	112.4	123.8	115.8	**352.0**
011: pw	119.8	122.8	120.4	**363.0**
111: vpw	116.8	125.3	116.5	**358.6**
Total	**939.3**	**968.3**	**963.9**	**2871.5**

Stage I Analysis

CF = $(2871.5)^2 / 24$ = 343563.0104

Total SS = $[(122.8)^2 + (108.2)^2 + \ldots + (116.5)^2]$ – CF = 1174.6196

Replication SS = 1/8 $[(939.3)^2 + \ldots + (969.9)^2]$ – CF = **61.0634**

Treatment SS = 1/3 $[(376.6)^2 + \ldots + (358.6)^2]$ – CF = **810.659**

Error SS = **302.8966**

Stage II Analysis

Sum of Squares for main effects and interactions are calculated using factorial effect totals which are obtained by any one of the methods specified earlier. Here, we use Algebraic Method:

Factorial effect	Treatment combinations and their totals								Effect total
	(1) 376.6	**v 332.9**	**p 347.4**	**vp 348.4**	**w 392.6**	**vw 352.0**	**pw 363.0**	**vpw 358.6**	
G	+	+	+	+	+	+	+	+	2871.5
V	-	+	-	+	-	+	-	+	-87.7
P	-	-	+	+	-	-	+	+	-36.7
VP	+	-	-	+	+	-	-	+	80.9
W	-	-	-	-	+	+	+	+	60.9
VW	+	-	+	-	-	+	-	+	-2.03
PW	+	+	-	-	-	-	+	+	-9.3
VPW	-	+	+	-	+	-	-	+	-8.5

The effect total for factor v is:

V = -(1) + v – p + vp – w + vw – pw + vpw

= -376.6 + 332.9 – 347.4 + 348.4 – 392.6 + 352.0 – 363.0 + 358.6 = -87.7

Similarly, all the other effect totals are computed and are shown in the table above.

The steps in computing the factorial effect totals by Yates Algorithm are as follows:

Step 1: Write down the treatment combinations in the systematic order as in the table below.

Step 2: Add the treatment totals in pairs. These results will form the first half of the column (1). Then, subtract the first no. of each pair from the second. These results form the second half of the column.

Step 3: To obtain column (2), apply the same process as in step (2) to column (1).

Step 4: Continue the process until we reach column n, where n is the no. of factors. The values in the last column are the effect totals.

Computation of effect totals for the data using Yates Algorithm

Treatment Combinations	Total	Effect Totals		
		1	2	3
(1)	376.6	709.5	1405.3	2871.5
v	332.9	695.8	1466.2	-87.7
p	347.4	744.6	-42.7	-36.7
vp	348.4	721.6	-45.0	80.9
Sub total	-	2871.5	2783.8	2828.0
w	392.6	-43.7	-13.7	60.9
vw	352.0	1.0	-23.0	-2.3
pw	363.0	-40.6	44.7	-9.3
vpw	358.6	-4.4	36.2	-8.5
Grand total	2871.5	2783.8	2828.0	

Computations in the previous table can be checked in two ways. First, the total of the upper half of a column should be equal to the total of the lower of the previous column. Second, the first value in the last column should be equal to the grand total. The effect totals in the previous two tables can be compared to be the same.

Sums of squares are computed as below:

X SS = (effect total of X)^2 / r.2^n

where X represents a factorial effect

r.2^n = 3.2^3 = 24

V SS = $(-87.7)^2$ / 24 = 320.4704

P SS = $(-36.7)^2$ / 24 = 56.1204

W SS = $(60.9)^2$ / 24 = 154.5338

VP SS = $(80.9)^2$ / 24 = 272.7004

VW SS = $(-2.3)^2$ / 24 = 0.2204

PW SS = $(-9.3)^2$ / 24 = 3.6033

VPW SS = $(-8.5)^2$ / 24 = 3.0104

It can be verified that the sum of all the SS values is equal to the overall treatment SS **(810.6591).** The results are summarized in the ANOVA table:

Analysis of Variance for the Data				
Sources of variation	**Degrees of freedom**	**Sum of squares**	**Mean square**	**F value**
Replication	2	**61.0364**	30.5317	
V	1	320.4704	320.4704	**14.812****
P	1	56.1204	56.1204	2.594
W	1	154.5338	154.5338	**7.143***
VP	1	272.7004	272.7004	**12.604****
VW	1	0.2204	0.2204	<1
PW	1	3.6033	3.6033	<1
VPW	1	3.0104	3.0104	<1
Error	14	**302.8966**	21.6355	
Total	23	**1174.6196**		

Note: SS for replication and error are brought from Stage I analysis

Since F is significant for V, W, and VP only, we need to calculate CD for V, W, and VP only.

SE (d) for V = √2(21.6335) / (3x2x2) = 1.8989

CD for V = 2.365 x 1.8989 = 4.4909

CD for W is the same as for V.

SE (d) for VP = √2(21.6335) / (3x2) = 2.6855

CD for VP = 2.365 x 2.6855 = 6.3512

Based on the results, we can conclude that the new paddy variety IR 20 gives a significantly higher yield than the traditional variety ADT 31. Both plant protection methods are similar in their effect. New irrigation practice increases paddy yield significantly, compared to local practice. IR 20 gives a significantly higher yield than ADT 31 under the old plant protection method, but their performance is similar under the new plant protection method.

6.12.5 Advantages of Factorial Experiments

We can evaluate the combined effect of 2 or more factors. We can study both the individual effects of each factor and also effects of their interactions. The factorial approach will ensure in saving of both experimental materials and time, than which are required for separate experiments. So, when we have several factors, factorial experiments can only be used, as a single-factor experiment will be unsatisfactory.

6.12.6 Disadvantages of Factorial Experiments

When the number of factors and their levels are increased, then the number of treatment combinations will also increase, which will increase the block size. The increased block size will make it difficult to ensure homogeneity of experimental materials. This will then increase the experimental error and loss of precision in the experiment. Also, when several treatment combinations are involved, the execution of the experiment and statistical analysis become more complex.

6.13 ANALYSIS OF COVARIANCE (ANACOVA)

Analysis of Covariance (ANACOVA) is a statistical procedure in which the variability of a dependent variable is explained by both categorical and continuous independent variables. A continuous variable is called a covariate. The common application of ANACOVA is to adjust the treatment means for a known source of variability that can be explained by a continuous variable.

E.g., an experiment is designed to test the effects of 3 diets on the weight of animals. As we know, the different initial weights or the different ages at the beginning of the experiment will influence the animal performance and precision of the experiment. Hence, it is necessary to adjust the final weights to the initial weight or initial age. This can be done by defining the initial weight or the initial age as a covariate, which will improve the precision of the experiment. Because part of the unexplained variability is explained by the covariate. Consequently, the experimental error will be reduced.

Exercise

The effect of three diets on the daily weight gain of steers was investigated, using a CRD. Weight at the beginning of the experiment (initial weight) was recorded, but not used in the assignment of animals to diet. At the end of the experiment, the following daily gains were recorded:

Diet A		**Diet B**		**Diet C**	
Initial wt. (kg)	**Gain (g / day)**	**Initial wt. (kg)**	**Gain (g / day)**	**Initial wt. (kg)**	**Gain (g / day)**
350	970	390	990	400	990
400	1000	340	950	320	940
360	980	410	980	330	930
350	980	430	990	390	1000
340	970	390	980	420	1000

To show the efficiency of including initial weight, a CRD without a covariate is to be first fitted. Then, the ANOVA model will be:

Source of variation	Sum of Squares	Degrees of freedom	Mean Sum of Squares	Computed F value
Treatment	173.333	2	86.667	**0.16**
Residual	6360.000	12	530.000	
Total	6533.333			

The tabular value for the treatment effect is $F_{0.05, 2, 12} = 3.89$. Since the computed F value is smaller than the tabular F value, the effect of the treatment is not significant. However, when the initial weight is included as a covariate, the ANOVA model will be:

Source of variation	Sum of Squares	Degrees of freedom	Mean Sum of Squares	Computed F value
Initial weight	4441.253	1	4441.253	**46.92**
Treatment	1050.762	2	525.381	**5.55**
Residual	1041.319	11	94.665	
Total	6533.333	14		

The critical (tabular) value for the treatment effect is $F_{0.05, 2, 11} = 3.98$. The critical (tabular) value for the regression of daily weight gain on the initial weight is $F_{0.05, 1, 11} = 4.84$. Since the calculated F values of 46.92 and 5.55 are higher than the tabular values, the effects of both initial weight and treatment are significant. That is, while the first model was not adequate, a significant difference between treatments was found by including initial weight in the model.

6.14 SPLIT-PLOT DESIGN

When some factors (independent variables) are difficult to be changed in an experiment, using a CRD is not adequate. In such cases, a split-plot design can be used, which has a mixture of hard-to-change and easy-to-change factors. The "Plot" part of the split-plot originally comes from a plot of land in agriculture. Split-plots were invented by Fisher (1935) and it has been suggested that all agricultural experiments are split-plot designs (Box *et al.*, 2005). Although these designs are commonly seen in industry, they can also be used across a wide variety of disciplines. In fact, any experiment where one of the factors is difficult to be changes is fit for a split-plot design.

Example

Suppose we want to study the effects of two irrigation methods (factor 1) and two different fertilizer types (factor 2) on four different fields (whole plots). However, we will run into a practical problem with randomization. While a field can easily be split into two for two different fertilizers, the field cannot easily be split into two for irrigation: One irrigation system normally covers a whole field and the systems are expensive to replace.

Step 1: Randomize the fixed or hard-to-change factor (in this e.g., it is the irrigation method) among the four fields:

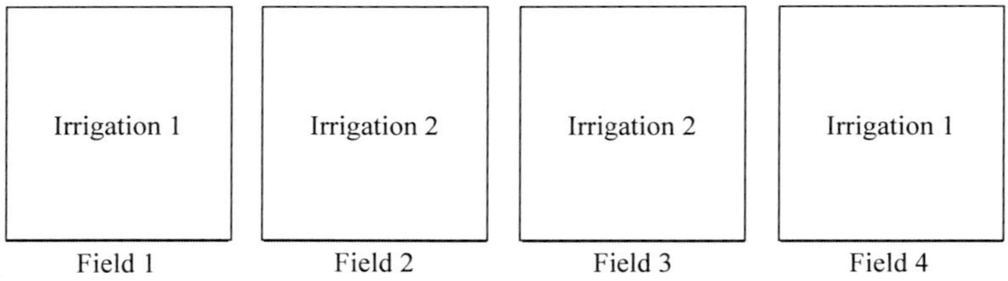

Step 2: Split the plots into two.

Step 3: Randomize the non-fixed or easy-to-change factor within each plot (in this e.g., it is the fertilizer):

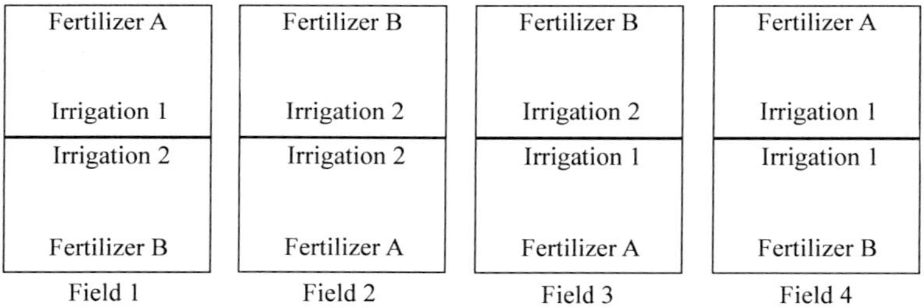

Compare the above with the one we would get from a complete randomization — where both the irrigation and fertilizer are randomly allocated between the 8 subplots:

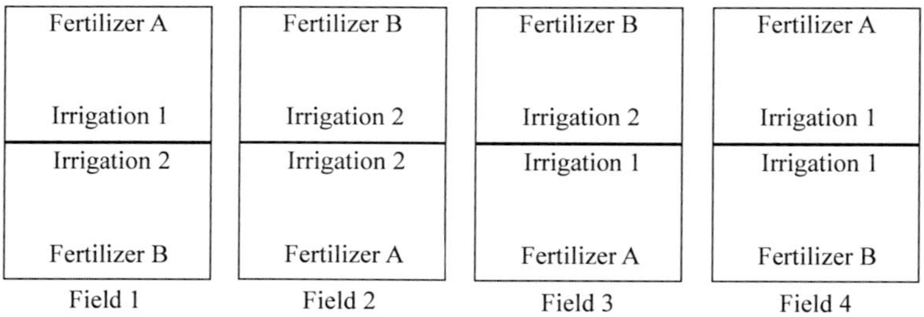

6.14.1 Advantage and Disadvantage of Split-plot Designs

Compared to CRDs, split-plot designs are cheaper to run and more efficient statistically, with increased precision.

Implementing the split-plot design is difficult and also it requires advanced knowledge of a specific discipline (e.g., agriculture, epidemiology, etc.).

7

Epidemiological Approaches to Animal Disease Investigation

Veterinary epidemiology is the study of disease within a livestock population, dealing with the investigation (including identification, quantification, and examination), of the direct and indirect determinants of disease distribution in animal populations. Any epidemiological investigation starts with whether there is an animal health problem in a population, which requires data collection on animal, management, economic, and environmental factors. These data are then analyzed descriptively to assess the frequency of disease occurrence. The results are then used to decide whether investigations of causal relationships between disease occurrence and potential risk factors are necessary for the development of control or prevention policies. Once the relationships are understood, necessary interventions for the disease are then planned and their impacts assessed. Hence, the goal of epidemiological investigations is the control and prevention of animal disease problems by integrating the available pieces of evidence into the decision-making process for disease control policy development.

Epidemiological study is conducted at the level of an animal population, like individual animals, herds, farms, regions, or countries. There are two reasons why an epidemiologist performs population-level research, by looking at a sample of a population. First, he wants to quantify a characteristic of that population, e.g., the prevalence of a disease. This type of research is called descriptive research, undertaken through surveys. Secondly, the epidemiologist wishes to test an association between a disease and exposure to a suspected causal factor. This research is called analytical research. Both descriptive research and analytical research are observational, because the researcher simply observes the events, without intervention or experimentation. Because of this non-intervention, observational epidemiology is different from experimental epidemiology in which the epidemiologist tries to know the effect of an intervention, like vaccination or therapy.

Irrespective of the type of observational research, any population is usually too large to observe all the units. Further, estimates of the association can be obtained to an acceptable degree of precision by selecting and observing only a few animals (called samples) much smaller than the population.

The basis for most of the epidemiological investigations is the assumption that disease does not occur randomly. A disease is usually influenced by multiple risk factors or determinants, which can be time, place, and animal characteristics. Epidemiological investigations focus on measuring these determinants for groups of animals selected from animal populations, and both healthy and diseased animals are examined to know the differences in the determinants. The parameters that are usually investigated include the health status of the animal and the factors that can potentially affect its health status, such as age, breed, body condition, vaccination status, pregnancy status, season, spatial and temporal locations, etc.

The key issue is that many animals suffer from the disease with different manifestations of symptoms. That is, those animals that have died or developed severe disease are usually detected, while those with mild illness are left undetected. However, the animals of both groups transmit infection, thus becoming an important factor in the transmission dynamics of an infectious disease, which varies between diseases and depends on a range of risk factors.

Temporal patterns of disease can be categorized into epidemic and endemic patterns. An epidemic is defined as a disease occurrence that is higher than normal, while an endemic refers to a disease normally present in a population. Pandemic disease occurrence refers to widespread epidemics occurring globally, like COVID-19 in 2019-2020. Outbreaks involve a sudden increase in the number of cases, and they describe unusual occurrences at the herd level. Sporadic disease occurrence is characterized by individual cases or clusters of disease that are normally not present in an area.

7.1 VETERINARY EPIDEMIOLOGY AND ECONOMICS

The two disciplines - animal health economics and veterinary epidemiology, although separate, are complementary and supplementary in animal health management. Epidemiological studies are used to identify the factors contributing to the development of disease conditions, the magnitude and directions of the contributions, and the relationships between diseases and other animal conditions. However, the epidemiological information is not enough to make decisions for disease control, unless some economic meaning is infused into it.

Hence, veterinary epidemiologists cannot limit their work purely to technical areas, but should also enter into the socio-economic aspects of animal health. Economic analysis is a natural progression from epidemiology, as it adds values to the estimates of productivity effects and relates the level of disease in a population with its cost to a farmer or society. Therefore, veterinarians should also practice as economists, especially while working on animal health policy formulation and evaluation, and the economics of interventions, and should be proficient in economic theory and methods.

7.2 COMPONENTS OF VETERINARY EPIDEMIOLOGY

1.	**Data Collection**	
2.	**Qualitative investigations**	
a.	*Natural history of disease*	
•	Ecology, transmission, pattern of occurrence, field observations	
b.	*Causal factors*	
•	Host, agent, environment	
3.	**Quantitative investigations**	
a.	*Surveys*	
•	Cross-sectional, longitudinal (prospective, retrospective), screening	
b.	*Monitoring and surveillance*	
c.	*Studies*	
•	Experimental	Clinical trials, intervention studies
•	Cross-sectional	Groups of animals based on characteristics (age, disease, etc.)
•	Case-control	Comparing diseased and healthy groups concerning exposure to factors
•	Cohort	Comparing the group exposed to the factor with the group not exposed
d.	*Modelling*	
e.	*Disease control*	

7.3 VETERINARY EPIDEMIOLOGICAL SURVEYS AND STUDIES – A SUMMARY

1.	**Quantitative**	
a.	*Observational*	
i.	Analytical	
•	Longitudinal	• Case-control study • Cohort study
•	Cross-sectional	• Exploratory survey
ii.	Descriptive	
•	Longitudinal	• Incidence study
•	Cross-sectional	• Descriptive study
b.	*Experimental (Field trials / Laboratory studies)*	
2.	Qualitative	

7.4 APPROACHES TO VETERINARY EPIDEMIOLOGICAL INVESTIGATIONS

Veterinary epidemiology aims to 1. Determine the origin of a disease whose cause is known; 2. Investigate and control a disease, whose cause initially is unknown; 3. Acquire data on the ecology and natural history of a disease; 4. Plan and monitor the disease control programmes; and 5. Assess the economic effects of disease and analyze the economic costs and benefits of alternative disease control programmes.

Accordingly, the approaches to veterinary epidemiological investigations are i). descriptive, ii). analytical, iii). experimental and iv). theoretical. Descriptive epidemiology involves observing and recording the diseases and the possible causal factors. Analytical epidemiology deals with the analysis of observations using suitable diagnostic and statistical tests. Experimental epidemiology involves the observation and analysis of data from groups of animals from which the epidemiologist can select and in which he/she can alter the factors associated with the groups. An important component of this approach is the control of the groups. Lastly, theoretical epidemiology consists of a representation of disease using mathematical models that can simulate natural patterns of disease occurrence.

7.5 DETERMINANTS OF A DISEASE

Understanding the potential risk factors that lead to the occurrence of disease and the cause-effect relationships will help to control or prevent the occurrence of the disease. Because not every animal in a given situation is affected by the disease. The term epidemiological triangle describes the interrelationships between agent, host, and environment as the determinants of a disease.

7.5.1 Agent Determinants

Agent determinants include pathogenicity, which is the ability of an infectious agent to cause disease in the hosts in different environmental conditions. The relationship between the host and the agent is a major component of the epidemiology of any infectious process. The occurrence of a disease is the result of the balance between the resistance mechanisms in the host, and the infectivity and virulence of the disease-causing agent. The presence of an agent may cause a latent infection, clinical disease, carrier state, or immunity in the host or death of the host. The infected host in a carrier state or latent infection, not showing any symptom of a clinical disease, will start disseminating the disease agent. The disease-causing agent may be transmitted through ingestion, aerial transmission, physical contact, inoculation, or coitus, the identification of which will help in finding and implementing specific measures for preventing disease transmission. Vectors or intermediate hosts are required for some infectious agents to survive in an ecosystem.

7.5.2 Host Determinants

The factors such as species, breed, age, and sex of animals are called the host determinants. Animals of a particular species may be the natural reservoirs of certain infection and such infection is maintained within the population, not requiring periodic re-introduction. This type of epidemiological scenario can extremely complicate the control or eradication of a disease. This is the case for Rabies where infection circulates in specific wild animals resulting in repeated introductions of infection into domestic animal populations.

7.5.3 Environmental Determinants

Environmental determinants of disease include positional, climatic, and husbandry factors. The geographical position is whether a farm is in the vicinity of an area with a high density of wild species, acting as a reservoir of infection. Climatic factors also affect the distribution of vectors and hence influence the status of infection in a population.

7.6 DESIGNING A VETERINARY EPIDEMIOLOGICAL STUDY

Describing the health status of animal populations, explaining the etiology of diseases, predicting the disease occurrence, and controlling the distribution of diseases are the key aims of veterinary epidemiology. All these aims require access to the data for further analysis. The data may be already available from a disease surveillance programme, or they may need to be collected through a specific study. If the data are not available, one needs to be clear about what the target population or source population is. The target population is one for which the results from the study are to be generalized. The source population is the one from which the actual units of study, like the animals or herds, have been selected.

Epidemiological studies can be descriptive studies or analytical studies. Case studies and surveys are examples of descriptive studies. Experimental and observational studies are analytical or explanatory studies, that involve the comparison of groups of animals concerning the association between one or more risk factors and the outcome of interest, like a disease, which will ultimately allow us to draw inferences on cause-effect relationships. In analytical studies, we need to keep in mind that all phenomena within the biological systems are interrelated, which complicate the situation for an investigator. An experimental study may not be able to represent the real world, because of intangible magnitudes inherent in a biological system. However, an observational study allows some control over the study conditions and measurement, and hence more likely to represent the real world.

7.6.1 Descriptive Studies

Case studies focus on individual sick animals. They are based on direct personal observation of anatomical structures and physiological functions, which can be quantified, but usually are largely qualitative. While observations can be intensive and detailed, their main disadvantage is that they do not involve comparison for assessing the cause-effect relationships. Surveys are also descriptive and involve the random selection of a sample from a population, aiming at describing the disease frequency, but they do not collect data on risk factors.

7.6.2 Experimental Studies

An experimental study usually involves manipulation of some parameters (for e.g., introducing an intervention like a new therapy, a vaccine, or a management factor), and is conducted either in a controlled environment, such as a laboratory, or in the natural environment (farmers' field). If conducted in a laboratory, great precision in the measurement of parameters and optimal control of influencing variables can be achieved. However, the disadvantage is that it may not be possible to represent the factors affecting the disease occurrence in farmers' fields and to work with sufficient numbers of animals to represent the true variations between animals in the natural population. If the experimental study is conducted in the natural environment, it is called an experimental field study (also a controlled trial, clinical trial, or intervention study). In contrast to the laboratory experiment, the animals will be exposed to all known and unknown factors present in the natural environment. These studies are usually used to evaluate the therapeutic or preventive effects of specific interventions.

Experimental studies involve dividing a group of animals into at least two subgroups, one to which an intervention is applied and another to the so-called control or comparison group that does not receive the intervention. The decision to apply an intervention to a particular animal within the study or not is based on random allocation, called as randomization. After a period of time, the status with respect to the outcome variable (e.g. disease status) is assessed for each animal. Summary measures of the response (e.g. incidence risk) are then compared between the subgroups.

7.6.3 Observational studies

An observational study is conducted in the natural environment of animals to measure or observe naturally occurring events. Being one of the most frequently used techniques in epidemiological research, they are conducted using the data collected prospectively or retrospectively. In a prospective observational study, after designing the study, the data are collected and used, beside the existing (the already collected) data. In a retrospective study, the data about the outcome and the risk factors already available are considered. The most important observational study designs are the cohort, the case-control, and the cross-sectional study.

7.6.4 Prospective and Retrospective Studies

7.6.4.1 Prospective Study

A prospective study observes the outcomes, like the development of a disease, during the study period. It usually involves taking a cohort of subjects and observing them over a long period. Efforts are made to avoid sources of bias such as the loss of individuals to follow up during the study. Prospective studies usually have fewer sources of bias than retrospective studies. These studies are done in the present to observe and analyze the outcome in the future. In a prospective study, the data are required to be gathered and are not available before the start of the study. An example of a prospective study is to follow up with a group of silage-eating cows to identify whether silage-eating for 5 years is linked to abortions. It is to be noted that none of the subjects included in the study should have earlier had the outcome of interest, i.e., abortion, before the start of the study. Follow-up is an important and inherent property of the prospective study and the absence of it may affect the outcome of the study.

A prospective study can help in analyzing the risk factors for new diseases, for which the data are not available, to help in the effective management of new diseases. Because of the good study design and more accurate gathering of data, the results provided by prospective studies are relatively more authentic. Detailed analysis can be done in prospective studies. Not only that, exposures to the risk factors can be measured before the disease and the disease process can also be determined. As the prospective study does not require any data recollection from old data, the risk of recall bias and its disadvantages can be eliminated. Other advantages are that the disease outcomes and prevalence are easy to calculate and many disease conditions can be studied at the same time. However, cohort studies are usually expensive and time-consuming, since sample sizes required for a prospective study are usually large.

7.6.4.2 Retrospective Study

Retrospective, as the term indicates, is to look back. Hence, a retrospective study analyzes the events that had already happened in the past. The one who does a retrospective study collects the data from past records. An example of a retrospective study is to compare the occurrence of mastitis in dairy cows that are exposed to good or bad floor and udder hygiene. A retrospective study looks backward and examines the exposures to the suspected risk or protection factors concerning an outcome (the disease) that is established at the start of the study. There could be some errors due to confounding and bias in retrospective studies, compared to prospective studies.

Many of the advantages and disadvantages of retrospective studies are similar to those of prospective studies. Retrospective studies are usually constructed from the previously collected data, in contrast to a prospective study. However, an advantage to both study designs is that the exposure to the risk factors can be recorded before the outcome occurs. Since the retrospective study uses the previously collected data, it is relatively inexpensive, quick, and easy to conduct. However, in a retrospective study, not all relevant risk factors can be identified and recorded. Despite this fact, retrospective studies are cheaper and require less time to complete, as the data related to the study are already available and the researcher has to only compile and compare the data, besides providing early results. Further, the retrospective study is effective in rare diseases, as the data related to the rare diseases are available only from a few centres. Retrospective studies use the data already available in the literature and hence there is a risk of loss of follow-up.

7.6.4.3 Advantages and Disadvantages

- In a prospective study, the data are gathered by the veterinarian / researcher after the enrolment of animal subjects, while in retrospective studies, he / she makes use of the already available data.
- The prospective study has more control over the subjects and data generation, as compared to the retrospective studies.
- More accurate results are obtained in prospective studies due to fewer biases.
- Prospective studies are time-consuming and costlier, compared to retrospective studies.
- The problem of recall bias is not there in prospective studies.
- Prospective studies are both observational and interventional, while retrospective studies are only observational.
- Prospective studies are useful in cases of emerging new exposures, while retrospective studies are not of much use in such scenarios.

7.7 CROSS-SECTIONAL, CASE-CONTROL AND COHORT EPIDEMIOLOGICAL STUDIES

Let us use the following illustration:

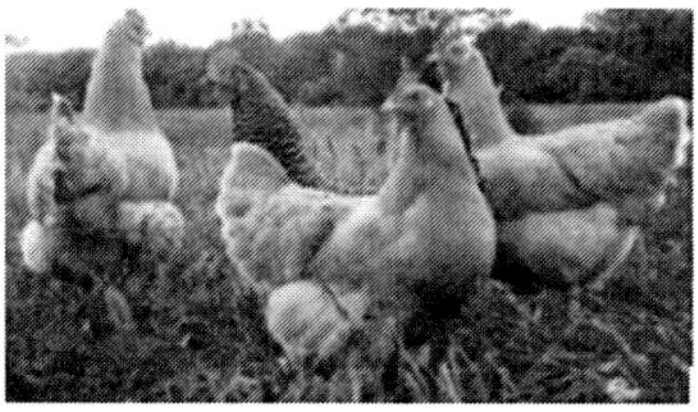

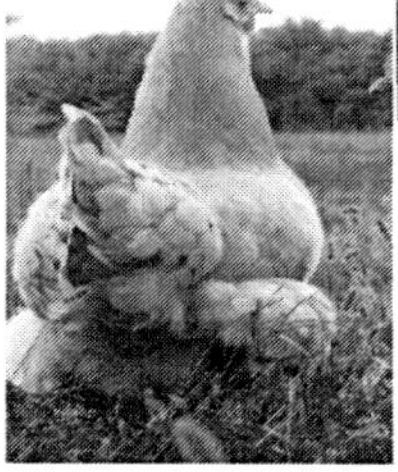

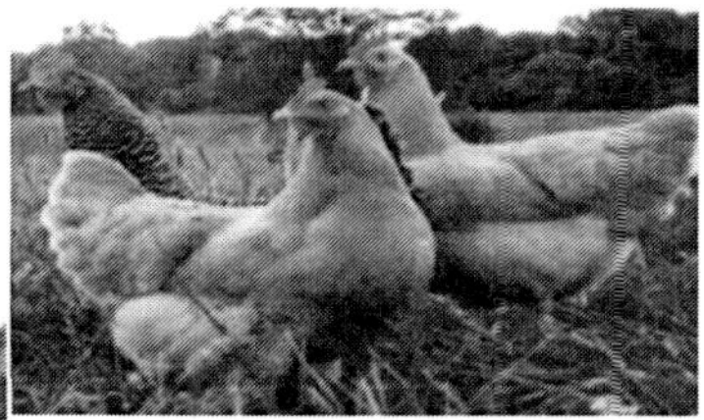

Population

Population Unexposed

Population exposed

There is a poultry farm in which there are 2,000 layers, of which 800 are exposed to a factor of interest that may predispose to a particular disease problem. Of the 800 exposed birds, 200 develop the disease and 600 birds remain free of the disease. Of the 1,200 unexposed birds, 200 develop the disease and 1,000 remain unaffected.

7.7.1 Cross-sectional studies

In cross-sectional studies, the individual birds are tested for the presence of the disease and for the exposure status at the same time. A cross-sectional study takes a picture of the situation at a specific moment. The measure of association calculated in this study is the Prevalence Ratio (PR) which is the ratio of the fraction diseased (A) among the birds exposed (A+B) to a risk factor and the fraction diseased (C) among the unexposed (C+D):

$$PR = [A / (A+B)] / [C (C+D)]$$

If the prevalence ratio equals 1.0, then there is no association between the disease and the assumed risk factor, if it is greater than 1.0, then the exposure factor can be called a risk factor, and if it is less than 1.0, then the exposure factor can be called a preventive factor. E.g., if a cross-sectional study is performed on a random sample of 100 birds chosen from the population, a 2x2 table can be formed as below:

	Disease	**No Disease**	**Total**
Exposed	30 (A)	10 (B)	40 (A+B)
Unexposed	20 (C)	40 (D)	60 (C+D)
Total	50 (A+C)	50 (B+D)	100 (A+B+C+D)

The Prevalence Ratio, PR = [A / (A+B)] / [C (C+D)], is hence (30/40) / (20/60) = 2.27. This indicates that the prevalence in exposed birds is 2.27 times higher than that in unexposed birds.

Cross-sectional studies are less suitable for identifying relationships between transient exposures and the disease because the current exposure might be too recent to be etiologically meaningful. However, for exposures that are there throughout the individual's life (like blood group, breed, sex, and housing system), cross-sectional studies are very useful. The disadvantage of cross-sectional studies is that diseases with low incidence or short duration will show low prevalence.

7.7.2 Case-Control Studies

In case-control studies, animals with the disease of concern (called cases) and animals without that disease (called controls) are selected. The frequency of exposure to the potential risk factors that are believed to predispose to the disease is measured retrospectively for both groups. The relative frequency of the exposure to the risk factor(s) is then compared between the two groups. All the cases may be selected to be included, or if the number of affected animals is extremely large, then it may be easier to choose a sample of cases. But, enough care should be taken to randomly select them, so that the sample chosen adequately represents the animal population being studied. A key requirement in case-control studies is that controls need to have had a similar exposure to risk factors, as that of cases. Though this process may be a little difficult to achieve, extra caution should be exercised to achieve at least the maximum possible. In other words, controls are a random sample of non-cases from the same population from which the cases are obtained. Hence, these studies are called population-based case-control studies.

Case-control studies are used more effectively for the study of low-incidence diseases and diseases that develop over a longer time. Because, case-control studies allow the investigation of preliminary causal hypotheses quickly, besides requiring relatively low cost, as compared to cohort studies. The disadvantages are that they allow studying single outcomes only and cannot provide information on the disease frequency in a population. Further, they are less suitable for the study of rare exposures and data collection is dependent on the quality of old records. It is also difficult to ensure an unbiased selection of the control group.

In a case-control study, the diseased (A+C) and the non-diseased (B+D) birds are purposively chosen as the units to be sampled. To measure whether or not the exposure is more common in the diseased group than in the control group, the (exposure) Odds Ratio (OR) is the measure of association that indicates the relative change in risk. The OR is calculated as:

ORexp = (A/C) / (B/D) = [A*D] / [B*C]

The numerical value of the odds ratio is interpreted in the same way as that of the prevalence ratio. If a case-control study is performed with 50 individuals in each of the two health status groups, then the frequencies in the example may be, for e.g.:

	Disease	No Disease	Total
Exposed	30 (A)	10 (B)	40 (A+B)
Unexposed	20 (C)	40 (D)	60 (C+D)
Total	50 (A+C)	50 (B+D)	100 (A+B+C+D)

The OR equals (30/20) / (10/40) which is equal to 6.0, which means that the exposure is six times more in the exposed birds than in the unexposed birds. This type of study is suitable for diseases with low incidence or short duration. The objective is to investigate whether or not a possible risk factor occurs more frequently in the diseased than in the control group.

Case-control and cross-sectional studies are more suited to screen for potential risk factors. The proof of causality is best known from cohort studies, starting with healthy individuals exposed or unexposed to the factor of interest.

7.7.3 Cohort Studies

A cohort is a group of individuals that either possess or do not possess a (risk) factor that may influence the occurrence of a disease. The group possessing the factor (the exposed group) is then observed over a period of time to ascertain if there is a change in health status. Another group (the unexposed group), comprising individuals that do not possess that specific factor or characteristic, but are otherwise very similar in other traits, is also selected and observed similarly. This study follows the effect of exposure on the change from the healthy status to the diseased state. A cohort study can be prospective and also retrospective. In a retrospective study, the allocation of animals/birds to the cohorts is based on the exposure experience in the past. In a prospective study, the allocation to cohorts is based on current exposure and we need to keep observing for the development of the disease in both cohorts.

A prospective cohort study (also called a longitudinal study) is done by selecting at least two groups of non-diseased animals with different exposure statuses in relation to the risk factors hypothesized to cause a disease. We select a sample of animals likely to be heterogeneous with respect to the risk factor levels and then determine their exposure status. The selected groups of animals (called the cohorts) are then followed over a period of time and any changes in the animals' disease status are recorded during the study period. On completion of the study, incidence measures are then compared between the exposure status groups.

As in experimental studies done for assessing the relationship between a risk factor and the disease, in a cohort study, the different exposure groups for a particular risk factor must be similar with respect to any other factors associated with that risk factor and the outcome, which are called as confounding factors. Though randomization is the best approach, it cannot be applied in an observational study. The disadvantage of this approach is that the findings may be less generalizable. A well-designed cohort study has many advantages. It is the most effective of the observational studies for the investigation of causal hypotheses with respect to disease occurrence. It provides disease incidence estimates which are more meaningful than prevalence data for assessing cause-effect relationships. The disadvantage is that cohort studies require a longer duration and hence affect the ability to demonstrate causality.

While the frequency of exposure in the population cannot be estimated in cohort studies, the frequency of disease in the population cannot be estimated in case-control studies. To estimate the relative change in risk, the Cumulative Incidence Ratio (CIR) is calculated, the incidence being the number of animals that developed the disease during the study divided by the total number of animals that were at risk at the start of the study. Synonyms for the CIR are the Risk Ratio and the Relative Risk (RR), with the relative risk being used as a general indicator for all types of relative measures of association.

CIR = [A / (A + B)] / [C / (C + D)]

The numerical value of the CIR is interpreted in the same way as those of the prevalence ratio and odds ratio. The (disease) odds ratio is calculated as below:

ORdis = (A/B) / (C/D) = [A * D] / [B * C]

Let us consider a cohort study with 100 animals per cohort:

	Disease	**No Disease**	**Total**
Exposed	70	30	100
Unexposed	25	75	100

The CIR = (70/100) / (25/100) = 2.8 and the OR = (70/30) / (25/75) = 7.0.

Summary of Observational Study Types

Observational Study Type	**Past**	**Present**	**Future**
Cross-sectional study		Disease / Exposure	
Case-control study	Exposure	Disease	
Prospective cohort study		Exposure	Disease
Retrospective cohort study	Exposure / Disease	Disease	Disease

7.8 ADVANTAGES AND DISADVANTAGES OF OBSERVATIONAL STUDIES

Cross-Sectional Study	**Case-Control Study**	**Cohort Study**
	Advantages	
• Estimations of the exposed and unexposed proportions possible • Require only a few animals/ birds and hence quick and less expensive to conduct • Existing or current records can be used • No risk to subjects (animals/ birds) during the study • Allow study of multiple potential causes of disease	• Suited for rare diseases or those with long incubation periods • Require only a few animals/ birds and hence quick and less expensive to conduct • Existing or current records can be used • No risk to subjects (animals/ birds) during the study • Allow study of multiple potential causes of disease	• Calculation of incidence in exposed and unexposed possible • Flexibility in the choice of variables to be recorded
	Disadvantages	
• Moderate sample sizes required to study rare diseases • Incomplete control of extraneous variables • Not possible to estimate incidence in exposed and unexposed individuals	• Not possible to estimate exposed and unexposed proportions in the population • Relying on recall or records for data on past exposures • Difficulties in the validation of data • Incomplete control of extraneous variables • Difficulties in the selection of comparison group	• Not possible to estimate the exposed and unexposed proportions in the population • Large numbers of subjects required for rare diseases • Longer duration for follow-up • Expensive to conduct • Incomplete control of extraneous variables

8

Measuring Animal Disease Frequencies

8.1 NEED FOR ANIMAL DISEASE FREQUENCY MEASURES

The very essence of veterinary epidemiology is to measure animal disease occurrence and to make comparisons between the animal population groups. The animal disease frequency measures help us to understand the distribution of diseases in animal populations. Hence, the principal role of veterinary epidemiology is to describe and explain differences in the distribution of animal diseases between the populations.

The health problems measured in veterinary epidemiological studies include:

1. Morbidity
2. Mortality
3. Incidence
4. Prevalence
5. Birth defects
6. Disability
7. Vaccine efficacy

Measures of the disease frequencies are used to describe how common an illness is concerning the size of the population (the population at risk) at a particular point in time. The major reason for determining the morbidity is to assess the extent of a disease problem in a population. This assessment is possible only when the number of diseased animals is calculated and compared with the total number of animals in the population. A report of 10 cases of mastitis in a dairy herd does not indicate the true extent of the disease problem, unless the report also indicates the total number of dairy animals in the herd or population. Thus, it is important to relate the number of cases of a disease to the population at risk of developing that disease.

Disease frequencies are measured at the population level for the reasons listed below:

1. We may be interested in the presence or absence of a disease in the population. E.g., in some countries, all dairy herds are routinely screened for FMD infections to maintain the status of FMD-free dairy animals.

2. Knowledge about the level of a disease in an animal population is important in deciding how the optimal design of the disease control or eradication programme should be. If the disease level is low, we may decide to use a stamping-out (or culling) policy, while at the higher levels, we may decide to use a vaccination programme as an initial measure to reduce the disease level first.
3. Disease levels may vary between regions or herds, giving indications that environmental or management factors play a key role in the transmission of infectious agents. Also, for calculations of economic losses due to a specific disease, it is necessary to have an estimate of the level of that disease.

Whatever may be the reason to investigate the frequency of a disease, the main principle is that the number of diseased animals is estimated. Because epidemiologists normally like to make comparisons between different populations, it is better to express the specific numbers of the diseased in relation to the population in which they remain. Hence, the counts are expressed as a fraction of the number of animals experiencing the event of interest (the disease), with the whole population being called the population at risk.

To determine the frequency of a disease, the disease status of individual animals is assessed, preferably through a diagnostic test meant for that. Such a test may detect the antibody or pathogen in the animal, detect an abnormal level of blood parameters, enzymes, or hormones, or a diagnosis by a clinician by looking at the physical and or physiological symptoms.

8.2 QUANTIFYING DISEASE OCCURRENCES

The occurrence of a disease can be measured in a static way (like assessing, did the cow have mastitis at the moment of measurement?) or in a dynamic way (like, did the cow get mastitis during the study period?). Both measurements have a time component, which may be a day, a year, or a season, in which the study is performed. Measurements of static situations may not appear to have a time component, because the length of the study period is small. If the occurrence of disease is measured as a dynamic event, then there is a time component, which may be equal to the length of the study period. An essential element is that the event of interest, like disease, can only occur once per period. So, if we want to study the occurrence of mastitis and count the event more than once per cow, we should choose that particular time, not the whole lactation period. The combination of the population at risk and the time component provides the basis for the calculation of denominators such as animal months or animal years at risk. For any disease, prevalence is the static situation analogue, and incidence is the dynamic analogue.

Quantifying animal disease occurrence is fundamental to any epidemiological study to provide a clear definition and description of the population in which the disease occurs. Counts, ratios, proportions, and rates are the quantities used for describing the disease occurrence. While the count is an enumeration of the number of cases, the ratio is a mathematical expression relating one quantity to another. A proportion is a ratio in which the numerator is included within the denominator. It has no units, ranges from 0 to 1, and is expressed as a percentage. Rate is also a ratio to express the change in the quantity of one to the change in quantity of another. The rate has a unit, maybe a number, e.g., heart rate.

A count is the number of animals infected, infested, diseased, or dead, which can also be expressed as a proportion of the number of animals that can pick up infection, disease or death, and is used to calculate the cost and facilities essential to provide the required animal health care. The risk is defined as the probability of the disease developing in an individual animal during a specific period and is calculated as a proportion. There are two main measures of disease frequency: 1). Prevalence, which measures the *existing cases* of disease, expressed as proportion, and 2). Incidence, which measures the *new cases* of the disease, expressed in animal–time unit.

8.2.1 Prevalence

Prevalence, also known as prevalence rate or prevalence proportion, is defined as the proportion of a population affected by a disease at a given point in time. Point prevalence describes the disease occurrence at a single point in time, while period prevalence describes the disease occurrence over a period of time. Unlike the incidence rate, the prevalence is interpreted as the probability of a randomly selected individual animal from a population having the disease at a particular point in time. The prevalent disease cases used in the numerator include old as well as new cases. This means that diseases with low incidence rates, but long survival, may result in relatively high prevalence values, and vice versa. Prevalence is of limited use in etiologic research of diseases associated with long duration, as it cannot differentiate between the factors that affect the disease occurrence and the survival of diseased animals.

Let us take a case where blood samples are taken from a herd of 300 dairy cows to assess the frequency of a disease. If 30 of these animals test positive, the prevalence can be calculated as 30 / 300, which will be equal to 0.10 (or 10%). It indicates that the randomly selected 300 dairy cows from the herd have a 10% chance of getting infected at that point of time.

Prevalence measures the proportion of individual animals in a population that has a disease or other health outcomes of interest at a specified point in time (point prevalence) or during a specified period (period prevalence). For e.g., Of 10,000 cows in Taluk A on 1st January 2024, 1,000 suffer from milk fever. The prevalence of milk fever among the cows in Taluk A on this date is calculated as 1,000/10,000 = 0.1 or 10%.

However, prevalence is not useful for establishing the determinants of disease in a population. It refers only to the amount of the disease in a known population, at a particular time, without distinction between old and new cases. It is commonly expressed as point prevalence, that is, the amount of disease in a population at a particular point in time. Prevalence represents the fraction (proportion) of existing cases in a population and is defined as the ratio [a / (a + b)] between the number of diseased animals (a) at a particular point in time and the total number of animals at risk including the diseased ones (a + b) at that time. In other words, prevalence is described as the probability that a randomly selected animal suffers from that disease at a certain time. If the prevalence of a disease is 0.01%, then 1 out of every 10,000 animals is affected and the probability of a randomly selected animal being affected at that time equals 0.0001.

8.2.2 Incidence

The incidence or incidence rate is the number of diseased cases expected per unit of animal time. The incidence rate is also called the incidence density, or hazard rate. Since it is not a measure of risk, the incidence rate does not have an interpretation at the individual animal level. On the contrary, it is the value calculated to express the rate at which the cases are occurring at a point in time. E.g., it is similar to the heart rate expressed in number per minute, at a particular time. Thus, the incidence rate is calculated using the number of new cases observed over time in the numerator and the sum of all individual's time at risk in the denominator. The time at risk contributed by each animal is the time from the start till the disease occurs.

The denominator is based on the sum of all the animal time units during which each animal was at risk. It uses the total number of disease-free animals at the start of the period, from which ½ of the diseased animals, ½ of the withdrawn animals and ½ of the added animals in / from / into the farm or herd are subtracted. The incidence rate has some disadvantages – 1). it allows the calculation of average rates over a time period, and hence temporal patterns may not be known, and 2). the same numeric quantity can be obtained from different size groups, leading to some complications in interpreting the results. That is, an incidence rate of one diseased case per 100 animal weeks can be obtained by following 100 animals for one week or from two animals for 100 weeks together.

For calculating the incidence rate, let us imagine 12 months to determine the mortality of cows in a village that has a total of 100 cows at the beginning. The number of cows that died at different periods may be as below:

- Seven cows died after four months, i.e., there were 7 * 4 = 28 animal months at risk.
- Two cows died after five months, i.e., there were 2 * 5 = 10 animal months at risk.
- Three cows died after eight months, i.e., there were 3 * 8 = 24 animal months at risk.

That is, a total of 12 cows died in a total of 62 animal months at risk. However, 88 cows survived the study period in 88 * 12 months = 1056 animal months at risk. Therefore, the incidence rate of cow mortality using the exact denominator method is 12 / 1056 = 0.011 deaths per animal month, or 11 deaths per 1000 animal months.

There are two main measures of incidence: 1). *Risk (or Cumulative Incidence - CI)* – The cumulative incidence is related to the population at risk at the beginning of the study period; and 2). *Rate* – Rate is related to a more precise measure of the population at risk during the study period and is measured in animal-time units.

Risk is the proportion of individuals in a population (initially free of disease) which develop the disease within a specified time interval. Incidence risk is expressed as a percentage (or if small as per 1000 animals). It assumes that the entire population at risk at the beginning of the study period is followed for the specified time for the development of the disease under investigation. However, in a cohort study, some animals may be lost during follow-up, as they may migrate, die, or enter the study sometime after it starts. To account for these variations during follow-up, a more precise measure, Incidence Rate (IR), is calculated. The incidence rate also measures the frequency of new cases of disease in a population. However, the incidence rate takes into account the sum of the time that each animal remained under observation and at risk of developing the disease. That is, IR = No. of new cases of the disease in a given time / Total animal time at risk during the follow-up period.

8.2.2.1 Cumulative Incidence and Incidence Rate

Two essential components of an incidence value are: 1). number of new cases and 2). time over which the new cases occur. There are also two parameters describing incidence: 1). *Cumulative Incidence (CI)* and 2). *Incidence Rate (IR)*. The CI is the ratio between the number of animals that contracted the disease in a period and the number of healthy animals at risk in the population at the start of that period. Thus, the CI is a proportion and can be regarded as the average risk of animals developing a specific disease in a certain period. CI takes values between zero and one and has no dimension. E.g., 20 out of 100 initially uninfected pigs develop pseudorabies in a week. The CI in that week is 20/100 = 0.2. If in the subsequent week, another 15 pigs get pseudorabies, the CI over the 2 weeks amounts to 0.35. Similarly, in the 3rd, 4th and 5th weeks, 10, 5 and 1 pig(s) develop the disease. Hence, if we calculate the CI over the entire 5-week period, it is 0.51. That is, the chance of a randomly chosen pig contracting the disease in those 5 weeks is 51%.

That is, the length of the period has a large influence on the CI. The longer the period, the higher the CI. The animals, all initially healthy, should enter the study at the same time. If animals are lost during the period (due to mortality or culling), we should use the average number of animals in the denominator (number of animals at risk at start plus animals at risk at end divided by 2, which is identical to the number at risk at start minus half the number of withdrawals).

The IR is defined as the ratio between the number of new cases of disease in a population during a certain period and the sum of the time units at risk for all animals in the population at risk. The time units can be represented as animal years, animal months, animal weeks, etc. In the above example, there were 51 new cases. The number of weeks at risk can be calculated as follows:

The 20 animals that were infected in the first week contribute 20 times 0.5 = 10 animal weeks, assuming that on average they contracted the disease halfway through that week. The 15 animals that contracted the disease in the second week contributed 15*1.5 = 22.5 animal weeks, those from week 3: 10*2.5 = 25, those from week 4: 5*3.5 = 17.5, and those from week 5: 1*4.5 = 4.5 animal weeks. The 49 animals that remained healthy throughout contributed 49*5 =245 animal weeks. In total, there were 324.5 animal weeks at risk. It should be noted that only healthy animals contribute to the denominator because only they were at risk of getting the disease. The incidence rate is thus equal to 51/324.5 = 0.157 animals per animal week at risk. This rate is also called the *force of morbidity*, which is the *velocity* with which new cases arise in the population and its dimension is per time unit. In contrast to other parameters, the incidence rate cannot be interpreted in terms of the probability of having or contracting a disease, because it has no upper limit. For instance, expressing 0.157 animals per animal week at risk every year will give a value above unity: 0.157 * 52 = 8.164.

The relation between Cumulative Incidence (Cl) and Incidence Rate (IR) is:

$$CI(t) = 1 - e^{(-IR*t)}$$

where e is the base of the natural logarithm, and t is the time unit of concern. When the expected Cl is smaller than 0.10, then the formula is approximately equal to:

$CI(t) = -IR*t$

E.g., We have a population of 1000 healthy animals at the start. Each week, 10% of the (remaining) healthy animals contract a disease and the study period is 5 weeks. Let us try to answer the questions - What is the Cl? What is the number of animal weeks at risk? What is the IR? What are the real and via IR estimated Cl per week? How do we explain the fact that real and estimated Cl are the same?

The number of cases in 5 weeks will be 410 (= 100 + 90 + 81 + 73 + 66). Hence, the Cl is 410/1000 = 0.41, which is the chance of a randomly selected animal contracting the disease in 5 weeks. The number of animal weeks at risk is 3890 (= 590*5 + 100*0.5 + 90*1.5 + 81*2.5 + 73*3.5 + 66*4.5). The IR is hence equal to 410/3890 = 0.1054 animals per animal week at risk. The comparison between real and estimated Cl is:

Week	No. of New Cases	Real CI	Estimated CI*
1	0.1 x 1000	0.100	0.100
2	1.1 x 900	0.190	0.190
3	0.1 x 810	0.271	0.271
4	0.1 x 729	0.344	0.344
5	0.1 x 656	0.410	0.410

** 1 – (e - 0.1054), 1 – (e - 0.2108), 1 – (e - 0.3162, and so on. Because the frequency of disease occurrence (10%) is constant per week, there is no difference between real and estimated Cl.*

The relationship between IR and prevalence (P) is:

$$\frac{P}{1-P} = IR * D$$

The term P / (1 - P) represents the proportion of cases expressed against the healthy population (1 - P: as only healthy animals can get the disease). When an animal contracts a disease, it is designated as diseased in D time units, where D is the duration of the disease. So, new cases contribute to P during only D periods. When P is small (<0.05), the formula reduces to:

$P = IR * D$

8.2.3 Period Prevalence

Prevalence and incidence values are at times combined as period prevalence (Pp). Pp is a measure of the existing total number of cases of a disease in a population during the period of study. It is the sum of the point prevalence at the beginning of the period (P) and the incidence (Ip) during the period of study:

$Pp = P + Ip$

However, this measure does not have much value, because we usually need to distinguish between old and new cases. Hence, whenever we use the term prevalence, it only refers to point prevalence.

8.2.4 Prevalence Vs. Incidence

Incidence has a temporal sequence and hence includes new cases too, while prevalence does not distinguish between old and new cases. Incidence predicts what will happen in the future, i.e., it gives the probability of similar animals developing the disease. Thus, the measure of prevalence is useful for making decisions about preventive measures such as vaccination. However, prevalence describes the probability of having the disease in a group of animals, at a point in time. Both measures are used to make comparisons between risk factors, but the measure of incidence is more appropriate, as it is not affected by the duration of the disease. The table below presents a comparison of the parameters used to calculate the incidence rate, incidence risk, and prevalence for expressing the disease frequency:

8.2.4.1 Measures of Incidence and Prevalence – A Comparison

	Incidence Rate	**Incidence Risk**	**Prevalence**
Numerator	No. of new cases occurring during a period in a group of animals, which is initially free of disease		All the animals developing the disease counted
Denominator	The sum of the periods during which individual animals develop the disease	All susceptible animals present at the beginning of the period	All animals examined, including diseased and non-diseased
Time	For each animal from the beginning of the period till the development of a disease	Duration of the period	Single point of time
Interpretation	No. of new cases per unit of time	Risk of developing the disease over a given period	Probability of having the disease at a particular point of time

Let us see an example of calculating prevalence and incidence. Say, we have a population of 10 healthy animals at the start, which are observed for 12 months. The animals that are diseased or culled in a given month and the time at risk are given in the following table. For e.g., animal 1 showed the disease in March and therefore had been at risk from January to February. Animal 5 was culled from the farm in September which means that it was at risk of becoming diseased from January to August. In total, 6 animals developed the disease and 2 were culled and hence, withdrawn from the study.

Animals	Months												Time at risk in months
	January	February	March	April	May	June	July	August	September	October	November	December	
1			Disease										2
2								Disease					7
3					Disease								4
4											Disease		10
5									Culled				8
6													12
7						Culled							5
8						Disease							5
9													12
10				Disease									3

The prevalence of the disease is calculated by dividing the number of animals diseased by the number of animals that were at risk of developing the disease. For e.g., if we calculate the prevalence of the disease in May, it will be the number of diseased animals in April divided by the number of animals that could develop the disease in May and beyond, which is equal to 2 / 8 = 0.25 and this expresses the probability of an animal being diseased in the respective month. This means that the numerators and the denominators will vary from March, when the first case occurs.

Incidence risk is calculated using the exact denominator where only the animals available are included for the complete study period, and using an approximate denominator where half of the culled animals are subtracted. That is, when we calculate the incidence for the year, we will have the exact denominator as 6 / 8 = 0.75, where 6 represents the diseased animals in the whole year and 8 represents the total animals (10) minus culled animals (2). The approximate denominator is 6 / (10 – 0.5*2) = 0.667. That is, some animals are culled from the farm, and hence we only take half of it. Since 2 animals have been culled, we take half of it and put it in the denominator. The incidence rates (in this example, 0.75 and 0.667 cases per year) do not express a risk or probability, but only the number of cases expected per year.

Similarly, the incidence rate per animal year can also be calculated by dividing the number of diseased animals from the average monthly risk. i.e., 6 / [(2 + 7 + 4 + 10 + 8 + 12 + 5 + 5 + 12 + 3)] / 12 = 6 / [68/12] = 1.059, using the exact denominator and 6 / [(10 – 0.5*2 - 0.5*2] = 0.600, using the approximate denominator, where the first 2 indicates the number of culled animals and the second 2 is the number of animals not affected in the year under study.

While Taneja *et al.* (1989) studied the incidence of mastitis in crossbreds, Saini *et al.* (1994) observed the prevalence of subclinical mastitis among crossbred cows and buffaloes in Punjab (India). Surveying in both government/university and private dairy farms in Tamil Nadu (India) during 1993-94 and 1994-95, Thirunavukkarasu and Prabaharan (1999a) reported a prevalence of mastitis of 13.01 percent in cows and 7.37 percent in buffaloes. Thirunavukkarasu *et al.* (2008) identified the factors influencing the prevalences of milk fever and ketosis in Tamil Nadu as the breed, age, lactation order, milk yield, season, and history of attack.

8.3 RATES, PROPORTIONS AND RATIOS OF DISEASE OCCURRENCE

Other measures of disease frequency include the attack rate, which is defined as the number of new cases divided by the initial population at risk. It is in fact an incidence risk and however, it is a probability and not a rate. The attack rate is used when the period at risk is short. Mortality rates are applied using several different interpretations and often do not represent true rates. The crude mortality rate has death as the outcome of interest and is calculated similarly to the incidence rate. The cause-specific mortality rate is estimated for specific causes of death and is also calculated similarly to the incidence rate. Case fatality rate represents the proportion of animals with a specific disease that die of it. It is a risk measure, not a rate, and is used to describe the impact of epidemics or the severity of an acute disease. Morbidity and mortality are the main categories of events for which the rates are calculated, besides others like culling, survival to culling, and pregnancy. All the rates have a time component that refers to a period or a point in time (often called the study period). The morbidity rate describes the level of a clinical disease in a population, which may be crude, cause-specific, or attribute-specific. The rates calculated in epidemiological studies are:

Rates / Proportions / Ratios	Method of Calculation
Crude Incidence Rate	No. of animals developing the disease during the period / No. of animals at risk during that period
Crude Prevalence Proportion	No. of animals with disease at a point of time / No. of animals at risk at that point of time
Attack Rate	No. of animals developing the disease during the period following exposure / No. of animals exposed

Rates / Proportions / Ratios	Method of Calculation
Crude Mortality Rate	Total no. of deaths in the period / Average population at risk in the period
Cause-specific Mortality Rate	Total no. of deaths from the disease in the period / Average population at risk in the period
Case Fatality Rate	No. of deaths from the disease in the period after diagnosis / No. of animals that acquired the disease
Foetal Death Ratio	No. of foetal deaths / No. of live births
Age-Specific Death Rate	No. of animal deaths in a specified age group / Average no. in the specified age group
Calf Mortality Rate	No. of deaths under a specified age / No. of live births
Neonatal Mortality Rate	No. of deaths under a specified age / No. of live births
Proportional Mortality Rate	No. of deaths from a specified cause / Total no. of deaths
Maternal Mortality Ratio	No. of deaths in dams from puerperal causes / No. of live births
Zoonosis Incidence Ratio	No. of new cases of a zoonotic disease in an area in a period / Average human population in the same area during the same period
Area Incidence Ratio	No. of new cases in a period / Unit geographic area

8.3.1 Survival or Time-to-Event

An important parameter of interest in epidemiological research is the time until the occurrence of events such as death, infection, or recovery from a clinical disease. The term survival is often used for this type of data, mainly because the methods were first developed for investigating mortality. It can be estimated if repeated measurements on the same group of animals are available, and one characteristic of such data is usually that some animals will not develop the event of interest during the follow-up period, which is a process called right censoring. There are several options for quantifying time-to-event for a group of animals. If one were to use the average of the time-to-event, the animals that did not experience the event of interest could not be included.

The following figure presents an example of such data. In the figure, they are the ones that were sold or alive at the end of the study period. This method has the disadvantage that the estimate will depend on the length of the period over which data were collected. If the interval is too short, survival time is likely to be underestimated, and if it is very long, a small number of animals with long time-to-event may have a strong influence on the mean estimate. It is also possible to calculate the incidence rate, but this calculation assumes that the rate at which the event occurs is constant throughout the period of study which very often is not the case. An example of time-to-event (event = becoming sick) can be picturised as below:

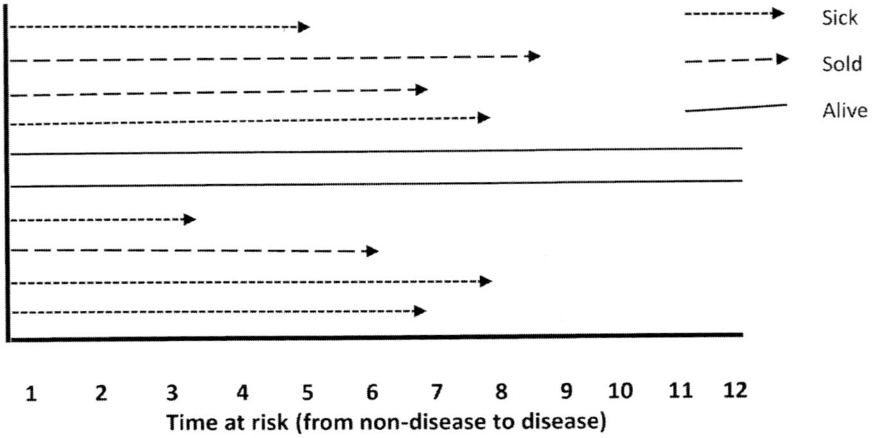

8.3.2 Calculation of Prevalence, Incidence, Mortality, and Case Fatality Rates

Suppose we investigated a disease that ran a clinical course ending in either recovery with permanent immunity, or death in a dairy herd. On July 1, 2023, the disease was already present. We investigated on July 1, 2024 and observed the following details:

Total herd size on 1 July 2023	:	600
Total number clinically ill on 1 July 2023	:	100
Total number becoming ill between 01.07.23 and 01.07.24	:	200
Total number dying of disease from 01.07.23 to 01.07.24	:	120
Calculations		
Prevalence on 1 July 2023	:	100 / 600 = 0.167 (16.7%)
Cumulative incidence (01.07.23 to 01.07.24)	:	200 / 500 = 0.4
Mortality rate (01.07.23 to 01.07.24)	:	120 / 600 = 20% per year
Case fatality rate (01.07.23 to 01.07.24)	:	120 / 300 = 40%

Selvam *et al.* (2003) estimated the disease frequencies of Infectious Bursal Disease, Ranikhet Disease, *E. coli* infection, and Coccidiosis in commercial layer farms in Tamil Nadu, using measures such as prevalence, cause-specific mortality rate, cohort incidence, and the true incidence.

8.3.3. Factors Influencing the Prevalence and Incidence of Diseases in Livestock

After measuring the prevalence and incidence of both infectious and non-infectious diseases in livestock, we come to know they are not usually similar in all the animals or herds and they differ probably due to the animals' inherent factors and the factors of the environment they are reared in. It is wise to identify these factors which will be very useful to control and prevent the diseases. Hence, almost all the studies aiming to estimate the losses due to animal diseases also study the prevalence and incidence of diseases and their predisposing factors (or the factors influencing them). We will know about these influencing factors for some diseases.

Thirunavukkarasu and Prabaharan (1998a) found that the incidence of clinical mastitis in bovines of Tamil Nadu (India) was significantly associated with animal factors such as breed, milk yield, stage, and order of lactation and udder morphology and environmental factors such as season and sanitation measures. Senthilkumar *et al.* (2006a) identified the factors influencing the prevalence of sheep pox, while Jeyakumari *et al.* (2006) found that the incidence of postpartum reproductive disorders in bovines was significantly associated with the management factor, milk yield, order of lactation, and birth weight of calf. Thirunavukkarasu and Kathiravan (2009) found dairy farm size, land holding, age, milk yield, stage and order of lactation, history of reproductive disorder, season, and distance to insemination centers as the factors affecting conception rates in bovines. Thirunavukkarasu *et al.* (2011) reported the factors influencing the prevalence of ketosis in dairy animals.

8.4 EPIDEMIOLOGICAL ASSOCIATIONS OF LIVESTOCK DISEASES

8.4.1 Assessing Epidemiologic Measures of Association in Animal Diseases

Statistical significance is a function of the magnitude of the difference, the variability of the difference, and the sample size. Once the decision is made that sampling variation (chiefly a function of sample size) is not a probable explanation for the difference observed, epidemiologic measures of association can be applied which are independent of sample size and include the strength of association, the effect of the factor in exposed individuals and the importance of the factor in the population. In other words, the factors that are found to be significantly associated with the incidence of a particular disease, say through χ^2 analysis, can be used to find the epidemiological measures of association between these factors and the disease. The results of any epidemiological study can be summarized as below:

		OUTCOME		
		Positive	**Negative**	**Total**
EXPOSURE TO THE FACTOR	**Exposed**	a	b	a + b
	Not Exposed	c	d	c + d
	Total	a + c	b + d	a + b − c + d

where a is the number affected in the exposed group, b is the number unaffected in the exposed group, c is the number affected in the unexposed group, and d is the number unaffected in the unexposed group; a + b + c + d = n (size of population).

8.4.1.2 Risk, Risk Factors, and Exposure

Risk is the probability of an event in a specified time, with the event being usually a disease or death. But risk can be applied equally to favourable events such as conception or parturition. The risk factor is a factor associated with a changed risk of the event occurring. Usually, the risk factors are associated with an increased risk. The factors that reduce the risk may be called as the protective factors or negative risk factors. Exposure is the contact with a risk factor before the occurrence of the event. If the risk factor is assumed to influence the occurrence of the event, then only the relevant exposure precedes the event.

Once a study has been carried out, the investigator has to determine the effect that a risk factor or intervention had on the event (disease). The two main methods are to assess the *strength of the association* between exposure to the risk factor (or intervention) and the risk of acquiring the disease, and the *effect of exposure* to the risk factor (or intervention) in either the exposed group or the general population.

8.4.1.3 Epidemiological Measures of Association between Predisposing Factors and Disease

The table below describes the epidemiological measures of association (Martin *et al.,* 1993) commonly used and how they can be derived from the 2 X 2 table shown above:

Epidemiological Measures of Association between Predisposing Factors and Disease

RISK MEASURE	DESCRIPTION	FORMULA
	Strength of Association	
Relative Risk (RR)	It is the strength of the association between a factor and a disease. It is the rate of the disease in the exposed group divided by the rate of the disease in the unexposed group.	[a / (a + b)] / [c / (c + d)]
Odds Ratio (OR)	It is the measure of association that indicates the relative change in risk. It is useful when the disease is relatively infrequent.	[a * d] / [b * c]
	Effect on the Exposed Group	
Attributable Risk (AR)	It is the rate of disease in the exposed group minus the rate in the unexposed group.	[a / (a + b)] – [c / (c + d)]

RISK MEASURE	DESCRIPTION	FORMULA
Attributable Fraction (AF)	This indicates what proportion of the disease in the exposed group is due to the factor.	(RR - 1) / RR
Total effect (Importance in population)		
Population RR (RRpop)	This indicates the relative impact of the factor in the population.	[(a + c) / n] / [c / (c + d)]
Population OR (ORpop)	This also indicates the relative impact of the factor in the population.	[d (a + c)] / [c (b + d)]
Population AR (ARpop)	It gives the importance of a causal factor in the population and is determined by multiplying its effect (AR) by the prevalence of the factor.	AR * [(a – b) / n]
Population AF (AFpop)	It is the proportion of the disease in the population that is attributable to the factor.	(RRpop – 1) / RRpop

Thirunavukkarasu and Prabaharan (1998a) identified factors such as species, breed, milk yield, stage of lactation, lactation order, and season of calving which predisposed to mastitis in bovines. Though the factors such as species, breed, milk yield, stage of lactation, lactation number, udder abnormalities, season, stall hygiene, and milking hygiene were found to be significantly associated with mastitis, the analysis could not be carried out for all of the variables, except species, breed, udder abnormalities, stall hygiene, and milking hygiene, as the other variables could not be presented in 2 X 2 contingency table with mastitis. Accordingly, Thirunavukkarasu and Prabaharan (1998b) assessed the epidemiological measures of association between the incidence of mastitis in bovines and the predisposing factors to mastitis, and the results are presented in the following table:

Epidemiological Measures of Association between Predisposing Factors and Mastitis

Measures of Association	**Factors**				
	Cow	**Exotic blood in cows**	**Udder/teat abnormalities in cows**	**Less hygienic stalls for cows**	**Less hygienic milking of cows**
Strength of the Factor					
Relative Risk (RR)	1.757	∞	1.407	1.297	1.287
Odds Ratio (OR)	1.880	∞	4.614	1.347	1.334
Effect of the Factor					
Attributable Rate (AR)	0.056	0.133	0.257	0.035	0.033
Attributable Fraction (AF)	0.431	1.000	0.289	0.238	0.223

Measures of Association	Factors				
	Cow	**Exotic blood in cows**	**Udder/teat abnormalities in cows**	**Less hygienic stalls for cows**	**Less hygienic milking of cows**
Total effect (Importance)					
Population Relative Risk (RRpop)	1.602	∞	1.075	1.149	1.127
Population Odds Ratio (ORpop)	1.684	∞	1.233	1.171	1.146
Population Attributable Rate (ARpop)	0.044	0.130	0.047	0.017	0.015
Population Attributable Fraction (AFpop)	0.376	1.000	0.070	0.130	0.115

Source: Thirunavukkarasu and Prabaharan (1998b)

As seen from the above table, the Relative Risk (RR) with respect to the cow factor was 1.757. If there was no association between the factor and the disease, the RR will be 1. The greater the departure (either larger or smaller) of RR from 1, the stronger the association between the factor and the disease. Hence, since the RR was 1.757 for the cow factor, it can be concluded that the rate of mastitis in cows was 1.757 times greater than the rate of mastitis in buffaloes. The Odds Ratio (OR) calculated of 1.880 can also be interpreted similarly. Since there was also some disease in the factor-negative group (i.e., buffaloes), not all of the disease in cows was due to the cow factor. Hence, only the difference between the two rates was attributable to the factor. The larger the Attributable Rate (AR), the greater the effect of the factor (cow) in the cow group. The calculated AR for the was 0.056 which implies that the rate of the disease in cows that might be attributed to cow factor was 5.60 percent. Attributable Fraction (AF) was 0.431 indicating that 43.10 percent of mastitis in cows was attributable to cow factor.

The calculated Population Attributable Rate (ARpop) was 0.044, indicating that the rate of mastitis in the milch animal population that can be attributed to the cow factor was 4.40 percent. That is, the rate of mastitis would decrease by 4.40 percent, if the animal was not a cow. Population Attributable Fraction (AFpop) provides a direct estimate of the rate of disease in the population due to the factor – cow. Hence, the AFpop of o.376 for the cow factor implies that 37.60 percent of all mastitis in the milch animal population could be attributed to the cow factor. RR, RRpop, OR and ORpop calculated as measures of association between the exotic blood factor and mastitis were all infinitives, because the incidence in the other group (non-descript cows) was zero. These results indicate that the incidence of mastitis in cows would increase by an infinite proportion if the cow had 'exotic' blood in it. The rates estimated for other factors can be interpreted in the same way as done for the cow factor.

Also, Jeyakumari *et al.* (2003) estimated the epidemiological measures of association between the incidences of postpartum reproductive disorders in dairy animals and their predisposing factors, as below, which can also be interpreted as above:

Epidemiological Measures of Association between Predisposing Factors and Postpartum Reproductive Disorders in Dairy Animals

Measures of Association	**Factors**				
	Breed	**Milk yield in the last lactation**	**Calf birth weight**	**Farm management (Organized / Unorganized)**	**Lactation order**
Strength of the Factor					
Relative risk (RR)	2.3059	1.7069	22.2515	1.6302	1.5069
Population relative risk (RRpop)	2.1375	1.1866	17.2561	1.3472	1.3041
Effect of the Factor					
Attributable rate (AR)	0.1728	0.1686	0.3464	0.1324	0.1100
Attributable fraction (AF)	0.5663	0.4143	0.9551	0.3866	0.3364

Thirunavukkarasu *et al.* (2010d) assessed the epidemiological measures of association between the prevalence of milk fever in dairy animals and its predisposing factors, respectively. Relative Risk (RR) with respect to the breed factor for the disease - milk fever was found to be 2.969. If there was no association between the factor and the disease, the RR should be equal to 1. The greater the departure of RR from 1 (either larger or smaller), the stronger the association between the factor and the disease. Hence, since the RR was 2.969 here, it can be concluded that the rate of milk fever in exotic purebred / crossbred cows and Murrah / graded buffaloes was 2.969 times greater than the rate of milk fever in native pure / non-descript cows and buffaloes. Odds Ratio (OR) too offered similar result and should be interpreted in the same way. The larger the Attributable Rate (AR), the greater the effect of the factor, i.e., exotic purebred / crossbred / Murrah / graded group, in causing milk fever in dairy animals. The calculated AR for the breed factor was 0.106, which implied that the rate of milk fever in dairy animals that might be attributed to exotic / crossbred / upgraded germplasm was 10.60 percent. The Attributable Fraction (AF) calculated of 0.663 indicated that 66.30 percent of milk fever in superior / upgraded breeds could be attributable to the exotic / crossbred / graded breed factor.

Later, Thirunavukkarasu *et al.* (2010d) also assessed the epidemiological measures of association between the prevalence of ketosis in dairy animals and its predisposing factors.

9

Economic Impacts of Animal Diseases

9.1 ECONOMIC LOSSES DUE TO ANIMAL DISEASES

Economic considerations are increasingly forcing their way forward in the decision-making processes of animal health management. With the continuing intensification of livestock production systems, the economic implications of livestock diseases have become increasingly important at both farm and national levels, as they represent avoidable waste of scarce resources (McInerney, 1988). From an economic point of view, an animal disease either destroys the basic resources, reduces the attainable output, dwindles the efficiency with which the resources are converted into products, or decreases the economic value of products (McInerney, 1995).

The effects of a disease present in an animal or herd may be manifested by stunted growth, lowered production, delayed maturity, delayed conception, mortality, reduced resource (especially feed) use efficiency, etc. These negative impacts of a disease demand more resource(s) than usual, resulting in higher expenditures for the same output and reduced farm income. Apart from these negative effects at the farm or herd level, animal diseases lead to economic losses at the regional, national, and global levels too by increasing animal mortality, reducing productivity, increasing disease control costs, swelling losses in animal trade, decreasing the market values of livestock and their products, and ultimately ending at food insecurity. These economic impacts of livestock diseases, besides their social impacts, have now been recognized globally, in both developed and developing countries, necessitating quantification of the economic impact of animal diseases as an urgent and important step to support the prevention and control decisions for improved animal health to ensure better rural and global economy.

9.1.1 Estimation of the Economic Impact of a Disease

Measuring the economic impact of an animal disease is not a simple task, as it may be believed, because the effects of any animal disease are not always obvious and well-pronounced, are influenced by other factors such as management and environment, have a temporal dimension adding to the complexity of evaluating their impacts at different stages of time, and often manifest themselves with other diseases making it more complex to evaluate.

Disease loss estimation is not just a problem of measurement by itself, it is a problem of disease-making. In other words, quantification of economic losses due to diseases is not very important in itself, but it is done to help us to provide a better overall view of the impact of disease and to contribute to estimating the extent of the losses to be avoided. More aptly, disease loss data are required as information to guide in decision-making process for allocating resources to disease control and prevention. Quantification of losses due to animal diseases usually follows the earlier disease investigation works undertaken. Once the disease prevalence or incidence and the nature and magnitude of the losses experienced have been defined, then the economic analysis of the disease losses incurred is done by classifying and presenting the data/information on the direct losses, quantifying the direct losses in monetary terms, and identifying and quantifying the indirect losses attributable to a disease, to the extent possible.

The majority of the disease effects are many times conveniently calculated in terms of lowered output and a few above-mentioned negative effects. Also, for effects like delayed maturity or conception, the loss may be assessed in terms of wasted inputs, by estimating the time value of the delay in reaching maturity or achieving conception by using a discounting measure to obtain the present value of the future costs and earnings involved in such delays. However, quantifying the indirect effects of a disease is a complex procedure, although it is not impossible.

9.1.2 Disease Losses of a Disease – Direct Vs. Indirect

The economic losses due to (or the costs of) animal diseases can be either direct or indirect. These losses including those that are caused due to zoonotic diseases have been estimated at least theoretically to be huge across the world. While the direct disease costs are important and affect a wide range of sub-sectors of the rural economy, indirect costs are also of much concern, as the losses due to animal diseases do not end at the farm gate and go on to affect the economies outside the livestock sector. Despite this fact, not many studies had/have been attempted to evaluate the detailed economic costs of animal diseases even in developed countries. Further, even the few studies attempted had considered only the costs at farm levels and indirect impacts have largely been excluded, for they are difficult to estimate. This issue of failing to capture the indirect costs associated with animal diseases usually underestimates the true costs of an animal disease. Hence, it is important to understand the full economic cost of animal diseases, and to achieve this, the economic frameworks of animal disease costs should include the indirect costs too. Estimating both the direct and indirect costs of a disease is essential to make and support an all-inclusive decision-making of animal disease prevention and control strategies.

At the same time, the definitions of direct and indirect costs of animal diseases widely vary in the literature. Some studies do not categorize economic costs as either direct or indirect at all, while others do not distinguish clearly the direct and indirect costs. A kind of inconsistency in the definition of direct and indirect costs does exist, making it difficult to quantify all the economic impacts of livestock diseases. Sometimes, the disease prevention and control costs are considered as direct costs, and at another, as indirect costs, probably based on the individual researcher's understanding and interpretation. Overall, the distinction between direct and indirect economic losses from animal diseases is still unclear and subjective. The lack of data and the absence of suitable analytical tools to capture indirect costs may be one of the reasons for this problem. Hence, there is a need for a more systematic framework to categorize direct and indirect costs more objectively and to estimate the complete economic impact of animal diseases.

9.2 ECONOMIC FRAMEWORK OF A LIVESTOCK DISEASE

McInerney *et al.* (1992) developed a framework for the economic analysis of disease in livestock to explain the total economic cost of a disease in terms of two distinct components: (i) output losses following disease occurrence; (ii) expenditures made to treat disease or prevent its occurrence, then to develop the general relationship between these two components, calling it the loss-expenditure frontier, and to use it to define the economically optimal level of disease costs.

9.2.1 Economic Effects of a Livestock Disease

Generally, the economic effects of a livestock disease include production losses and the resulting additional expenditures, as below:

- Requiring more resources (expenditures) for the same level of production, due to
    - Use of drugs and medicines for cure
    - Fees to the veterinarians
    - Need for additional labour
    - Additional costs due to preventive measures like vaccination, deworming, etc.

- Resulting in reduced production with the same resources, which may result due to
  - Decreased production
  - Discarded milk / egg / other products, because of poor quality
  - Reduced prices of milk / egg / other products, because of reduced quality
  - Forced culling due to reduced productivity

Animal diseases reduce the efficiency with which inputs are converted into outputs, i.e. they decrease productivity. They affect the livestock resource transformation process and result in extra resource use and / or fewer animal products than before (direct effects). These direct effects may be immediately visible (death, abortion) or unnoticed (reduced milk / egg yield) initially. Animal diseases may also affect other parts of the economic system, thus decreasing benefits to people (indirect effects). These indirect losses can be divided into those that are tangible (drops in export trade), and those that are intangible (constraints on livestock developments). The following figure shows the economic implications of diseases on livestock farming (Modified from Rushton *et al.,* 1999):

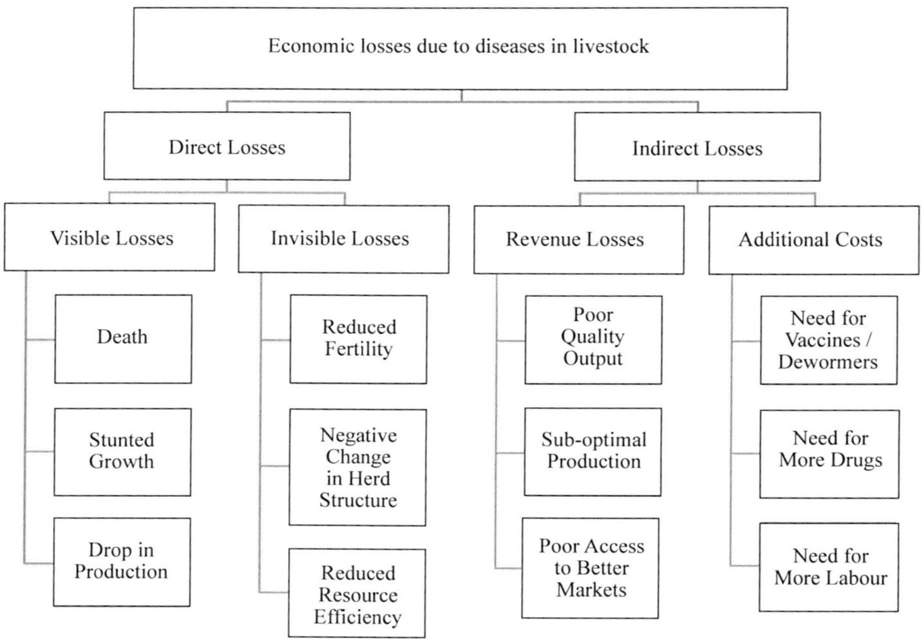

9.2.2 Ways in which a Disease Affects the Animal Productivity

Effect on feed intake and feed digestibility	• Altered feed intake, with the feed being not fully used by animals • Altered feed digestibility, with the nutritive value of feed not fully used
Effect on the physiological process	• Altered nutrient utilization (Energy, protein, minerals, etc.) • Altered respiratory efficiency • Body material excreted abnormally
Effects on livestock productivity	• Premature death • Reduced value of animals / birds • Reduced body weight • Reduced yield and or quality of milk, eggs, wool, etc. • Reduced capacity to work • Altered production of dung and urine • Wasted body materials, being diverted for use by disease agent • Reduced productive life of animals / birds • Reduced fertility and fecundity
Effects on herd maintenance and improvement	• Need for quick animal / herd replacement • Reduced capacity for genetic improvement
Effects on human welfare	• Reduction in supply of quality protein to humans • Reduction in supply of services like traction and dung • Reduction in supply of non-nutrition services like games • Negative effect on human health due to spread of zoonotic diseases animal welfare

The above table summarizes various ways by which a disease adversely affects the productivity of a livestock herd or a poultry flock and the direct and indirect ways through which a disease influences the productivity of livestock and poultry. In infectious and parasitic diseases, the disease agents are in constant competition with their host for access to their nutrient supply. The disease agents divert the nutrients for their use and multiplication, which the animals / birds would have otherwise used for their growth and production. Not all the diseases will have all of the effects listed, but an economic study should consider all possibilities and select those that are relevant to the disease chosen.

9.2.3 Direct Losses or Direct Effects of a Disease

The direct losses due to or the direct effects of animal disease are:

1. Destruction of the basic resource (animal or bird) of the livestock production process through mortality of productive stock;
2. Lowering the efficiency of the production process and the productivity of resources used (e.g. reduced feed use efficiency); and
3. Reduction in the quantity and or the quality of output.

Of all the economic losses caused by the diseases in livestock and poultry, the death of animals / birds causes great concern, as this loss is not only huge but also requires the farmers to replace them at a considerable cost. The value of dead stock alone cannot be considered as a cost, but also the costs of feed, fodder, labour, etc. used so far to bring them up to this production stage, which should also to taken into consideration while working out the economic loss due to disease.

The other important economic losses that arise from diseases are infertility, unsoundness, cessation of growth, and reduced production. Failure to produce fertile sperm or eggs, failure to accomplish fertilization, failure to breed, failure of the foetus to mature (abortion), and increased breeding intervals (repeat breeding) due to diseases also cause severe economic losses. Cessation of milk or egg production, and production of abnormal milk or eggs caused by diseases also contribute to losses. Diseases may also cause inappetence, malabsorption, diarrhoea, fever, stunted growth of animals, reduction in weight, permanent disability, delayed maturity, etc. which all will reduce the attainable production, resulting in economic loss to the farm / farmer. Diseases in draught animals (used for tilling or transport) will cause losses to their owners.

Hence, the direct economic losses caused by a disease can be divided into four categories:

1. Cost of resources (feed, etc.) consumed by animals/birds that died of the disease;
2. Cost of treatment (medicine cost and veterinary fees);
3. Excess expenditure due to poor feed conversion efficiency; and
4. Loss due to inefficient production.

Taneja *et al.* (1989) studied the production losses due to mastitis in crossbreds and observed that the milk yield showed a large decline in animals affected by mastitis in the first stage of lactation and the lactation length decreased accordingly. McInerney *et al.* (1992) stated that the economic cost of the disease is the sum of the losses and expenditures, defining losses as a benefit that has been taken away (such as discarding mastitic milk) or a potential benefit not realized (such as reduced output yield), and expenditures as the resources allocated to counteract the disease threat (such as veterinarian treatment). Tambi *et al.* (1999a) assessed the economic impact of the Pan-African Rinderpest Campaign (PARC), which commenced in 1986 to control and eradicate Rinderpest from Africa. From 35 countries that participated in PARC, 10 countries were selected for the analysis, based on data availability. Yang *et al.* (1999) reported a devastating outbreak of FMD, serotype O, that occurred in pigs in Taiwan, during March - July 1997. A total of 6,147 pig farms with more than 4 million pigs were infected, and 37.7 percent of the pigs either died (0.18 million pigs) or were killed (3.85 million pigs). The cost of the epidemic was estimated to be US$ 378.6 million, including affected production, vaccines, carcass disposal, environmental protection, and loss of market value. Owing to the ban on exports of pork to Japan, the total economic loss to Taiwan's pig industry was about US$ 1.6 billion.

Thirunavukkarasu and Prabaharan (1999b) estimated the economic impact of mastitis on dairy farms in a randomly selected sample of five organized government / university dairy farms and 25 private dairy farms during the years 1993-94 and 1994-95, including the direct losses such as production losses (milk yield loss and discarded milk), veterinary expenses (costs of medicines and veterinarians' fees), mastitis prevention costs (costs for maintaining shed hygiene and milking hygiene including udder hygiene) and animal replacement / culling costs. They found that each mastitis-affected cow caused a monetary loss of INR 536.25 and each mastitis-affected buffalo INR 404.73. Awa *et al.* (2000) found that PPR and gastrointestinal helminthiasis are important causes of economic losses in small ruminants in Cameroon.

Tambi *et al.* (2006) estimated the economic cost of CBPP and the benefits of its control in 12 sub-Saharan African countries using a spreadsheet economic model developed in MS Excel. The value of morbidity and mortality losses was estimated to be 30 million euros (2.5 million per country), while the total economic cost (direct and indirect production losses plus disease control costs) was 44.8 million euros (3.7 million euros per country). An investment of 14.7 million euros to control CBPP would prevent a loss of 30 million euros, with the financial return on investment in CBPP control being positive, with benefit-cost ratios ranging from 1.61 (Ghana) to 2.56 (Kenya). Thirunavukkarasu and Kathiravan (2006) studied the FMD-affected animals in four districts of the Cauvery Delta zone of Tamil Nadu (India) where there were 213 FMD outbreaks during the period from November 2002 to December 2003, of which 75 outbreaks were randomly selected. The estimated losses due to mortality and culling were INR 3.17 million in large and small ruminants. Besides, Thirunavukkarasu and Kathiravan (2007) estimated the monetary losses due to reproductive failures in FMD-affected bovines. Of 76 abortions resulting due to FMD, 70 were in cattle and 6 in buffaloes. The total loss due to abortions, infertility, and repeat breeding (including lost milk and unborn calves) due to FMD was estimated to be INR 1.75 million in the sampled animals. Extrapolating this to all the outbreaks, the total loss due to reproductive failures was INR 4.96 million.

Pritchett *et al.* (2005) reviewed the literature on animal disease impacts. Pendell *et al.* (2007), by demonstrating the local economic impact of an FMD outbreak in southwest Kansas, the US, estimated the expected economic impact of the disease. Whatford *et al.* (2022) attempted to systematically review the literature on the economic impact of endemic disease in UK sheep and cattle.

9.2.3.1 Estimated Economic Losses due to some Animal Diseases in Tamil Nadu (India)

Livestock economists in Tamil Nadu initiated research in 1993 in the emerging field of animal health economics. Several studies were done thereafter either by Thirunavukkarasu and/or Prabaharan or by their guidance to analyze the economic consequences of diseases in livestock and poultry in Tamil Nadu State as detailed below:

S. No.	Disease / Disorder	Year	Estimated Annual Loss (INR. Million)	Source
1	Clinical mastitis in dairy animals	1996	56	*Thirunavukkarasu and Prabaharan (1999b)*
2	Metritis in bovines	2002	1156	*Jeyakumari et al. (2003b)*
3	Retained placenta in bovines	2002	63	
4	Conception failures in dairy animals	2003	2066	*Thirunavukkarasu and Kathiravan (2006c)*
5	RD, IBD, Colibacillosis, and Coccidiosis in layers	2003	16.23 / million layers	*Selvam et al. (2006)*
6	Foot and Mouth Disease	2004	127	*Thirunavukkarasu and Kathiravan (2006a and 2007)*
7	Enterotoxaemia in sheep	2004	419	*Senthilkumar et al. (2008)*
8	Sheep pox	2004	967	*Senthilkumar and Thirunavukkarasu (2010)*
9	Milk Fever in milch bovines	2008	406	*Thirunavukkarasu et al. (2010b)*
10	Ketosis in milch bovines	2008	253	*Thirunavukkarasu et al. (2011b)*

(RD - Ranikhet Disease; IBD - Infectious Bronchitis Disease)

The direct loss components included for the above diseases / disorders at the farm level are as follows:

1. ***Clinical mastitis*** – Production loss (yield loss and discarded milk), Veterinary expense (Medicine cost and Veterinarian's fee), and Disease control cost (Cost for maintaining Stall hygiene and Milking hygiene).

2. ***Metritis and Retained placenta*** – Yield loss, Veterinary expense, Extra labour, and Extended calving interval.
3. ***Conception failures in bovines*** – Unattained milk and calf, Costs of additional inseminations and labour, and Extended calving interval.
4. ***Diseases in layers*** – Mortality in birds, Vaccination and disinfection cost, Medicine cost, and Extra labour
5. ***Foot and Mouth Disease*** – Yield loss, Drop in draught power, Infertility, Mortality, Culling, and Replacement cost.
6. ***Sheep pox*** – Mortality, Forced sale at less price, Vaccination cost, Medicine cost, Extra labour, and Replacement cost.
7. ***Enterotoxaemia*** – Mortality, Forced sale at less price, Vaccination cost, Medicine cost, Extra labour, and Replacement cost.
8. ***Milk fever*** – Production loss (yield loss and discarded milk), Veterinary expense, Extra labour, and Extended calving interval.
9. ***Ketosis*** - Production loss (yield loss and discarded milk), Veterinary expense, Additional labour, and Extended calving interval.

9.2.3.2 Factors Influencing Economic Losses due to Animal Diseases

After measuring the economic losses due to animal diseases, both infectious and non-infectious, we often notice that losses are not similar in all the animals or herds and they differ probably due to the animals' inherent factors and the factors of the environment they are reared in. It is valuable to identify these factors which may be useful in designing disease control and prevention measures. Hence, almost all the studies aiming to estimate the losses due to animal diseases also study the factors influencing the losses. Let us know about these loss-influencing factors for some diseases:

Thirunavukkarasu and Prabaharan (2000) used a multiple linear regression analytical technique to assess the factors that influence the losses due to clinical mastitis in bovines of Tamil Nadu (India) and found that the variables *viz.*, milk yield before infection, number of quarters affected, number of days of treatment, and reduced lactation length were significantly influencing the losses. Selvam *et al.* (2004) used a multiple linear regression analysis to assess the factors influencing the losses due to diseases in layer farms and found that the number of birds affected, health care expenses and farm size were significantly influencing the disease losses. Jeyakumari *et al.* (2004) found that the losses due to postpartum reproductive disorders in bovines were significantly associated with the management factor, milk yield, order of lactation, and duration of illness. Thirunavukkarasu and Kathiravan (2006) found breed, order of lactation, and health expenses as the factors affecting the losses due to conception failures in bovines. Thirunavukkarasu *et al.* (2010c) reported the factors influencing the economic losses due to milk fever in dairy animals as milk yield, order of lactation, and duration of illness, through a multiple linear regression model fitted, while Thirunavukkarasu *et al.* (2011c) found the same factors as influencing the losses due to ketosis in dairy animals.

9.2.4 Negative Effects of Animal Diseases at Different Levels

Level	Prevalence of a Disease in Farms	Outbreak of a Contagious Disease	
		Trade Restrictions	No Trade Restrictions
Farms and the Sector	Negative effects on farm and sectoral income	Huge loss to the farmers, sector, and traders due to dropping prices and falling demand	Considerable loss to the farmers and sector
Input industries	Less demand for their products	Huge, as there would be less demand for their products like feed	
Processing industries	Less supply of raw materials to them, Less demand for their products due to rising prices	Considerable losses due to less supply of raw materials and increased prices of their products which might bring down the demand much	
Consumers	Loss due to rising prices	Advantage, due to falling prices	Disadvantage, due to rising prices
National economy	Loss due to inefficient use of resources	Severe loss due to drops in export earnings	Reduced national output and income
Global economy	-	Severe price rise in importing countries and drop in revenue in exporting countries	-

The losses accruing due to the diseases may differ considerably, as above, across different levels of the economy. For e.g., in the case of common diseases that the farmers can control (e.g., mastitis), it is the farmer who loses considerably due to reduced milk yield and or production of poor-quality milk unable to find the market. However, in case of contagious diseases like FMD, market prices of output will drop very fast and foreign trade will be seriously affected due to the import restrictions imposed by many developed countries.

9.2.5 Indirect Losses or Indirect Effects of a Disease

Indirect losses or effects of an animal disease normally include:

1. Incurring extra costs to avoid or reduce the disease itself through vaccination, quarantining the affected animals, etc.;

2. Bringing in some negative effects of the antibiotics, anthelmintics, insecticides, chemicals, etc. that need to be used to treat affected animals and or to prevent / control the diseases, which may cause health hazards both in animals and humans that may many times go unnoticed or become immeasurable;
3. Causing substantial drops in export earnings due to the undesirable effects of antibiotics, anthelmintics, insecticides, chemicals, etc., as many importing countries could have banned such chemicals;
4. Banning of imports of livestock and poultry and their products by many countries from the country where some serious contagious diseases like FMD are prevalent, thus causing huge drops in export earnings;
5. Posing serious threats to human health through the spread of zoonotic diseases;
6. Causing Anti-Microbial Resistance (AMR) in animals and thus in humans too, which is of serious concern nowadays in recent times;
7. Resulting in serious reductions in export earnings for countries like India, due to the imposition of WTO and SPS regulations further reduce the attainable export earnings.

Understanding how an animal disease negatively impacts livestock farmers and the livestock products marketing channel is a complex phenomenon. A more accurate assessment of losses due to animal diseases should include all these indirect effects too for the administrators and policymakers to effectively plan for the prevention and control of animal diseases. To summarize, the indirect losses due to animal diseases include:

- Disease control costs;
- Revenue foregone due to the restricted local market access;
- Revenue foregone from trade restrictions and export losses; Berentsen *et al.,* 1990 analyzed the negative effects of FMD on export;
- Losses beyond the farm gate in the supply chain like post-production and processing sectors;
- Additional expenditures by the governments to formulate and implement disease control and prevention policies;
- Losses to other sectors like tourism (E.g., Blake *et al.* (2003) found that the FMD outbreak significantly reduced tourism expenditures in the UK); and
- Reduced economic welfare of the producers, processors, and consumers

9.3 SECONDARY EFFECTS OF ANIMAL DISEASES AND EXTERNALITIES

Economic impacts of livestock diseases can be observed across all the related systems (Whatford *et al.,* 2022), e.g., human health expenditures through zoonoses (Zinsstag *et al.*, 2007, Martins *et al.*, 2014) and environmental impact through the increased use of drugs leading to residues and resistance in nature (Boxall, 2004).

9.3.1 Secondary Effects

What we have seen under direct effects and indirect effects of animal disease can be called as primary effects of diseases, as they are seen in the sector itself. However, some negative effects could be seen in the related sectors too, as could be seen in sectors that have some linkages with the livestock sector. These effects are called as secondary effects arising due to both the forward and backward linkages that the livestock sector has with the other sectors. For e.g., the livestock sector has a forward linkage with the sectors that deal with post-production activities like processing and marketing of livestock and poultry products after they leave the farm gates. Similarly, there is a backward linkage with the sectors that deal with the production and supply of inputs to the livestock sector like the feed industry. These linked industries too suffer, because of the disease issues in livestock and poultry. Unfortunately, these secondary effects in the other linked sectors are not usually assessed, though the reduced or uneconomic activities in these secondary sectors also cause significant losses to the society and the nation, by pulling down the income and employment that otherwise could have been generated in these industries.

9.3.2 Externalities

Apart from the secondary effects, the diseases also cause some externalities or outward effects which are almost difficult to estimate and include in disease losses. This outwardness or externality in disease losses occurs when the activities of one group of farmers or consumers affect another group, without the former group paying for what has been lost by the latter. What has to be paid may be a cost or a receipt. This externality part of loss can be better explained by a few examples, for the external costs and external receipts:

1. We know that the effluents coming out of a tannery are usually drained into the nearby lands or water sources like rivers. These effluents containing hazardous chemicals, if left untreated before being drained out, would make the surrounding lands uncultivable and water sources unusable either for drinking or for agricultural uses. As a result, the crop farmers and water consumers living around tanneries would be buying

water at some price. Had the effluents been treated according to the rules stipulated by the Government or local bodies, the cost would have been absorbed by the tanneries themselves. However, if the effluents are untreated and drained into public or private lands or water bodies, then it is the farmers and common people who pay for it by buying water at a cost or dispose of their lands made uncultivable by the effluents of tanneries at a much lower price. This occurs because the tanneries had not borne the cost of treating the polluted effluents. This is the typical case of the cost not being paid for by the concerned firms, but borne by others.

2. Let us imagine a situation wherein a few farmers have not vaccinated their livestock against a particular disease (for e.g., FMD), despite the strict instructions given by the authorities concerned. These farmers put not only their animals but also the animals of nearby farms or even the whole community at risk of picking up the infection during an outbreak. This is another example of cost not being paid for by the few farmers who had not vaccinated their animals, but the cost of mild to moderate levels of infection is borne by others, despite having vaccinated their stock, in the community.
3. Let us have another situation wherein a few youths of some villages in a district plant tree saplings in the wastelands and other common areas and continue to water them and maintain them. This positive approach of a few youths is expected to provide shade, bring in more rain, and prevent soil erosion. These benefits expected to result from the efforts of a few people would be now enjoyed or shared by all the people in those communities without paying anything for the benefits. This is an example of benefits being reaped without paying for the same.

Like the above, there could be many externalities in terms of costs and benefits. However, quantifying them precisely is not so easy. One possibility to measure an externality is to first “internalize” the externality. For e.g., the tannery must be made, by enacting suitable laws, to install a treatment plant to render the effluents harmless, before draining them out. The livestock farmers may be imposed with suitable penalties by the Government, local body, or community, for failing to vaccinate their livestock. The communities for the benefit of whom the trees were planted may charge a reasonable fee from the people of the villages concerned to effectively manage the trees and to further propagate such initiatives in more areas. These are a few suggestive ways of internalizing the externalities that seem to be present, so that the relevant costs and benefits can be accounted.

9.4 INTANGIBLE LOSSES DUE TO ANIMAL DISEASES

Apart from the above secondary effects and externalities of animal diseases, certain other negative effects result from animal diseases, which are less tangible or intangible. They are:

9.4.1 Zoonoses

Although the effects of zoonotic diseases spreading from animals to humans can be quantified in terms of the reduced working capability of the affected human population, reduced income earned, and the costs of treatments to a certain extent, it is very difficult to evaluate objectively the costs of human mortality and human suffering. Also, the fear of contracting diseases from animals (like Rabies, Brucellosis, Parasitic infestations, etc.) itself can be a negative effect of animal diseases on human activities. In all, the economic impact of zoonotic diseases on human beings is by itself intangible. Economic impacts of livestock diseases can be observed on human health expenditures through zoonoses (Zinsstag *et al.*, 2007, Martins *et al.*, 2014). and environmental impact through the increased use of drugs leading to residues and resistance in nature (Boxall, 2004)

Roth *et al.* (2003) estimated the economic benefit, cost-effectiveness, and distribution of benefits of improving human health through the control of Brucellosis by mass vaccination of livestock in Mongolia. Estimated intervention costs were US$ 8.3 million, and the overall human health benefit was US$ 26.6 million, which resulted in a Net Present Value of US$ 18.3 million and an average benefit-cost ratio for the society of3.20. Hence, although industrialized countries were able to contain outbreaks of zoonotic diseases, as reported by Zinsstag *et al.* (2007), many resource-limited countries could not react adequately. Cross-sectoral assessments of interventions such as mass vaccination for Brucellosis in Mongolia or vaccination of dogs for Rabies in Chad considered human and animal health sectors from a societal economic perspective. Combining the total societal benefits, the intervention in the animal sector would save money and open new approaches for controlling zoonoses in resource-limited countries through contributions from multiple sectors.

9.4.2 Rising Anti-Microbial Resistance (AMR)

With the rising antibiotic-resistant microbes in human medicine, there are increasing concerns over the less controlled use of antibiotics in livestock and poultry. These are believed to further worsen the antibiotic-resistant microbes in the human food chain, especially in the last few decades. Although steps are being taken to regulate the use of antibiotics in animals in developed countries, a majority of other countries especially developing countries are yet to take initiatives in this regard. This is true and there is a long way to go, even though initiatives for better regulation of veterinary medicines are underway following the directions of the World Organization for Animal Health (*Office International des Épizooties* - OIE), especially in many developing countries. Further, the live animals and animal products imported or exported are believed to carry antibiotic-resistant bacteria across countries. Otte, *et al.* (2004) assessed the socio-economic impacts of transboundary animal diseases and based on them, suggested some institutional responses to control them. Economic impacts of livestock diseases can be observed in the environment through the increased use of drugs, which leads to residues and resistance in nature (Boxall, 2004).

To conclude, there would be difficulties in estimating the costs of animal diseases due to the secondary effects and intangible effects of animal diseases, more so for an entire country or the whole world. Hence, necessary analytical tools need to be developed so that we can capture all the impacts of animal diseases, overcoming the challenges of disease impact assessment. Because of the complexities in estimating animal disease losses, often loss estimates are made at farm, national, and regional levels, rather than more precise calculations. Not long ago, the World Bank, in cooperation with OIE, produced a study detailing the impact of animal diseases. However, such studies need to be regularly updated to document the total costs of animal diseases. Though national data may be available for some animal diseases and if feasible they may be extrapolated to the whole world for a better understanding of animal disease losses.

10

Economic Methods of Estimating Disease Losses

After assessing the prevalence or incidence of the disease concerned, the next step is to quantify the economic losses due to that disease by classifying and presenting all the information available on the losses, expressing these in monetary values, and identifying and quantifying the indirect losses attributable to a disease, to the extent possible. Usually, most of the negative effects of diseases can be conveniently estimated in terms of reduced output, mortality, reduced weight, delayed maturity, and treatment cost, directly. However, quantifying the indirect effects of the disease will be complex, but it is not impossible.

As we saw earlier, the economic impacts of animal diseases can be measured using statistical / epidemiological methods and economic methods. Economic methods of disease loss estimation include the Gross Margin Analysis, Enterprise Budgeting, Equi-Marginal Principle, Partial Budgeting, Cost-Benefit Analysis, and Decision Analysis.

10.1 GROSS MARGIN ANALYSIS & ENTERPRISE BUDGETING

Gross margin analysis and enterprise budgeting are done to evaluate the economic viability of a farm as a whole. The gross margin is the value of farm output minus the variable costs. Fixed costs like sheds and equipment are not included in this analysis. Farm output includes livestock and livestock products sales and the net change in the herd. However, the enterprise budget measures the profit from the farm enterprise. That is, the fixed costs are also included to calculate the profit. Hence, the enterprise budget is equal to the value of farm output minus the variable costs minus the fixed costs. In short, enterprise budget = output – variable costs – fixed costs or simply, enterprise budget = gross margin – fixed costs. For e.g., the Gross margin and enterprise budget (per year) table for a dairy herd will be as below (Figures are only hypothetical):

Item	Costs / Value (in INR) of outputs in the farm	
	Not following vaccination	**Following vaccination**
	Output	
Milk sales	9,000	10,000
Animal / calf sales	4,000	5,000
Net value change in herd	2,000	2,500
Total Output (TO)	**15,000**	**17,500**
	Variable Costs	
Feed	1,800	2000
Fodder	800	900
Labour	500	500
Veterinary expenses	400	250
Vaccine costs	0	250
Total Variable Costs (TVC)	**3,500**	**3900**
Gross Margin (GM) = TO - TVC	**11,500**	**13600**
Fixed Costs		
Rent for buildings	250	250
Interest on investment	100	100
Depreciation of durable assets	100	100
Electricity charges	50	50
Total Fixed Costs (TFC)	**500**	**500**
Enterprise Budget (EB) = TO – TVC - TFC = GM - TFC	**11,000**	**13100**

10.2 EQUI-MARGINAL PRINCIPLE

The equi-marginal principle works by allocating the available resources to get optimum benefits, by maximizing the utilization of inputs, productivity, and profitability in a farm. This principle is applied in farm budgeting for allocating resources to such enterprises that yield maximum profit. The very basis of the term 'equi-marginal' means that the farmer needs to stop adding inputs when the marginal product (MP) becomes equal to the marginal cost (MC). The term 'marginal' means 'additional'. This can be explained using an example.

Suppose a farmer has five cows in his farm, which are in different stages of lactation. The farmer is feeding different levels of a particular concentrate feed to his cows according to their milk yield. To increase the yield, the farmer may try to add more feed which may increase the milk yield. In this process, the farmer will not only get additional milk yield, but also incur additional cost due to increased feed usage. Unfortunately, the farmer cannot keep on adding more and more feed, thinking that he will reap more and more output. What happens at a stage is that the added cost or additional cost or marginal cost (MC) will be equal to added revenue or additional revenue or marginal revenue (MR). This is the point at which the farmer should stop increasing the feed further, because beyond this point of production wherein MC = MR, the MC will keep rising above MR, which means that the additional cost incurred will be more than the additional revenue the farmer reaps.

10.2.1 Economic Optimum Production

Total revenue (TR) in a farm is the revenue obtained by selling the farm products, while marginal revenue (MR) is the quantity of revenue added to the Total Revenue (TR) when the farmer produces one more unit of output. That is, MR is the price of the output per unit that is added to the total revenue when one more unit of product is produced and or sold. Hence, MR = P_Q (Price of the product). We draw the total revenue curve and the total cost curve to see the zone of profit and zone of loss, besides the break-even point of production, which is the point at which the farmer would cover at least the cost of production. Whatever that is produced above this point would yield profits, while the production below this breakeven point would result in loss.

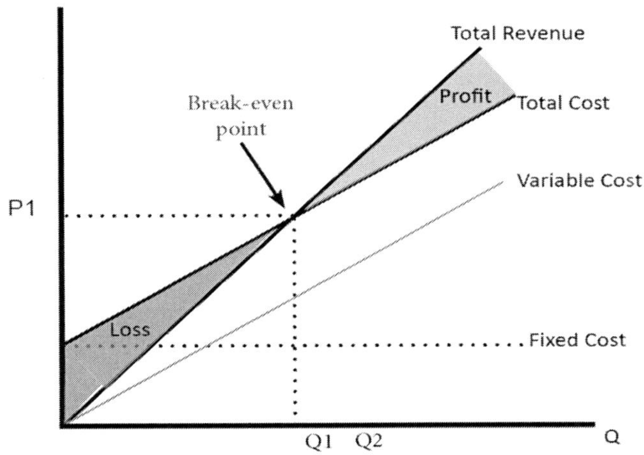

In the following graph, we notice ATC and AVC which are average total cost and average variable cost, respectively. Now, we introduce the MR (P_Q) curve in the unit cost curves graph to find out the level of maximum profit giving optimal output. The maximum profit giving optimal output will be the point of production where the MR curve intersects the MC curve, i.e., when MR = MC. When we look at the levels of production below this point, MC < MR, which means the addition to the total cost is less than the addition to the total revenue when one more unit of output is produced. That is, the farmer can keep increasing the level of production till he reaches the point where MR

= MC. This point is the optimum level of production. Because, if the farmer produces more than what is produced at this point, what is added to the total cost (MC) will be more than that will be added to the total revenue (MR), thereby incurring loss in the farm. One more important concept we have in the graph called the shut-down point wherein the level of production just covers the variable cost of production and not the fixed cost. To continue to operate the farm business, the farmer should at least produce at least this much; otherwise, it is better to shut the farm down as the production below this point would only lead to loss.

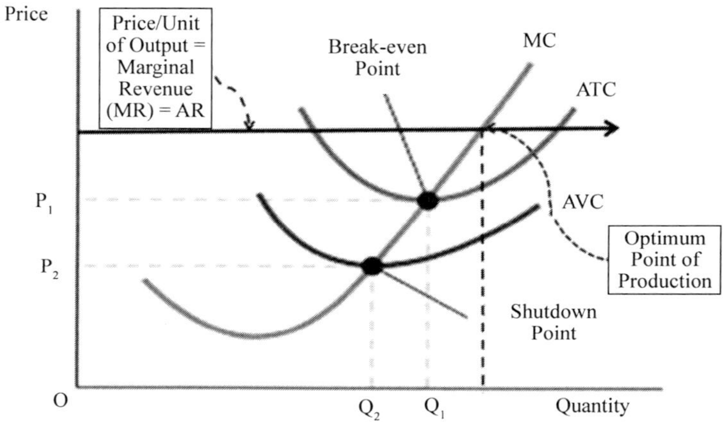

10.3 PARTIAL BUDGETING

Partial budgeting is an economic decision-making tool used to compare the costs and benefits of alternative methods available and choose the better method for implementation by a farmer. Unlike the whole farm (enterprise) budgeting which calculates all the costs and returns in a farm business, partial budgeting takes into account only a specific intervention the farmer is trying to introduce in his farm. It looks into the changes in income and expenses that would result from the introduction of a particular alternative strategy or input.

Partial budgeting is used to analyze several farm decisions, like, introducing a new technology (for e.g., using weedicide instead of manual removal of weeds, leasing in some tools instead of buying them, rearing goats instead of sheep, etc.) or modifying a different production practice like machine milking rather than hand-milking. In partial budgeting, a few key steps are performed before implementing a new decision proposed on the farm:

1. Listing the increased returns we expect because of this change (For e.g., if we plan to introduce a milking machine, the increased milk extraction, and the reduced possibility of teat infection in monetary terms);

2. Listing the reduced costs because of this new intervention (For e.g., wages paid so far to the labourers for hand milking and cost of disinfectants and antiseptics having been applied to teats and udder during hand milking will be now saved);
3. Listing the added costs of the proposed new item (For e.g., interest on investment we make in buying the machine, and maintenance and electricity charges, etc., arising);
4. Listing the reduced returns, if any; and
5. Finally, finding the total of S. Nos. 1 and 2 to get added returns and 3 and 4 to get added costs, and then subtracting the added costs from the added returns to get the net returns of introducing the new alternative.

If the net returns are positive, then we can decide that the new intervention has an economic advantage and we can introduce and use this proposed technology in our farm to get more benefits. If the net returns are negative, then we continue the same old hand-milking method.

10.3.1 General Format of Partial Budget

OUTCOME OF THE PROPOSED INTERVENTION			
POSITIVE OUTCOME		NEGATIVE OUTCOME	
Increased Returns	**INR**	Increased Costs	**INR**
a.		a.	
b.		b.	
Total Increased Returns		Total Increased Costs	
Reduced Costs	**INR**	Reduced Returns	**INR**
a.		a.	
b.		b.	
Total Reduced Costs		**Total Reduced Returns**	
TOTAL POSITIVE OUT-COME (Increased Returns + **Total Reduced Costs**)		TOTAL NEGATIVE OUT-COME (Total Increased Costs + **Total Reduced Returns**)	

10.4 COST-BENEFIT ANALYSIS

The Cost-Benefit Analysis is an analytical tool used to estimate the costs and benefits of the decisions made by the farmer to identify the most cost-effective option to implement the same on his farm. Normally, a Cost-Benefit Analysis evaluates all the possible costs and benefits involved in a farm business. While the costs include costs such as direct costs, indirect costs, and intangible costs, the benefits would include direct benefits and indirect benefits.

Direct costs are the costs that directly relate to the production of output, like animal, feed, fodder, labour, tools, and implements, etc., while indirect costs are the expenses that are not directly related to the production like rent, transport cost, etc. Intangible costs are the ones that cannot be quantified, like a change in the consumer taste or preference which may bring down the demand for the product. Direct benefits are the benefits arising from the farm. E.g., revenue obtained from the sale of products from the farm. Indirect benefits are the ones that we can only perceive but not realized in monetary terms like preferences shown by the consumers to farm products.

After totaling the costs and benefits separately, we arrive at the total costs, total benefits, and then the net benefits, which may be positive, zero, or negative. Using cost-benefit analysis, besides evaluating the costs incurred and the benefits reaped in the farm business, we assess the Net Present Value or Worth (NPV or NPW), Benefit-Cost Ratio (BCR), and Internal Rate of Return (IRR).

10.4.1 Net Present Value (NPV) or Net Present Worth (NPW)

Net Present Value (NPV) or Net Present Worth (NPW) is calculated by finding the difference between the present value or present worth of the benefits and the present value or present worth of the costs and subtracting the latter from the former. That is, NPV or NPW is equal to the Present Worth of Benefits minus the Present Worth of Costs. Mathematically,

$$\text{NVP} = \sum_{t=1}^{n} \frac{B_n}{(1+i)^n} - \sum_{t=1}^{n} \frac{C_n}{(1+i)^n} = \sum_{t=1}^{n} \frac{B_n - C_n}{(1+i)^n}$$

where Bn = Benefits in each year of the project, Cn = Costs in each year of the project, n = number of years in the project, i = interest (discount) rate, and Bn – Cn = Net Cash Flow in n^{th} *year of the project.*

The investment for the farm will be profitable, if the NVP calculated is positive; not worth investing if the NPV is negative.

10.4.2 Benefit – Cost Ratio (BCR)

Benefit – Cost Ratio (BCR) is the ratio of the Present Worth of the Benefits to the Present Worth of the Costs. That is, BCR = Sum of the present worth of benefits / Sum of the present worth of costs. Mathematically,

$$\text{BCR} = \sum_{t=1}^{n} \frac{B_n}{(1+i)^n} / \sum_{t=1}^{n} \frac{C_n}{(1+i)^n}$$

where Bn = Benefits in each year of the project, Cn = Costs in each year of the project, n = number of years in the project, and i = interest (discount) rate.

The investment for the farm will be profitable, if the BCR calculated is greater than one; not worth investing if the BCR is less than one.

Let us use an example of a farm business for which the expenses and returns are available for five years:

Year	Cash Outflow or Expenditures (Rs.)	Cash Inflow or Returns (Rs.)
1	75,000	25,000
2	75,000	30,000
3	50,000	54,000
4	50,000	92,000
5	25,000	92,000

We will assume that the interest (discount) rate is 12 percent per annum and calculate the NPV and BCR as below:

Year	Cash Outflow	Cash Inflow	Discount factor $[1/(1+i)^n]$	Incremental Cash Outflow (Rs.)	Incremental Cash Inflow (Rs.)
1	75,000	25,000	0.89	66,750	22,250
2	75,000	30,000	0.80	60,000	24,000
3	50,000	54,000	0.71	35,500	38,340
4	50,000	92,000	0.64	32,000	58,880
5	25,000	92,000	0.57	14,250	52,440

For the first year, the discount rate is calculated as $1 / (1.12)^0 = 0.89$, for the second year, it is $1 / (1.12)^1 = 0.80$, and so on. Then, the annual cash outflows and cash inflows are multiplied by the respective discount rates to arrive at the incremental cash outflows and incremental cash inflows, respectively. Once this is done, we add all the incremental cash outflows and incremental cash inflows, separately, which work out to Rs.2,08,500/- and Rs. Rs.1,95,910/-, respectively. Now, the NPV = Rs.2,08,500/- minus Rs.1,95,910/- = Rs.12,950/- and the BCR = Rs.2,08,500/- divided by Rs.1,95,910/- = 0.94.

Now, although the NPV is positive, the BCR is less than one and hence, this project is not economically viable. Hence, it is not worth investing in this farm business which will result in loss, considering the time value of money, meaning that had the amount been invested in the bank, the interest accrued (at 12 percent per annum) would be more than the income earned in this farm business.

10.4.3 Internal Rate of Return (IRR)

Internal Rate of Return (IRR) is the discount rate which just makes the net present value (NVP) of the cash flow equal to zero. IRR is considered to be the most useful measure of project worth. Mathematically, IRR is that discount rate 'i' such that:

$$\sum_{t=1}^{n} \frac{B_n - C_n}{(1+i)^n} = 0$$

i.e., NPV = 0

where Bn = Benefits in each year of the project, Cn = Costs in each year of the project, n = number of years in the project, i = interest (discount) rate, and Bn – Cn = Net Cash Flow in n^{th} year of the project.

An enterprise is profitable or feasible for investment when the internal rate of return is higher than the opportunity cost of capital. The computation of IRR for the project involves a trial-and-error method. Here alternative discount rates are used for the cash flow streams of the project under consideration till the NPV of the project reaches zero. However, it is not always possible to get a discount rate which makes the NPV exactly equal to zero through this trial-and-error method. We may get the discount rate, which makes the NPV nearer to zero, i.e., either positive or negative.

Internal Rate of Return is the rate of return per rupee invested in a farm business over its life span. If the IRR is 30 percent in a livestock project - this project gets an average annual return of Rs.30 per Rs.100 invested in the project over its life span. It is the rate of return at which the present value of total cash flows in a project is equal to zero. It is the discount rate at which the NPW of the project is zero.

$$\text{IRR} = \begin{matrix}\text{Lower}\\ \text{discount}\\ \text{rate}\end{matrix} + \left\{ \begin{matrix}\text{Difference}\\ \text{in}\\ \text{discount rate}\end{matrix} \left(\frac{\text{Present worth of cash flow at lower discount rate}}{\text{Total of present worth of cash flow of both discount rates}} \atop \text{(Ignore the signs)} \right) \right\}$$

A viable project will have an IRR of more than the opportunity cost (i.e., bank interest).

We will solve such a problem and find the IRR for it. A small dairy farm has the following cash outflows (expenses) and cash inflows (returns) over a period of five years. Find out the Internal Rate of Return for the farm:

Year	Cash outflow (Rs.)	Cash inflow (Rs.)
1	55,000	25,000
2	38,000	28,000
3	15,000	33,000
4	12,000	36,000
5	13,000	40,000

Solution

What we need to do is to calculate the following measures for the problem:

Year	Cash outflow (Rs.) Cost	Cash inflow (Rs.) Benefit	Incremental Net Benefit (INB)	Discount factor @ Lower Discount rate	Discount factor @ Higher Discount rate	Present Value of INB @ Lower discount rate	Present value of INB @ Higher discount rate
1							
2							
3							
4							
5							

First let us calculate the incremental net benefit, by subtracting the absolute costs from the absolute benefits for each year and present them in a table:

Year	Cash outflow (Rs.) - Cost	Cash inflow (Rs.) - Benefit	Incremental Net Benefit - INB (Benefit – Cost)
1	55,000	25,000	- 30,000
2	38,000	28,000	- 10,000
3	15,000	33,000	18,000
4	12,000	36,000	24,000
5	13,000	40,000	27,000

After this, we need to find the number of years in which the INB is negative, number of years in which the INB is positive, average annual INB for the positive INB years, total sum of INB for the INB negative years, average annual INB for the positive INB years and total sum of INB for the negative INB years and present them in another table to find lower and higher discount rates.

S. No.	Parameters	Solution
1	Number of years in which the INB is negative	2
2	Number of years in which the INB is positive	3
3	Average annual INB for the positive INB years	Rs. 69,000 / 3 = Rs.23,000
4	Total sum of INB for the INB negative years	= Rs.40,000
5	Average annual INB for the positive INB years / Total sum of INB for the negative INB years	= Rs.23,000 / Rs.40,000 = 0.57

With the above parameters worked out, we need to refer to the IRR Table, which is given below:

First Determine: No. of years in which INB is negative	**Second Determine:** No. of years in which INB is positive	**Third divide:** **Average annual positive incremental net benefit** / **Total Negative incremental net benefit** Use the result worked out above to select the column to find the initial estimate opposite to the appropriate no. of years for negative and positive INB streams							
		0.1	**0.2**	**0.3**	**0.4**	**0.5**	**0.6**	**0.8**	**1.0**
1	5	-	0	12	22	30	38	>50	>50
	10	0	12	21	28	34	40	50	>50
	20	7	16	23	28	34	38	47	>50
2	**5**	-	0	10	19	**25**	**30**	40	49
	10	0	11	18	24	29	34	42	48
	20	6	14	20	25	29	33	40	46
3	5	-	0	9	15	21	25	33	40
	10	0	10	16	21	26	29	36	41
	20	6	13	18	23	26	29	35	40
4	5	-	0	7	13	18	22	28	34
	10	0	9	15	19	23	26	31	36
	20	6	12	17	21	24	26	31	35
5	5	-	0	7	12	16	19	25	29
	10	0	8	13	17	21	23	28	32
	20	5	12	16	19	22	24	28	31

Since the number of years in which INB is negative is 2, we select 2 in the first column. Now, the number of years in which INB is positive is 3, however, we are not able to select the appropriate column (2nd column) since it starts from only 5. Hence, we can select the nearest number of years in which INB is positive, i.e., 3. We now move on to the third step, in which we have to see where our Average annual INB for the positive INB years / Total sum of INB for the negative INB years, i.e., 0.57 lies. Since it is between 0.5 and 0.6, we select both and these two columns indicate the discount (interest) rates of 25 percent and 30 percent.

We now move further and incorporate these discount (interest) rates of 25 percent and 30 percent in the following table:

Year	INB	$DF_L = 1 / (1+0.25)^t$	$DF_H = 1 / (1+0.30)^t$	INB * DF_L	INB * DF_H
		Discount Factor (DF) @ Lower Discount Rate (LDR of 25%)	Discount Factor (DF) @ Higher Discount Rate (HDR of 30%)	Present Value of INB at LDR	Present value of INB at HDR
1	-30,000	0.80	0.77	- 24,000	- 23,077
2	-10,000	0.64	0.59	- 6,400	- 5,917
3	18,000	0.51	0.46	9,216	8,193
4	24,000	0.41	0.35	9,830	8,403
5	27,000	0.33	0.27	8,,847	7,272
Total				**- 2,506**	**- 5,126**

Now, we will use the formula to calculate the IRR in the farm:

$$\text{IRR} = \begin{matrix}\text{Lower}\\ \text{discount}\\ \text{rate}\end{matrix} + \left\{ \begin{matrix}\text{Difference}\\ \text{in}\\ \text{discount rate}\end{matrix} \left(\frac{\text{Present worth of cash flow at lower discount rate}}{\text{Total of present worth of cash flow of both discount rates}} \right) \right\}$$

(Ignore the signs)

IRR** = 25 + 5 {-2506 / (2506 + 5126)} = 25 + (5 * -0.33) = 25 – 1.65 =* ***23.35%.

What we infer from this result of IRR of 23.35% is that the rate of interest on the investment made in the dairy farm is 23.35%. Since it is more than the nominal bank interest rate of 14% (maximum), investing money in this farm enterprise is highly profitable.

James and Ellis (1978) used benefit-cost analysis to evaluate the benefits of control measures on the production of FMD-affected animals. Awa *et al.* (2000) collected data on reproduction and mortality over one year from 5,100 sheep and 13,300 goats that were vaccinated and or treated for PPR and control flocks and fitted a benefit-cost analysis model. At a 7% discount rate, the benefit-cost ratio of the PPR vaccine ranged from 2.26 to 3.27 in goats and 3.01 to 4.23 in sheep. Barasa *et al.* (2008) conducted a benefit-cost analysis of vaccination for FMD in South Sudan and reported a benefit-cost of 11.5 for FMD vaccination and the need for mass and strategic vaccination. A few selected applications of benefit-cost analysis to animal diseases were derived from Rich *et al.* (2005) and presented below:

Authors	**Level(s)**	**Time**	**Disease(s)**
Horst *et al.* (1999)	Herd, aggregated to multiple regions	5-year simulation period	Foot and Mouth Disease and Classical Swine Fever
Meuwissen *et al.* (1999) and Nielen *et al.* (1999)	Herd, sector, meat industry	Single period	Classical Swine Fever
Perry *et al.* (1999), Disney *et al.* (2001), and Randolph *et al.* (2002)	Herd, aggregated to nation	Discounting to alternative time horizons	Foot and Mouth Disease
Bates *et al.* (2003)	Herd, aggregated to three countries	Single period	

10.5 DECISION ANALYSIS

Unlike endemic diseases, some diseases are sporadic in nature, making it difficult to predict the incidence. This method requires various tools such as decision trees and expected value calculations to understand all aspects of the problem we are trying to solve. By doing so, we compare several options against one another for a more comprehensive decision. In the process, we look at all the relevant information related to each decision, along with the probabilities. We then use the data visuals to determine which option gives the best possible outcome. This analysis also examines potential uncertainties attached to a particular decision. We assess our decisions based on the likelihood of their success and their ensuing potential value, as well as the likelihood of their failure and the corresponding loss.

Decision analysis allows farm businesses to evaluate the potential outcomes of various decisions to determine the correct course of action. While making decisions to improve the income from the farm, we are likely to encounter certain uncertainties. There may be different courses of action to achieve the objective of maximizing the income, each of which may have different probabilities of occurrence and different expected outcomes. Taking into account various goals, outcomes, uncertainties involved, and their probabilities, the tool of decision analysis measures the expected outcomes of various possible decisions.

10.5.1 Decision Tree

After creating a framework to evaluate a problem, a decision tree is developed to evaluate the outcomes of various decisions. The decision tree is a visual representation of the expected outcomes and is used to illustrate the possible decisions in comparison to other alternatives. By modeling various expected outcomes and their probabilities using the decision tree, a farm or firm can then select the decision that gives a favourable outcome. A decision tree is a tree-shaped model with branches that represent potential outcomes from different alternatives.

10.5.2 Expected Value (EV)

After a decision tree model is constructed, it is important to find the expected value (EV) to evaluate which decision results in the most favourable outcome. By calculating the expected value, we can observe the average outcomes of different decisions and then make a viable decision. To calculate the expected value, we require the probability of each outcome and the resulting value. The formula for the expected value is:

*EV = (Probability A * Expected Payoff A)+(Probability B * Expected Payoff A)*

The above formula assumes that a farm's or firm's decision has two outcomes – success or failure. Each outcome can be represented by Probability A or B. The Expected Payoff refers to the gain or loss expected with each outcome. If there are multiple decisions possible, we need to calculate the expected value for each decision to determine the most favourable outcome.

10.5.3 Steps in Decision Analysis

1. First, we identify the problem to be solved or the decision to be made. After that, we list out the options or solutions available. For e.g., we have some money which can be invested. We may have several investment options to choose from and decision analysis can help us to choose the best one.
2. After this, we analyze the options available. This analysis looks at the costs involved, risks to be faced, possible benefits, and the probabilities of attaining them.
3. While analyzing different options, we develop a framework to study the outcomes too. While making an investment, we focus on getting the highest possible return and hence, choose the option that is more appropriate to meet our goal(s).
4. Then, we can combine our framework with a decision to evaluate the options.
5. Using the analysis and the decision tree picture, we begin calculating the Expected Values (EVs) of all our options. The EV represents the average outcome of each of our decisions. Finally, we assign monetary or numerical values to each outcome, simultaneously determining the probability of each outcome. However, finding the probability may be difficult.

10.5.4 Decision Analysis Examples

Example 1

A milk processing firm had developed two new milk products, A and B. The firm has two options: 1. to produce and sell product A and 2. To produce and sell product B, because the firm has limited capacity to produce both. The firm performs a study to find out the probability of success for both options, along with the potential revenue from each. It also learns the probability of failure and corresponding losses for each.

Option 1: Producing and marketing product A has a 65% probability of success with potential revenue of Rs.1,75,000 in a year. However, this option has also a 35% probability of failure with a potential loss of Rs.1,00,000.

Option 2: Producing and marketing product B has a 50% probability of success with potential revenue of Rs.2,25,000 in a year. However, this option has also a 30% probability of failure with a potential loss of Rs.75,000.

These details can be more clearly explained in a table as below:

Decision	Success		Failure	
	Probability	**Potential Revenue (Rs.)**	**Probability**	**Potential Loss (Rs.)**
Product A	65%	1,75,000	35%	1,00,000
Product B	50%	2,25,000	30%	75,000

With the above outcomes of its study, the firm should calculate the expected value of each option using the formula:

Expected Value (EV) of Option = (Probability of its success x Potential revenue) - (Probability of its failure x Potential loss)

Expected Value (EV) of Option 1 = (65% x Rs.1,75,000) - (35% x Rs.1,00,000) = Rs.78,750.

Expected Value (EV) of Option 2 = (50% x Rs.2,25,000) - (30% x Rs.75,000) = Rs.90,000.

We can also construct a decision tree for the problem as below:

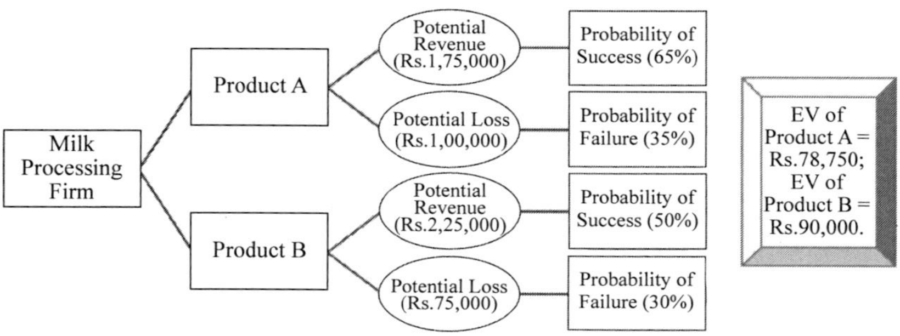

Based on the expected values of revenue calculated for options 1 and 2, the firm would decide to produce and market product B, as this product is expected to provide better revenue than product A for the time being.

While Parsons *et al.* (1986) assessed the economics of porcine parvovirus vaccination by decision analysis, Rodrigues *et al.* (1990) used this tool in their financial analysis of pseudorabies control and eradication in swine. Tomassen *et al.* (2002) developed a decision tree to support decision-making on the control measures after an outbreak of FMD to minimize the direct costs and export losses of FMD epidemics under several scenarios based on livestock and herd density in the outbreak region, the possibility of airborne spread, and the time between first infection and first detection.

Example 2

Suppose a veterinarian is called to examine and treat a sick male dairy calf born 3 days ago. The cost of rearing of the calf up to 15 days is Rs.300. This calf is expected to be sold at 15 days of age for Rs.1,600. The calf is diagnosed as diseased since it has been experiencing fever, diarrhoea, and dehydration for the past 24 hours. The veterinarian warns the farmer that the treatment cost would be about Rs.600. Given the current low market price of such a sick male calf, the owner wonders about whether or not to treat it. He asks the veterinarian to recommend to him the most profitable decision. The veterinarian uses decision tree analysis to answer.

The possible decisions are a). to treat the calf and b). to leave the calf untreated. Once a decision is made on this, what are the outcomes of such a decision? Here, we have the probability of survival in the case of treatment is 0.7. The likelihood of death in case of no treatment is 0.8. Hence, the probability of death after treatment is 1 – 0.7 = 0.3 and the likelihood of survival without treatment is 1 – 0.8 = 0.2.

The decision tree will be:

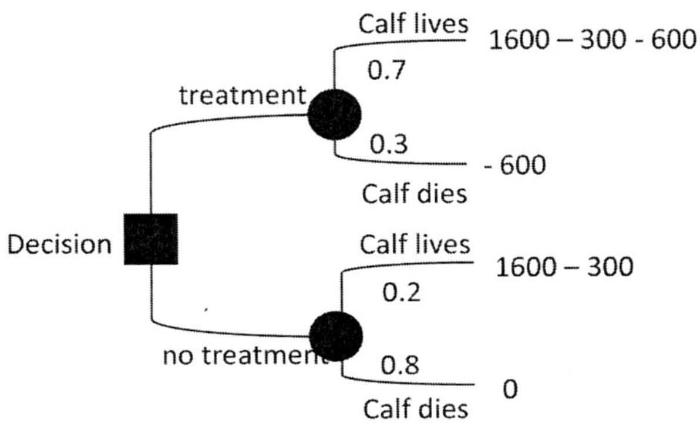

Expected value (calf treated, alive) = 0.7 * (1600 – 300 - 600) = Rs.490

Expected value (calf treated, dead) = 0.3 * (-600) = - Rs.180

Expected value (calf untreated, alive) = 0.2 * (1600 - 300) = Rs.260

Expected value (calf untreated, dead) = 0.8 * 0 = 0

Given the conditions set for this example, the most profitable action is to treat the calf because it is expected to fetch a maximum benefit of Rs.490 rather than leaving it untreated.

11

Regression Techniques for Assessing Factors Influencing Disease Frequencies and Losses

An animal disease is an economic process in the farming system, as it consumes a considerable amount of scarce economic resources that would have been otherwise productively utilized by the animals and results in negative benefits to society. Hence, while measuring the losses attributable to animal diseases, the manifestation of such losses and the factors influencing such losses may also be identified, which require modelling the ways by which the negative effects of the diseases are exhibited. A description of such models and their procedures is essential to understand the comprehensive effects of diseases. We will list and describe such models and tools in this chapter.

11.1 CORRELATION ANALYSIS

While simple descriptive statistical tools are adequate to estimate the economic effects of animal diseases, these tools cannot measure the nature and strength of the relationships between two or more variables. However, the statistical knowledge can effectively be used to understand Various statistical measures studied so far, like measures of central tendency and dispersion and skewness, relate to one variable only. However, there are many situations where there are several problems involving the use of two or more variables. Although correlation analysis is only a bivariate technique like t-test, ANOVA, and Chi-square test, we will briefly see about correlation in this chapter, as it is also a part of multivariate analysis. The first step is to determine which bivariate analytical tool we need to adopt to test the study hypothesis.

If two variables are related in such a way that the change (increase or decrease) in the value of one variable results in the change (increase or decrease) in the value of the other, then the two variables can be said to be correlated. If there is no relationship between two variables, they are said to be independent or uncorrelated. Correlation is an analysis between two or more variables.

11.1.1 Coefficient of Correlation

The coefficient of correlation is a measure of correlation free from units of measurement. It is denoted by 'r', which takes values from –1 to +1. When r = +1, the correlation is perfect and positive, when r = -1, the correlation is perfect and negative, and when r = 0, there is no correlation.

11.1.2 Types of Correlation

11.1.2.1 Simple, Partial and Multiple Correlations

When only two variables are involved in the study of correlation, it is called as the simple correlation. E.g., feed intake and growth of animals; and birth weight and number of piglets. When more than two variables are involved in the study, it is either partial or multiple correlation. In multiple correlation, the correlation of one dependent variable over other independent variables is studied. E.g., milk yield Vs. stage of lactation, feed, fodder, age of animal, etc. In partial correlation, we study the relationship between two variables (one dependent and one independent), assuming that other variables are constant. E.g., the correlation between the weight of broiler and feed intake, assuming other factors like birth weight, labour used, medicines used, etc. as constant.

11.1.2.2 Linear and Non-linear Correlations

Based on the degree of covariation, the correlation may be classified as linear or non-linear. When the correlation between two sets of variables is perfect with degree one (unity), meaning that they have an exact functional relationship, the correlation is said to be linear. The graphical depiction of a linear correlation presents a straight line, with its relationship represented by the function, y = a + bx, where x is the independent variable, y is independent variable, and a and b are constants.

A perfect linear correlation may be positive or negative. Thus, its numerical coefficient will be either +1 or –1. These are the limits of correlation. Thus, the coefficient of correlation cannot be greater than +1 or less than –1. If the correlation is imperfect, its graph will be non-linear, and it will not form a straight line. Non-linear correlation will always be less than unity, lying between -1 and +1.

11.1.3 Methods of Studying Correlation

11.1.3.1 Scatter Diagram

A scatter diagram (also called a scatterplot) graphically represents the relationship between two variables. Taking the independent variable on the X axis and dependent on Y axis, the points corresponding to each pair of observations are marked. This figure of the collection of the points is called a scatter diagram. The way in which the dots lie on the scatter diagram shows the type of correlation. If these dots show some trend either upward or downward, there is a correlation between the two variables. If the dots do not show any trend, there is no correlation between them.

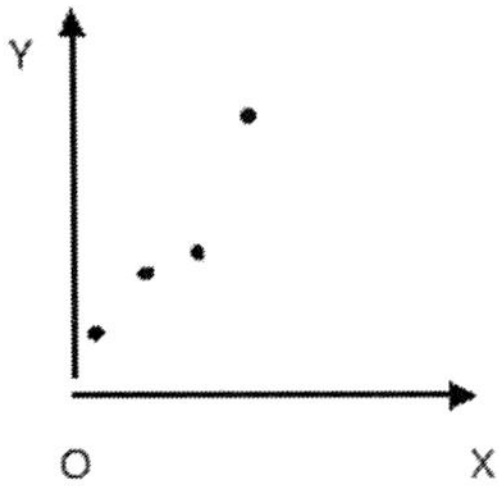

Perfect positive correlation

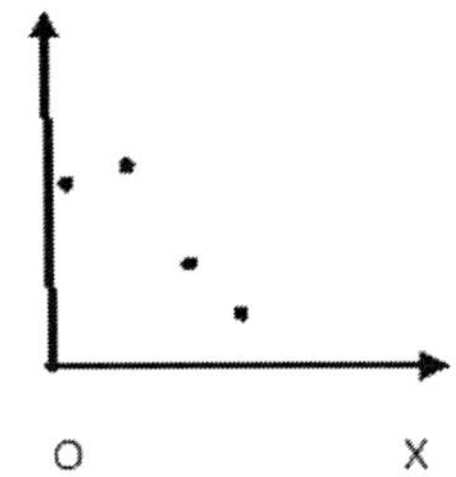

Perfect negative correlation

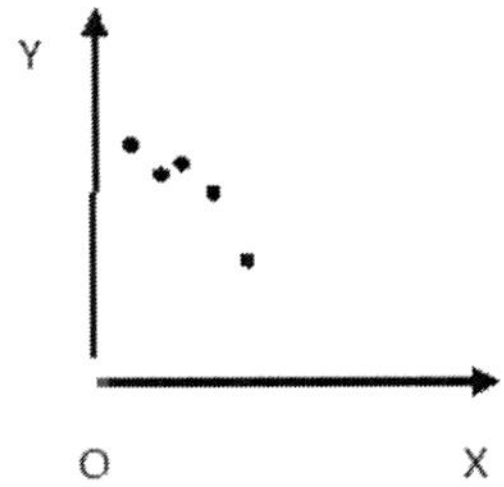

Moderately positive correlation

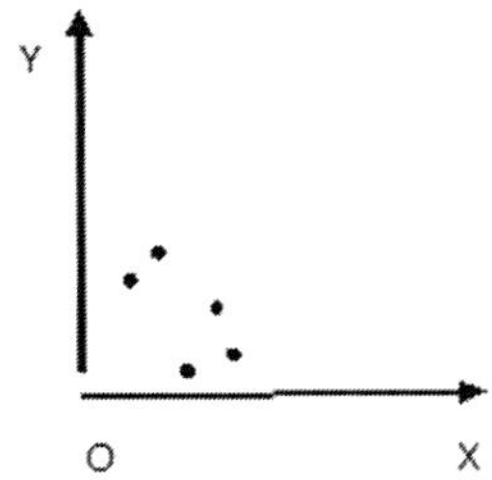

Moderately negative correlation

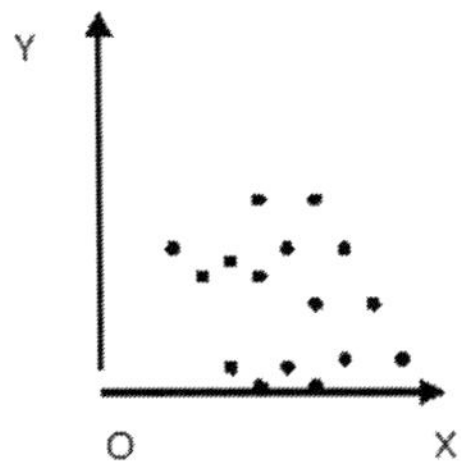

Absence of correlation

This method is not suitable when the number of observations is large. By this method, we can only know the existence of correlation and the direction of correlation, but we cannot obtain a measure of correlation.

11.1.3.2 Correlation Graph

Curves are plotted for the data on two variables. By examining the direction and closeness of the curves drawn, we can know whether the variables are related or not. If both the curves drawn move in the same direction (upward or downward), the correlation between them is positive. If they move in the opposite direction, the correlation is negative.

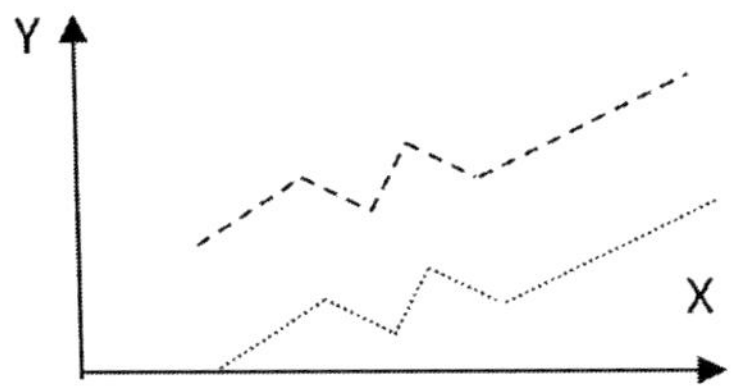

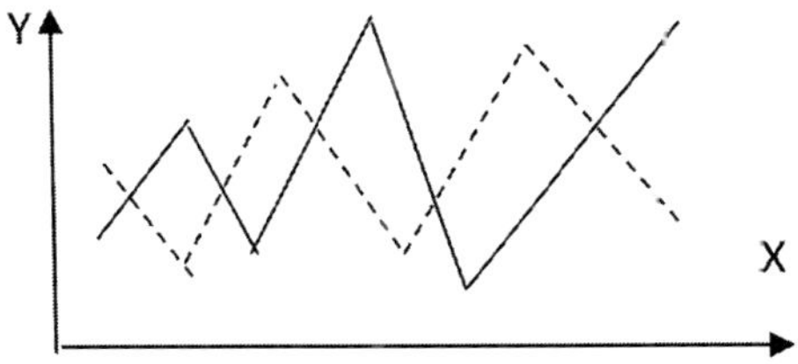

Like a scatter diagram, this method also does not offer any numerical value for the coefficient of correlation.

11.1.3.3 Karl Pearson's Correlation Coefficient

Both the above methods tell us only the existence and direction of correlation. But, to measure the correlation, we need to know the correlation coefficient. The Karl Pearson's method, popularly known as Pearsonian coefficient of correlation, is a mathematical method which measures the degree to which two variables are linearly related. If two variables are denoted by X and Y, the correlation coefficient between them is represented by r_{xy} or r.

The Karl Pearson's coefficient of correlation,

$$r = \frac{\Sigma\, dxdy}{\sqrt{\Sigma\, dx^2 * \Sigma dy^2}} \text{ (OR) } r = \frac{(XY * N) - (\sum X * \sum Y)}{\sqrt{\sum X^2 * N - (\sum X)^2}\sqrt{\sum Y^2 * N - (\sum Y)^2}}$$

where $dx = X - \overline{X}$, $dy = Y - \overline{Y}$, N is the number of paired observations.

Exercise

Calculate the coefficient of correlation between x and y from the following data:

X	1	2	3	4	5	6	7
Y	2	4	5	3	8	6	7

Solution

X	**$dx = X - \overline{X}$**	**dx^2**	**Y**	**$dy = Y - \overline{Y}$**	**dy^2**	**dxdy**
1	-3	9	2	-3	9	9
2	-2	4	4	-1	1	2
3	-1	1	5	0	0	0
4	0	0	3	-2	4	0
5	1	1	8	3	9	3
6	2	4	6	1	1	2
7	3	9	7	2	4	6
$\sum X = 28$ $\overline{X} = 4$		**$\sum dx^2 = 28$**	**$\sum Y = 35$ $\overline{Y} = 5$**		**$\sum dy^2 = 28$**	**$\sum dxdy = 22$**

Means $\overline{X} = \sum X/N = 28/7 = 4$; $\overline{Y} = \sum Y/N = 35/7 = 5$

Coefficient of correlation (by calculating the deviations from the mean)

$$r = \frac{\sum dxdy}{\sqrt{\sum dx^2 * \sum dy^2}}$$

= 22 / Sqr (28*28)

= 22/28

= **0.79**

Another method (This method will be useful when calculating deviations is difficult)

X	Y	X^2	Y^2	XY
1	2	1	4	2
2	4	4	16	8
3	5	9	25	15
4	3	16	9	12
5	8	25	64	40
6	6	36	36	36
7	7	49	49	49
$\sum X = 28$	**$\sum Y = 35$**	**$\sum X^2=140$**	**$\sum Y^2=203$**	**$\sum XY=162$**

$$r = \frac{\left(\sum XY * N\right) - \left(\sum X * \sum Y\right)}{\sqrt{\sum X^2 * N - \left(\sum X\right)^2} \sqrt{\sum Y^2 * N - \left(\sum Y\right)^2}}$$

$$r = \frac{(162 * 7) - (28 * 35)}{\sqrt{140 * 7 - 28^2} \sqrt{203 * 7 - 35^2}}$$

= (1134 - 980) / [sqrt (980-784) * sqrt (1421-1225)]

= 154 / sqrt (196) * sqrt (196) = 154 / 14 * 14

= **0.79**

Properties of Coefficient of Correlation

a) Coefficient of correlation is a measure of closeness between two variables.

b) The range of correlation coefficient (r) is from -1 to +1.

c) If r=+1, the correlation between two variables is perfect and positive.

d) If r=-1, the correlation between two variables is perfect and negative.

e) If there is a strong positive linear relationship between variables, r will be close to +1.

f) If there is a strong negative linear relationship between variables, r will be close to -1.

g) If r=0, there is no correlation between two variables. It means variables are independent.

11.1.3.4 Concurrent Deviation Method

This method of studying correlation is the simplest of all the methods. What is to be found in this method is the direction of change of x and y variables. The procedure is below:

Step I. Find out the direction of change of x variable, i.e. as compared with the first value, whether the second value is increasing or decreasing or constant. If it is increasing, put a + sign; if it is decreasing, put a – sign and if it is constant, put zero. Similarly, as compared to second value, find out whether the third value is increasing, decreasing or constant. Repeat the same process for the other values also. Denote the column as Dx.

Step II. In the same way, find out the direction of change of y variable and denote this column as Dy.

Step III. Multiply Dx with Dy and determine the value of c, the number of concurrent deviations or the number of positive signs obtained after multiplying Dx with Dy.

Step IV. Thenapply the formular $= \pm\sqrt{\pm\left[\frac{2c-n}{n}\right]}$ sign is taken as that of (2 c-n).

Exercise

Calculate coefficient of concurrent deviation for the following data:

Price	368	384	385	361	347	384	395	403	400	385
Imports	22	21	24	20	22	26	24	29	28	27

Solution

Price X	368	384	385	361	347	384	395	403	400	385
Direction of change of X = dx		+	+	-	-	+	+	+	-	-
Imports Y	22	21	24	20	22	26	24	29	28	27
Direction of change of Y = dy		-	+	-	+	+	-	+	-	-
Concurrent deviation dxdy		-	+	+	-	+	-	+	+	+

Hence, C = 6 (the no. of positive signs in concurrent deviations)

N = 9

Coefficient of concurrent deviation r_c = + sqrt {+ [2C-N)/N}

= + sqrt {+ [2*6-9)/9} = + sqrt {+ [12-9)/9}

= + sqrt 0.33 = 0.577

11.1.3.5 Spearman's Rank Correlation Method

Karl Pearson's method cannot be used when variables are qualitative. Hence, when variables are qualitative such as ranks, colours, etc., Spearman's Rank Correlation method, which is a non-parametric method, is used. Also, even the quantitative values can be ranked and correlation can be measured by this method, using the formula:

$$\rho = 1 - (6\Sigma d^2) / n(n^2 - 1)$$

where ρ is the correlation coefficient, d is the difference between the ranks of two datasets and n is the number of paired observations

11.1.3.6 Measuring Correlation from Covariance

If covariance between X and Y variables is 10 and the variances of X and Y are respectively 16 and 9, find the coefficient of correlation.

Covariance of X and Y = ∑xy / N = 10

Variance of X = 16, therefore σx = √16 = 4

Variance of Y = 9, therefore σy = √9 = 3

r = ∑xy / N σx σy = 10 / (4*3) = 0.833

Probable Error of Correlation Coefficient

The probable error of correlation coefficient is an amount which, if added or subtracted from the mean correlation coefficient, produces amounts, within which a correlation coefficient from a series selected at random is expected to fall. The probable error of correlation coefficient helps us to interpret the value of correlation coefficient.

$$\text{PE of r} = 0.6745\frac{\left(1-r^2\right)}{\sqrt{n}}$$

r + PE (r) denotes the limits of correlation in the population. If the observed value of r is less than its PE, the r is not significant. If the observed value of r is more than 6 times its PE, the r is significant.

E.g., If r = 0.79 and n is 7, then the probable error is 0.6745*((1 – (0.79)^2) / √7 = 0.6745*(1 – 0.6241) / 2.645 = **0.0958.** Since the r is very higher than the PE, r can be said to be significant.

Coefficient of Determination and Coefficient of Non-determination

The square of the correlation coefficient (r^2) is defined as the coefficient of determination. If r^2 = 0.85, it implies that 85% of the variation in the dependent variable is due to the independent variable studied. (1 – r^2) is defined as the coefficient of non-determination. If 1-r^2 = 0.24, we infer that 24% of the variation in the dependent variable is due to the other variables which are not studied. This is called unexplained variations.

11.2 REGRESSION ANALYSIS

The meaning of regression is the act of returning or going back in a phenomenon. We may be interested in studying the relationship between age and blood pressure, height and weight, feed and weight gain, etc. In such cases, we estimate the value of one variable, given the value of another. The nature of the relationship between variables such as these may be examined by regression analysis.

11.2.1 Objectives of Regression Analysis

1. Regression analysis helps to ascertain the probable form of relationship between variables and to predict or estimate the value of one variable to the value of the other variable.
2. The goal of regression is to find out equations of the lines (or curves) with functional relationship between two variables, independent or explanatory (x) and dependent or explained (y). That is, y depends on x. The simple linear regression is of the form $y = a + bx$, where 'b' represents the slope of the line (also called as regression coefficient) and 'a' the intercept of the line, where a and b are numerical constants, while the multiple linear regression is of the form $y = a + b1x1 + b2x2 + \ldots + bnxn$, where 'bi' represent the regression coefficient for variable xi.

11.2.2 Difference between Correlation and Regression

Correlation is merely a tool for ascertaining the degree of relationship between two variables and hence we cannot say that one variable is the cause and the other is the effect. However, in regression analysis, one variable is taken as dependent while the other is independent, thus making it possible to study the cause-and-effect relationship. In short, the presence of association does not imply causation, but the existence of causation always implies association, which can be studied only using regression.

11.2.3 Types of Regression Analysis

1. Simple regression: The regression analysis confined to the study of only two variables (one independent and one dependent) at a time is termed simple regression.
2. Multiple regression: The regression analysis for studying more than two variables (more than one independent variable and one dependent variable) is known as multiple regression.

11.2.4 Regression Line and Linear Regression

When observations from two variables are plotted as a graph, and if the points so obtained fall in a straight line, then the relationship is linear and it is said that there is linear regression between the variables. However, if the line is not a straight line, the regression is termed as non-linear regression.

In a study, where data on age and weight of animals are available, age is the independent variable, while weight is the dependent variable. It means that weight regresses with age. The regression line y = a + bx can be fitted, by estimating the coefficients a and b as below:

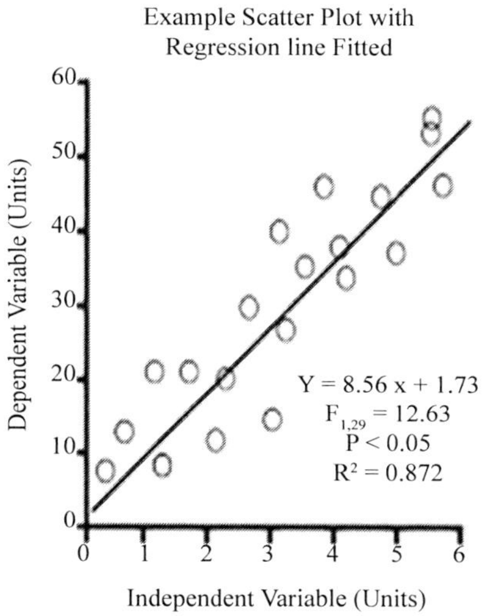

1. Using normal equations

For the regression line y = a + bx, the normal equations are:

$\sum y = na + b \sum x;$

$\sum xy = a\sum x + b\sum x^2$

When we find $\sum x$, $\sum x^2$, $\sum y$ and $\sum xy$, we will have two equations and two unknowns a and b. We can solve these equations to find the values for a and b. E.g.,

x	y	x^2	xy
1	1	1	1
3	2	9	6
4	2	16	8
6	4	36	24
8	6	64	48
9	8	81	72
11	8	121	88
14	9	196	126
$\sum x$=56	**$\sum y$=40**	**$\sum x^2$=524**	**$\sum xy$=373**

40 = 8a + 56b; 373 = 56a + 524b

Solving these equations, we get a = 0.072 and b = 0.704

Hence, y = 0.072 + 0.704x

2. Formula Method

In this method, we calculate the values of a and b directly by using the following formula, when the mean is known:

$$b = \frac{\sum(x-\bar{x})(y-\bar{y})}{\sum(x-\bar{x})^2} = \text{Covariance } (x, y) \,/\, \text{variance of } x$$

$$b = \frac{Sxy}{Sxx}$$

where Sxy = $\sum xy - [\sum x \sum y / n]$, and Sxx = $\sum x^2 - [\sum x]^2 / n]$

and a = $\bar{y}$ - b$\bar{x}$

Therefore Sxy = 373 – [(40*56)/8] = 93 and Sxx = 524 – [$(56)^2$ / 8] = 132

Hence, b = Sxy / Sxx = 93 / 132 = 0.704

Substituting b = 0.704 in a = $\bar{y}$ - b$\bar{x}$ we get

a = (40/8) – 0.704*(56/8) = 5 – (0.704*7) = 0.072

Thus the regression equation is **y = 0.072 + 0.704x**

Exercise

Calculate correlation and regression coefficients (Or fit a regression equation) from the following data:

X	*2*	*4*	*6*	*8*	*10*	*12*	*14*
Y	*4*	*2*	*5*	*10*	*4*	*11*	*12*

Solution

X	dx = X-8	dx^2	Y	dy = Y-7	dy^2	dx*dy
2	-6	36	4	-3	9	18
4	-4	16	2	-5	25	20
6	-2	4	5	-2	4	4
8	0	0	10	3	9	0
10	2	4	4	-3	9	-6
12	4	16	11	4	16	16
14	6	36	12	5	25	30
∑X=56 = 8	**∑dx=0**	**$\sum dx^2$=112**	**∑Y=48 = 6.86**	**∑dy=-1**	**$\sum dy^2$=97**	**∑dx*dy=82**

The regression coefficient of X on Y

$$bxy = \frac{\sum dxdy - \frac{\sum dx * \sum dy}{N}}{\sum dy^2 - \frac{\left(\sum dx\right)^2}{N}}$$

$$bxy = \frac{82 - \frac{0*(-1)}{7}}{97 - \frac{(-1)^2}{7}}$$

$= 82 / 96.86 = \mathbf{0.85}$

The regression coefficient of Y on X

$$byx = \frac{\sum dxdy - \frac{\sum dx * \sum dy}{N}}{\sum dx^2 - \frac{\left(\sum dx\right)^2}{N}}$$

$$byx = \frac{82 - \frac{0*(-1)}{7}}{112 - \frac{(0)^2}{7}}$$

$= 82 /112 = \mathbf{0.73}$

Correlation coefficient $r = \sqrt{bxy * byx}$

$= \sqrt{0.85 * 0.73} = 0.79$

Regression equation of Y on X

$Y - \bar{Y} = byx\ (X - \bar{X})$

$Y - 6.86 = 0.73\ (X - 8)$

$Y - 6.86 = 0.73X - 5.84$

$\mathbf{Y = 1.02 + 0.73X}$

The regression coefficient (b) gives the rate of change in the value of the dependent variable (y) for a unit change in the independent variable (x). The regression equation is useful in estimating the values of y by knowing the values of x.

11.2.5 Coefficient of Determination (R^2)

Whenever we find a regression equation, we should know how well the equation fits the data. One way to assess the goodness of fit is to check the coefficient of determination (R^2), which can be computed by the following formula:

$$R^2 = \frac{1/n \sum (x - \bar{x})(y - \bar{y})}{(\sigma_x * \sigma_y)}$$

where n – no. of observations, x is value for each x, is mean x value, y is value for each y, is mean y value, σ_x is SD of x, and σ_y is SD of y.

E.g., Computation for a sample problem is shown below:

x	y	$(x - \bar{x})$	$(x - \bar{x})^2$	$(y - \bar{y})$	$(y - \bar{y})^2$	$(x-\bar{x})(y-\bar{y})$
1	1	-6	36	-4	16	24
3	2	-4	16	-3	9	12
4	2	-3	9	-3	9	9
6	4	-1	1	-1	1	1
8	6	1	1	1	1	1
9	8	2	4	3	9	6
11	8	4	16	3	9	12
14	9	7	49	4	16	28
Mean = 7	**Mean = 5**		**$\sum(x - \bar{x})^2=132$**		**$\sum(y - \bar{y})^2=70$**	**$\sum(x-\bar{x})(y-\bar{y})=93$**

σ_x = sqrt[$\Sigma(x - \bar{x})2/N$] σy = sqrt[$\Sigma(y - \bar{y})^2/N$]

σ_x = sqrt(132/8) = sqrt(16.5) = 4.062 σy = sqrt(70/8) = sqrt(8.75) = 2.958

$$R^2 = \frac{1/n\sum(x-\bar{x})(y-\bar{y})}{(\sigma_x * \sigma_y)^2}$$

R2= (1/8)* 93/ (4.062* 2.958)2 = 11.625/ (12.015)2 = 11.625/144.370 = 0.08

The coefficient of determination for this equation is 0.08 which indicates that only 8% of the variation in the dependent variable is explained by the independent variable. That is, the coefficient of determination is the proportion of the variance in the dependent variable that is predictable from the independent variable.

The coefficient of determination is the square of the correlation (r) between predicted y scores and actual y scores; thus, it ranges from 0 to 1. An R^2 of 0 means that the dependent variable cannot be predicted from the independent variable. An R^2 of 1 means the dependent variable can be predicted exactly without any error from the independent variable. An R^2 between 0 and 1 indicates the extent to which the dependent variable is predictable. An R^2 of 0.10 means that 10 percent of the variance in *Y* is predictable from *X*; an R^2 of 0.20 means that 20 percent is predictable; and so on.

11.2.6 Multiple Linear Regression

What we have seen is the simple linear regression, wherein we tried to estimate the influence of one independent variable (X) on the dependent variable (Y). Whereas, in reality, a dependent variable does not usually depend on a single independent variable alone. For e.g., if we want to predict the milk yield (Y) in a dairy farm, the Y usually depends on many independent variables (Xi) such as species, breed, feed, fodder, season, etc. However, for simplicity, we might have considered only the quantum of concentrate feed given to the dairy animals as an independent variable, keeping other variables constant (*ceteris paribus*). This may not give an accurate prediction of milk yield, as other variables also might influence the yield. In such occasions, we need to use multiple linear regression, wherein we would consider all the possible independent variables. i.e., There is just one x variable and one y variable in a simple linear regression and there is one y variable and two or more x variables in a multiple linear regression.

Multiple linear regression, also known as multiple regression, is a multivariate statistical technique that uses several explanatory (independent) variables to predict the outcome of a response or explained (dependent) variable. It is the most widely used technique in all sciences for measuring the impacts of independent (or explanatory) variables on a dependent variable.

11.2.6.1 Assumptions in a Multiple Linear Regression

1. **Linear relationship between dependent and independent variables:** There is a linear relationship between the dependent variable and each of the independent variables. Linearity (Linear relationship) indicates that the line of best fit through the data points is a straight line, rather than a curve.
2. **Independent variables not correlated with each other:** The independent variables (explanatory variables) are not related or correlated to each other. i.e., independent variables are independent and there are no hidden relationships among them. If some of the independent variables are related or correlated, then that situation is called the presence of multicollinearity in the data. Hence, we assume that there is an absence of multicollinearity between any of the independent variables in the data. It is possible that some of the independent variables may be correlated with one another, so it is important to check these before developing the regression model. If two independent variables are correlated ($r^2 > \sim 0.6$), then only one of them should be used in the regression model.
3. **Constant variance of residuals:** The amount of error in the residuals is similar at each point of the linear model. This scenario is known as homoscedasticity. i.e., There should not be heteroskedasticity meaning that the amount of error in the residuals is dissimilar. In other words, there is **homogeneity of variance.** Homoscedasticity indicates that the size of the error in the prediction does not change significantly across the values of the independent variable.

4. **Independence of observation:** The observations should be independent of one another. i.e., The values of residuals are independent. i.e., There is no autocorrelation.
5. **Multivariate normality:** Multivariate normality occurs when residuals are normally distributed. Multivariate normality is that the data follow a normal distribution.

11.2.6.2 Multiple Linear Regression Form

A common multiple linear regression will be of the form:

Y = b0 + b1X1 + b2X2 + … + bnXn + ε

where, *Y = the dependent variable*

b0 = the Y-intercept (value of Y, when all other parameters (bi's) are set to 0)

b1X1 = the regression coefficient (b1) of the first independent variable (X1), i.e., the effect of increasing the value of X1 by one unit on Y

b2X2 = the regression coefficient (b2) of the first independent variable (X2), i.e., the effect of increasing the value of X2 by one unit on Y…

bnXn = the regression coefficient (bn) of the first independent variable (Xn), i.e., the effect of increasing the value of Xn by one unit on Y

ε = error (i.e., how much variation is there in the estimate of Y)

To find the best-fit line for each independent variable, multiple linear regression calculates four things:

- Regression coefficients (all bi's) that lead to the smallest overall model error
- *t* statistic for each of the regression coefficients; and the associated *p* value (how likely the *t* statistic would have occurred by chance if the H_0 of no relationship between the independent and dependent variables is true)
- F statistic for the whole regression model fitted
- R^2 (Coefficient of Multiple Determination)

11.2.6.3 Multiple Linear Regression in Disease Loss Estimation

Thirunavukkarasu and Prabaharan (2000) used a multiple regression analysis to assess the factors that determined the economic losses from mastitis in 301 dairy animals. They collected relevant data during 1993-94 and 1994-95 from five organized dairy farms and 25 private unorganized dairy farms selected randomly and fitted a linear regression function, as below:

$$EL_L = \alpha + \beta_1X_1 + \beta_2X_2 + \beta_3X_3 + \beta_4X_4 + \mu$$

where,

EL_L = Economic losses due to mastitis per lactation in INR;

X_1 = Average daily milk yield in litres in the preceding week before infection;

X_2 = Number of infected quarters;

X_3 = Number of days of treatment;

X_4 = Reduction in lactation length in days (calculated by subtracting current lactation length from average/previous lactation length);

α, β_i = Coefficients to be estimated; and

μ = error term.

The results of the linear regression function fitted were:

Independent Variables	Regression Coefficients
Constant (Intercept) (α)	-357.8727
Average daily milk yield in litres in the preceding week before infection (X_1)	28.9354** (4.3873)
Number of infected quarters (X_2)	141.9871**(17.0478)
Number of days of treatment (X_3)	23.0261**(3.1564)
Reduction in lactation length in days (calculated by subtracting current lactation length from average/previous lactation length) (X_4)	37.1886**(2.5336)
Coefficient of Multiple Determination (R^2)	0.8485
F Statistic	414.3853**
N (Sample size)	301

(Figures in parentheses indicate standard errors) ** Significant ($P < 0.01$)

The highly significant F value indicated that the fitted regression model was a good fit model. Generally, if none or only a very few of the independent variables chosen for the model are statistically significant, the F statistic also will be not significant. That is, all the four independent variables chosen and included in the model are able to explain well the variations in the dependent variable. Also, the R^2 of 0.8485 indicates that about 85 percent of the variations in the response variable could be explained by the independent variables. Hence, the estimated regression equation can be written as:

$$EL_L = -357.8727 + 28.9354\, X_1 + 141.9871\, X_2 + 23.0261\, X_3 + 37.1886\, X_4$$

Each coefficient is interpreted as the increase in the dependent variable for every unit increase in the concerned independent variable from its average, assuming that all other independent variables are held constant. For e.g., for each additional litre of milk yielded preceding infection, the expected increase in the loss due to mastitis would be INR 28.94, assuming that all the other variables are held constant. All the other coefficients estimated for the independent variables *viz.*, number of quarters affected (X_2), number of days of treatment (X_3), and reduction in lactation length (X_4) can also be interpreted in the same way that the loss due to mastitis would increase by INR 141.99, 23.03, and 37.19, respectively, for the one unit increase in these variables from their averages concerned. However, interpreting the intercept of a regression output in any way does not always make sense to do. For e.g., in this case, the intercept is negative, which does not have an obvious interpretation. This does not mean that the model is wrong, but it simply means that the intercept by itself should not be interpreted to mean anything. The standard error is a measure of the uncertainty surrounding the estimate of the coefficient for each variable. The t-statistic can be calculated by dividing the coefficient by the standard error.

Thirunavukkarasu and Prabaharan (2000) fitted a multiple linear regression model to identify the factors determining losses due to mastitis and found that 85 percent of the variation in losses per mastitic lactation could be explained by the chosen explanatory variables. While Selvam *et al.* (2004) fitted linear regression models to explain the variations in the losses due to RD, IBD, *E. coli* infection and Coccidiosis in layer farms, Jeyakumari *et al.* (2004 and 2006) fitted linear regression models to explain the variations in the losses due to metritis and retained placenta, and to explain the variations in the incidence of postpartum, respectively, in dairy animals. Thirunavukkarasu and Kathiravan (2006) fitted six linear regression models, one each for six agroclimatic zones in Tamil Nadu to identify the factors influencing economic losses due to conception failures in artificially inseminated bovines and found that all the fitted models were significant, indicating that all were good fits. Thirunavukkarasu *et al.* (2010c and 2011c) assessed the factors influencing economic losses due to milk fever and ketosis, respectively, in dairy animals using linear regression models.

11.3 LOGISTIC REGRESSION ANALYSIS

We have seen in the above linear regression analysis that the dependent variable Y would take any value. However, there would be some occasions in scientific studies where Y may take only two values, for e.g., the presence or absence of a disease in an animal. It means that the dependent variable Y is binary in nature. In such occasions, we use logistic regression which is the statistical technique used to predict the relationship between the dependent variable (Y) and the independent variables (Xi), where Y may be Success/Failure, 0/1, True/False, or Yes/No. In short, linear regression is used for continuous Y variables, and logistic regression is used for categorical Y variables, such as survival and death. Eyduran *et al. (2005)* carried out a study to examine the effects of environmental factors on different growth factors in sheep using logistic regression.

When economic considerations of animal diseases are becoming more and more important in the farm business, decision-making with regard to the control or prevention of the factors that predispose to the diseases becomes vital. This underlines the need to assess the relationship of the animal and environmental factors with the disease incidence. In this regard, estimating the probability of an animal, characterized by its own attributes and the environment in which it is reared, getting affected by a particular disease is an issue of practical interest, as it is likely to provide information useful for determining the disease control / prevention measures.

11.3.1 Estimation of the Probability of Animals picking up Diseases

Thirunavukkarasu and Prabaharan (1999c) attempted to use the logistic regression technique to predict the probability of a milch animal picking up mastitis, by using the data collected during the years 1993-94 and 1994-95 from five organized and 25 unorganized dairy farms, randomly selected in the State of Tamil Nadu (India). In all, data on 301 mastitic animals (202 from organized farms and 99 from private farms) and 148 non-mastitic animals (99 from organized farms and 49 from private farms) were collected and analyzed.

11.3.1.1 Principle and Method of Logistic Regression Technique

Predicting whether an event will occur or not, as well as identifying the variables in making the prediction, is important in the discipline of veterinary epidemiology. The most popular multiple regression technique poses difficulties when the dependent variable can take only two values – an event occurring or not occurring. Because, in this situation, the assumptions necessary for hypothesis testing in regression analysis are necessarily violated that the distribution of errors is non-normal and the predicted values are not constrained to fall in the interval of 0 and 1. However, the logistic regression technique can estimate the probability of occurrence of an event and is the technique of choice for analyzing binary response variable in veterinary and human epidemiology (Dyke and Patterson, 1952).

This technique was employed by Thirunavukkarasu and Prabaharan (1999c) to estimate the probability that an animal with a given set of attributes will pick up mastitis or not. The model used was:

$$\text{Prob (event) or Pi} = \sum (Y = \frac{1}{Vi}) = \frac{e^{\alpha + \beta 1V1 + \beta 2V2 + ... + \beta iVi}}{1 + e^{\alpha + \beta 1V1 + \beta 2V2 + ... + \beta iVi}}$$

or equivalently, $Pi = 1 / (1 + e^{-Z})$

where, i = 1, 2, 3, …, 14;

α and βi – coefficients to be estimated;

V1 – Species indicator (= 1 if cow; = 0 if otherwise);

V2 – Breed indicator 1 (= 1 if exotic purebred cow; = 0 if otherwise);

V3 – Breed indicator 2 (= 1 if crossbred cow / Murrah or graded buffalo; = 0 if otherwise);

V4 – Average daily milk yield in litres;

V5 – Lactation number;

V6 – Stage of lactation in days;

V7 – Season dummy 1 (= 1 if rainy; = 0 if otherwise);

V8 – Season dummy 2 (= 1 if summer; = 0 if otherwise);

V9 – Stall hygiene indicator (= 1 if less hygienic; = 0 if otherwise);

V10 – Udder hygiene indicator (= 1 if less hygienic; = 0 if otherwise);

V11 – Grazing dummy (= 1 if allowed for grazing; = 0 if otherwise)

V12 – Milking method (= 1 if manual; = 0 if manual);

V13 – Weaning dummy (= 1 if day old weaning; = 0 if otherwise);

V14 – Udder morphology (= 1 if pendulous / abdominal udder or lengthy / leaky teat(s); = 0 if otherwise);

e – The base of the natural logarithm, approximately 2.718; and

Z – The linear combination of the equation such that $Z = e^{\alpha + \beta 1V1 + \beta 2V2 + \ldots + \beta iVi}$

The probability of an event not occurring is estimated as:

Prob (no event) = 1 - Prob (event)

The probability estimates will always be between 0 and 1, regardless of the value of Z. In linear regression, the parameters of the model are estimated using the least squares method, in which the regression coefficients are selected so that they result in the smallest sums of squared distances between the observed and the predicted values of the dependent variable. However, when estimated through the Ordinary Least Squares (OLS) method, the logistic regression model suffers from the following problems:

1. The variance of the disturbance term will not be homoscedastic which is against one of the assumptions of OLS;
2. The assumption of normality is no longer tenable because like the dependent variable, the error term also takes only two values;
3. The estimated probabilities lie outside the range of 0 and 1; and

4. The estimation of probability by OLS procedure assumes that the probability increases linearly with the explanatory variable, i.e., the marginal effect of the explanatory variable remains constant throughout which may not happen in reality.

Given these limitations, the logistic coefficients are estimated using the Maximum Likelihood Technique, where the coefficients that make the observed values 'most likely' are selected. The Wald statistic with a $\chi 2$ (Chi-square) distribution is used in logistic models to test the hypotheses about the coefficients. Wald statistic is the square of the ratio of the coefficients to its Standard Error (SE). That is,

$$\text{Wald} = (\beta i \,/\, SEi)^2$$

As in the case of multiple regression, the contribution of the individual variable in the logistic regression is difficult to determine, because the contribution of each variable depends on the other variables in the model. A statistic that is used to look at the partial correlation between the dependent variable and each of the independent values is the *R* statistic, which can range from -1 to +1. A positive *R*-value indicates that the likelihood of the event occurring increases as the variable increases in value. If it is negative, the opposite is true. Small *R*-values indicate a small partial contribution in the model. The equation for the statistic is:

$$R = \pm\sqrt{\frac{(\text{Wald statistic} - 2K)}{-2LL(0)}}$$

where K is the degrees of freedom for the variable (Atkinson, 1990) and - 2LL (0) is the -2 times the log-likelihood of a base model that contains only the intercept.

If the Wald statistic is less than 2K, then *R* is set to 0.

A measure of how well the model fits is the goodness of fit statistic which compares the observed probabilities to those predicted by the model. This statistic is given as:

$$Z^2 = \Sigma\,[\text{Residual}_i^2 \,/\, Pi\,(1 - Pi)]$$

where residual is the difference between the observed value Vi and the predicted values Pi.

For interpreting the logistic coefficient, the logistic model is rewritten in terms of the odds of an event occurring. The odds of the event occurring are defined as the ratio of the probability that it will occur to the probability that it will not. The logistic model rewritten in terms of the log of odds, called as logit, is as follows:

$$\text{Log}\,[Pi / (1 - Pi)] = \alpha + \beta 1V1 + \beta 2V2 + ... + \beta iVi$$

where the logistic coefficient **βi** can be interpreted as the change in the log odds associated with one unit change in the independent variable. The logistic equation can also be written in terms of odds, instead of log odd, for easier interpretation, as below:

$$Pi\,(1 - Pi) = e^{\alpha + \beta 1V1 + \beta 2V2 + ... + \beta iVi}$$

$$= e^{\alpha}\, e^{\beta 1V1 + \beta 2V2 + ... + \beta iVi}$$

where e raised to the power βi is the factor by which the odds change when the ith independent variable increases by one unit.

Now, in the following table, the estimated coefficients of the variables in the logistic regression model fitted for understanding the probability of a milch animal being mastitic are presented:

Variable		Estimated coefficient	Standard error	Wald statistic	R statistic	Exp (β)
V1	Species indicator	1.2587	0.5102	6.0868*	0.0847	3.5208
V2	Breed indicator 1	8.8225	16.6658	0.2802	0.0000	6785.1050
V3	Breed indicator 2	8.7131	16.6529	0.2738	0.0000	6082.1560
V4	Average milk yield	0.6497	0.0875	55.0867**	0.3054	1.9149
V5	Lactation number	0.4542	0.1276	12.6619**	0.1369	1.5748
V6	Stage of lactation	-0.0178	0.0030	36.1001**	-0.2448	0.9824
V7	Season dummy 1	1.7268	0.5507	9.8319**	0.1173	5.6224
V8	Season dummy 2	1.9920	0.4527	7.0164**	0.0939	3.3176
V9	Stall hygiene	0.3376	0.5659	0.3560	0.0000	1.4016
V10	Udder hygiene	3.1993	0.6047	27.9872**	0.2137	24.5153
V11	Grazing dummy	-1.5401	0.8794	3.0672	-0.0433	0.2144
V12	Milking method	0.6671	1.1942	0.3120	0.0000	1.9485
V13	Weaning dummy	2.1630	0.9212	5.5127*	0.0786	8.6970
V14	Udder morphology	1.8410	0.6777	7.3790**	0.0972	6.3026
Constant (α)		-16.6723	16.7372	0.9923	-	-

* Significant at 1 percent level of probability;** Significant at 5 percent level of probability; and the degree of freedom for each variable is 1.

Wald Statistic

The Wald statistic values obtained indicated that the logistic regression coefficients for the independent variables – species, average milk yield, lactation number, stage of lactation, season indicators 1 and 2, udder hygiene, weaning dummy, and udder morphology are all significantly different from 0 at 1 degree of freedom (either $P < 0.05$ or $P < 0.01$). The coefficients for the variables breed 1 and 2 which are considered theoretically important in influencing the probability of mastitis occurrence are found insignificant, as per the Wald statistic. This is a very undesirable property of Wald statistic. When the absolute value of a coefficient is large, the estimated SE for the coefficient is also large, which produces a small Wald statistic leading to the rejection of H0 that the coefficient is 0 (when in fact it should be rejected).

R Statistic

The *R* statistic calculated is used to look out for the partial correlation between the dependent variable and each of the independent variables, which ranges from -1 to +1. The sign of the coefficient is attached to the *R* statistic. The positive values of *R* obtained for the variables - species, milk yield, lactation number, season indicators 1 and 2, udder hygiene, weaning, and udder morphology indicate that as these variables increase in value, the likelihood of mastitis increase by the value of the concerned *R* statistic. The negative values of *R* obtained for the variables – stage of lactation and grazing indicator indicate that as these variables increase in value, the likelihood of mastitis decreases by the value of the concerned *R* statistic. Small or zero values of *R* for the statistically insignificant variables like breed indicators 1 and 2, stall hygiene, and milking method indicate that these variables contributed very little to the model.

11.3.1.2 Logit Equation

The logit equation indicates that the logistic coefficients are the changes in the log odds associated with a one-unit change in the independent variables. Rearrangement of the logistic equation obtained in terms of the odds of the event occurring is done for interpreting the coefficients estimated. Hence, the logit, the logistic model estimated in terms of the log odds, is:

$$\text{Log}\,[Pi / (1 - Pi)] = \text{Log}\,[P(\text{mastitic}) / P(\text{non-mastitic}]$$

$$= -16.6723 + 1.2587V1 + 8.8225V2 + 8.7131V3 + 0.6497V4 + 0.4542V5 - 0.0178V6 + 1.7268V7 + 1.9920V8 + 0.3376V9 + 3.1993V10 - 1.5401V11 + 0.6671V12 + 2.1630V13 + 1.8410V14$$

That is, when the species indicator changes from 0 to 1 (from buffalo to cow), *ceteris paribus,* the log odds of the animal becoming mastitic increase by 1.2587. Similarly, when any of the other variables such as season 1, season 2, udder hygiene, weaning dummy, or udder morphology changes from 0 to 1, *ceteris paribus,* the log odds of the animal becoming mastitic would increase by 1.7268, 1.9920, 3.1993, 2.1630 and 1.8410, respectively. The log odds of the animal going mastitic would increase by 0.6497 and 0.4542, when the average daily milk yield and lactation number increase by one unit (one litre and one lactation), respectively. However, when the grazing dummy changes from 0 to 1, the log odds of the animal picking up udder infection would decrease by 1.5401. Similarly, the log odds would decrease by 0.0178 when the stage of lactation increases by a day.

11.3.1.4 Logistic Equation in terms of Odds

Since it is easier to think of the odds rather than log odds, the logistic equation can be written in terms of odds as:

$$Pi / (1 - Pi) = e^{-16.6723 + 1.2587V1 + 8.8225V2 + 8.7131V3 + 0.6497V4 + 0.4542V5 - 0.0178V6 + 1.7268V7 + 1.9920V8 + 0.3376V9 + 3.1993V10 - 1.5401V11 + 0.6671V12 + 2.1630V13 + 1.8410V14}$$

The e raised to the power βi is the factor by which the odds change when the ith independent variable increases by one unit. If **β**i is positive, this factor will be greater than 1 which means that the odds are increased; if **β**i is negative, the factor will be less than 1, which means that the odds are decreased. When **β**i is 0, then the factor will be equal to 1, which would leave the odds unchanged. Hence, as seen in the last column of the table where Exp (**β**i), when the species indicator, season dummy 1, season dummy 2, udder hygiene, weaning dummy, or udder morphology changes from 0 to 1, the odds of the animal picking up mastitis would decrease by 3.5208, 5.6224, 3.3176, 24.5153, 8.6970 or 6.3026, respectively. However, the odds would decrease by 0.2144, when the grazing dummy changed from 0 to 1. At the same time, the odds would increase by 1.9149 and 1.5748, when the average milk yield and lactation number increase by one unit (one litre and one lactation) from their mean levels, respectively, while the same would decrease by 0.9824 when the stage of lactation advances by a day.

Now, calculating the odds of being mastitis for an observation in the same study (a crossbred cow, yielding an average of 9 litres of milk per day, in 2nd lactation, 15 days postpartum, rainy season, less hygienic stall, less hygienic udder management, not allowed for grazing, milked manually, calf weaned when day old, with no udder/teat abnormalities) needs the computation of the probability of this animal turning mastitic:

$= \text{Estimated } (Pi = 1) / (1 + e^{-Z})$

where $\boldsymbol{Z}$ = -16.6723 + 1.2587(1) + 8.8225 (0)+ 8.7131 (1) + 0.6497 (9) + 0.4542 (2) - 0.0178 (15) + 1.7268 (1) + 1.9920 (0) + 0.3376 (1) + 3.1993 (1) -1.5401 (0) + 0.6671 (1) + 2.1630 (0) + 1.8410 (0);

i.e., $\boldsymbol{Z = 5.7147}$

Therefore, the estimated probability for this animal is 0.9967, showing that this animal is most likely to pick up udder infection. The probability of not picking up mastitis is 0.0033 (1 – 0.9967). The odds of having mastitis can be then calculated as Pi / (1 - Pi) = 0.9967 / 0.0033 = 302.03 and the log odds as 248.

11.3.1.4 Classification Table

One way to assess how well this model fits is to compare the model's predictions with the observations. The classification table below compares the model's predictions with the observations:

Category	Predicted	Observed	% Correctly predicted
Non-mastitic (0)	130	148	87.84
Mastitic (1)	283	301	94.02
Overall	413	449	91.98

It can be seen that 130 out of the total of 148 milch animals without mastitis (87.84 percent) have been correctly classified by the model not to have mastitis. Similarly, 283 animals with mastitis (94.02 percent of the total mastitic cases) have been correctly classified to have mastitis. Overall, 91.98 percent of the total 449 milch animals have been correctly classified, except 36 cases (8.02 percent) which are misclassified, by the model. Kristula *et al.* (1992) developed a repeated measures logistic regression model to identify cows with chronic mastitis, which could not accurately classify cows with chronic mastitis.

11.3.1.5 Use of -2 times the log of the likelihood (-2LL)

Another way of assessing the goodness of fit of the model is to examine how 'likely' the sample results are, given the parameter estimates. The probability of the observed results is known as the likelihood. Since the likelihood is a small number less than 1, it is customary to use -2 times the log of the likelihood (-2LL) as a measure of how well the estimated model fits the data. A good model results in a high likelihood of the observed results. This translates to a small value for -2LL. If a model fits perfectly, the likelihood is 1, and -2 times the log likelihood is 0. Let us look at the table below:

Particulars	Values
-2LL when constant alone is included in the model	569.251
-2LL when all the independent variables are included	178.751
Goodness of fit	734.382*
χ^2 (Chi-square) of the model	390.500*
Improvement of the square over the model with only constant	390.500*

* Significant at 1 percent level of probability (df = 14)

For the logistic regression model that contains only the constant, -2LL is 569.251. For the model with all the independent variables, the value of -2LL is 178.751 which is smaller than the -2LL for the model containing only the constant. The goodness of fit statistic is 734.382. The model χ^2 (Chi-square), the difference between -2LL for the model with only the constant and -2LL for the model with all the independent variables is 390.500 (569.251 - 178.751), which tests the H0 that the coefficients for all the variables included in the model, except constant, are 0. The degrees of freedom are the difference between the number of parameters in the two models. The 'improvement' is the change in -2LL between successive stages of model building, which tests the H0 that the coefficients for the variables added at the last step are 0. Since the study had only two models – the constant only model and the model with a constant and 14 independent variables, the χ^2 value for the model and the improvement are the same.

Earlier, in the parameters estimates table, we saw that the breed indicator variables 1 and 2 had larger coefficients and, as a result, larger SEs leading to the conclusion of the 'insignificant' contribution of these two theoretically important variables to the model, expressed in terms of small Wald statistic. To overcome this undesirable property, three other logistic models were tried – one without the variable breed indicator 1, another without the variable breed indicator 2, and the third without both and the resulting changes in the log likelihood were examined, as below:

Logistic model	**-2LL**
With constant and all the independent variables	178.751
With constant and all the variables except breed 1	188.093
With constant and all the variables except breed 2	191.111
With constant and all the variables except breed 1 and breed 2	191.734

A good model is one that results in a high likelihood of the observed results, leading to a small value for -2LL. However, when the variables in question are removed from the model, -2LL increases indicating that the H0 of zero coefficients of these variables should be rejected. That is, even though the Wald statistic failed to recognize the contribution of these variables to the model, basing the hypothesis test on the changes in log likelihood in the models with or without these variables demonstrated the significance of their contributions to the model.

Houben *et al.* (1993), using their logistic regression model, also made similar observations that the risk of mastitis was influenced by the stage of lactation (higher risk in early stage of lactation), lactation number (higher risk in higher parity), and milk yield (higher risk in high producing cows). A similar attempt was also made by Nielen *et al.* (1995) to develop a logistic model for detecting subclinical mastitis based on milk yield, parity, and days in milk among others which had a specificity of 90 percent for individual cases.

11.4 DISCRIMINANT ANALYSIS

Discriminant analysis is a multivariate analytical technique used to distinguish statistically between two or more groups of cases, using a set of discriminating variables that measure characteristics on which the groups are expected to differ. The objective of this technique is to weigh and linearly combine the discriminating variables in some fashion so that the groups are made as distinct as possible (Ngategize and Kaneene, 1985). In this analysis, a linear combination of the independent variables is formed to serve as the basis for assigning the cases to groups. The information contained in multiple independent variables is summarized into a single index and the weights are estimated so that they result in the best separation between the groups.

For example, a veterinarian may perform a discriminant analysis to identify cows at high or low risk for mastitis (Thirunavukkarasu, 1996), based on some animal and environmental variables/attributes (e.g., breed, stage of lactation, udder hygiene, etc.) There are several different ways to conduct a discriminant analysis. The approach described here is based on linear regression.

11.4.1 Two-Group Discriminant Analysis

A common research problem in veterinary epidemiology involves classifying the animals into two groups, based on two or more quantitative or qualitative dependent variables.

- The dependent variable is a dichotomous, categorical variable, that can take only two values like Yes or No, Present or Not present).
- The dependent variable is expressed as a dummy variable (having values of 0 or 1).
- Animals are assigned to either of the two groups, based on whether the dependent variable is 1 or 0.
- The regression equation is called as the discriminant function. The biggest difference between discriminant analysis and standard regression analysis is the use of a categorical variable as a dependent variable.

The key steps in the analysis include

- Estimating the regression coefficients;
- Assessing the fit of the discriminant (regression) equation to the data included;
- Assessing the ability of the discriminant equation to correctly classify the animals; and

- Assessing the relative importance of the independent variables considered.

11.4.2 Multiple Discriminant Analysis

Although discriminant analysis can be used for more than two groups, such an analysis will be complicated. Because, with more than two groups, there will also be more than two discriminant functions. For example, if we want to classify cows into three groups – high-risk, medium-risk, and low-risk groups to pick up mastitis, then we will need to have a two-group discriminant analysis, one discriminant function to classify cows as high-risk or medium-risk groups and another function to classify medium-risk or low-risk groups. Here, the goal will be to define discriminant functions that maximize differences between groups and minimize differences within groups. The calculations to do this will be very complex.

An Example

Thirunavukkarasu (2003b) used the discriminant analysis to distinguish statistically between mastitic and non-mastitic groups of milch animals, through a set of variables (both animal and environmental factors) on which the groups did differ, using SPSS® for Windows™: Release 6.0. The linear discriminant function used was of the following form:

Z = a + b1M1 + b2M2 + b3M3 + … + biMi

i = 1, 2, 3, …, 11

where

Z – Total discriminant score for mastitic and non-mastitic milch animals

M1 – Standardized species indicator (=1 if cow, =0 if otherwise)

M2 – Standardized breed indicator (=1 if non-descript cow/buffalo, =2 if graded/Murrah buffalo, =3 if crossbred cow, =4 if exotic purebred cow)

M3 – Standardized average daily milk yield in litres

M4 – Standardized lactation number

M5 – Standardized stage of lactation in days

M6 – Standardized season indicator score (=1 if winter, =2 if summer, =3 if rainy)

M7 – Standardized stall hygiene score (=1 if cleaning daily with disinfectants, =2 if cleaning daily only with water, =3 if occasional cleaning, =4 if no cleaning at all)

M8 – Standardized udder hygiene score (=1 if cleaning daily with disinfectants, =2 if cleaning daily only with water, =3 if occasional cleaning, =4 if no cleaning at all)

M9 – Standardized method of milking indicator (=1 if machine milking, =0 if hand milking)

M10 – Standardized weaning indicator (=1 if day-old weaning, =2 if weaning at first week, =3 if weaning at third months, =5 if no weaning)

M11 – Standardized udder morphology score (=1 if no udder/teat abnormalities, =2 if udder/teat abnormalities)

a, bi – Coefficients to be estimated

The variables were standardized (to a mean of 0 and a standard deviation of 1) to adjust for the unequal means and standard deviations, as the magnitude of unstandardized coefficients cannot be a good index of relative importance, when the variables differ in the units of measurement.

If a linear discriminant function is to distinguish the milch animals that pick up mastitis from those that do not, the groups must differ in their Z values. Therefore, the bi's are chosen so that the values of the discriminant function differ as much as possible between the groups, or so that the discriminant score, the ratio – *(between-groups sum of squares) / (within-group's sum of squares)*, called as eigen value, is maximum. The discriminant score for a particular observation is obtained by multiplying the standardized coefficients by the values of the variables and summing these products.

Wilk's lambda statistic, sometimes called as the U statistic, is the test for the univariate equality of group means. When variables are considered individually, lambda is the ratio of the *within-group's sum of squares* to the *total sum of squares.* A lambda of 1 results when all the observed group means are equal. Values close to 0 occur when within-group variability is small compared to the total variability - that is, when most of the total variability is attributable to the differences between the groups. Thus, large values of lambda indicate that group means do not appear to be different, while small values indicate that group means do appear to be different.

The Mahalanobis distance D^2 is a generalized measure of the distance between two groups. The Mahalanobis distance D^2 is:

$$D^2 = (n-g)\sum_{i=1}^{p}\sum_{j=1}^{p} w_{ij}(m_{ia}-m_{ib})(m_{ja}-m_{jb})$$

where,

n – sample size

g – number of groups

p – number of variables

w_{ij} – an element from the inverse of the within-groups covariance matrix

m_{ia} – mean for the ith variable in the group a

m_{ib} – mean for the ith variable in the group b

m_{ja} – mean for the jth variable in the group a

m_{jb} – mean for the jth variable in the group b

The discriminant function is to be tested for significance to examine whether the variables considered together could significantly discriminate between the two groups, using the following F statistic:

$$F = \left[\frac{n1n2(n1 + n2 - p - 1)}{p(n1 + n2)(n1 + n2 - 2)} \right] D^2$$

where,

D^2 – Mahalanobis statistic

p – number of variables

n_1 – number of mastitic cases

n_2 – number of non-mastitic cases

Using the discriminant score, it is possible to obtain a rule for classifying cases into one of the two groups, based on Bayes' rule. The probability that a case with a discriminant score of Z belongs to group i is estimated by:

$$P\left(\frac{Gi}{Z}\right) = \frac{P\left(\frac{Z}{Gi}\right) P(Gi)}{\sum_{i=1}^{g} P\left(\frac{Z}{Gi}\right) P(Gi)}$$

where,

P(Gi) is the prior probability, an estimate of the likelihood that a case belongs to a particular group when no information about it is available;

P(Z/Gi) is the conditional probability of Z given the group, the probability of obtaining a particular discriminant function value of Z if the case is a member of group 1 or group 2; and

P(Gi/Z) is the posterior probability, an estimate of how likely membership in various groups is, given the available information.

A case is classified based on the discriminant score, in the group for which the posterior probability is the largest. That is, it is assigned to the most likely group based on its discriminant score. The discriminant function is used to measure the net effect of the variables. It also helps to know the relative importance of the variables to discriminate between mastitic and non-mastitic milch animals. The method seeks to obtain coefficients such that the squared difference between the mean Z score for one group and the mean Z group for the other group is as large as possible in relation to the variation of the Z scores within the groups.

Stepwise variable selection

Instead of using a large number of potential variables to separate the groups without knowing which are important for group separation, it is better to identify the good predictor variables using the algorithm for variable selection - stepwise selection. Two criteria are usually used for this, *viz.*, minimization of Wilk's lambda and maximization of Mahalanobis distance (D^2). In this stepwise method, the first variable included in the analysis has the largest acceptable value and is selected. After the first variable is entered, the criterion is reapplied to all the other variables not included in the model and the variable with the largest acceptable criterion value is entered next. The selection of variables is terminated when no more variables meet the entry criterion. Entry of each variable is considered as a step. The maximum number of steps permitted is twice the number of chosen independent variables. That is, 22 steps were done in this case. The problem of multicollinearity was also tested before a variable was entered into the model by checking the tolerance of a variable, a measure of the degree of linear association between the variables. All the 11 variables had a high tolerance of 1, indicating the absence of multicollinearity.

11.4.3 Discriminant Function Fitted

$Z = 0.00125 + 0.12844\ M1 + 0.08898\ M2 + 0.60948\ M3 + 0.19991\ M4 - 0.47702\ M5 + 0.25698\ M6 + 0.10986\ M7 + 0.61047\ M8 + 0.01766\ M9 + 0.02127\ M10 + 0.20717\ M11$

The Mahalanobis D^2 statistic and F ratio calculated are 2.3498 and 20.7204, respectively, which imply that the F calculated based on D^2 shows a significant discriminating power between the two groups of animals. Hence, it can be concluded that the variables considered in the model fitted together are able to classify effectively the mastitic and non-mastitic milch animals.

The value of F is tested for its significance with p and $(n_1 + n_2 - p - 1)$ degrees of freedom. The results of the test for univariate equality of group means are presented below:

Variable		Wilk's lambda	F statistic	Significance
M1	Species	0.99358	2.8863	0.0900
M2	Breed	0.92049	38.6125	0.0000
M3	Milk yield	0.63751	254.1620	0.0000
M4	Lactation number	0.99807	0.8654	0.3527
M5	Stage of lactation	0.81200	103.4898	0.0000
M6	Season	0.92007	38.8316	0.0000
M7	Stall hygiene	0.92518	36.1515	0.0000
M8	Udder hygiene	0.68666	203.9754	0.0000
M9	Milking method	0.99651	1.5633	0.2118
M10	Weaning practice	0.99507	2.2153	0.1374
M11	Udder morphology	0.95511	21.0081	0.0000

A lambda of 1 or close to 1 indicates that all the observed group means are equal. Values close to 0 occur when within-group variability is small compared to the total variability. As could be seen in the significance column, the variables *viz.*, breed, milk yield, stage of lactation, season, stall hygiene, udder hygiene, and udder morphology, as the observed significance levels are less than 0.05 for these variables, have the means which are most different for the mastitic and non-mastitic milch animals and the hypothesis 'that all group means of these variables are equal' is rejected. The F values are nothing but those calculated from a one-way ANOVA for each variable.

To know the relative importance of each variable's power to discriminate between the two groups, the percentage contribution of each variable to the total distance measured is presented in the following table:

Variable	Estimated Coefficient (EC)	Mean Difference (MD)	EC X MD	% contribution
Species	0.12844	0.1702	0.02186	0.92378
Breed	0.08898	0.5992	0.05332	2.26203
Milk yield	0.60948	1.2794	0.77977	33.08077
Lactation number	0.19991	0.0934	0.01867	0.79205
Stage of lactation	–0.47702	-0.9214	0.43950	18.64524
Season	0.25698	0.6008	0.15438	6.54938
Stall hygiene	0.10986	0.5813	0.06386	2.70918
Udder hygiene	0.61047	1.1895	0.72615	30.80600
Milking method	0.01766	0.1255	0.00322	0.13660
Weaning practice	0.02127	-0.1492	-0.00317	0.13448
Udder morphology	0.20717	0.4502	0.09327	3.95686
		Total	**2.35717**	**99.99997 ≈100.00**

Interpretation of discriminant coefficients is similar to that in multiple regression. The variables with large coefficients do contribute more to the overall discriminant score. It can be seen from the table that the average daily milk yield (33.08 percent), udder hygiene (30.81 percent), stage of lactation (18.65 percent), season (6.55 percent) and udder morphology (3.96 percent) are the important factors that discriminated mastitic cases from non-mastitic cases and these variables collectively contributed to 93.05 percent of the total distance measured.

However, when the variables were selected using the stepwise procedure, the above percent contribution table shrunk, with a few variables getting eliminated, as below:

Variable	Estimated Coefficient (EC)	Mean Difference (MD)	EC X MD	% contribution
Species	0.58588	0.1702	0.0997	4.1740
Milk yield	0.63603	1.2794	0.8141	34.0827
Lactation number	0.20018	0.0934	0.0187	0.7829
Stage of lactation	–0.48329	-0.9214	0.4453	18.6427
Season	0.26483	0.6008	0.1591	6.6608
Udder hygiene	0.63836	1.1895	0.7593	31.7885
Udder morphology	0.20526	0.4502	0.0924	3.8684
		Total	**2.3886**	**100.00**

It can now be seen from the table that the average daily milk yield (34.08 percent), udder hygiene (31.79 percent), stage of lactation (18.64 percent), season (6.66 percent), species (4.17 percent) and udder morphology (3.87 percent) are the important factors that discriminated mastitic cases from non-mastitic cases and these variables now collectively contributed to 99.01 percent of the total distance measured. The convenience resulting from this step-wise analysis is that good results, if not better, are now obtained with a smaller number (only 7 out of 11) of variables, which also shows that only these variables have the power of discrimination. One more important point that should be noted is the entry of the variable – milk yield which was not contributing much to the total distance measured earlier. More useful information could also be derived from the results as presented in a Confusion Matrix (Classification of results):

11.4.4 Confusion Matrix (Classification of Results)

Actual group	No. of cases	Predicted membership	
		1	0
Mastitis: 1	301	276 (91.7%)	25 (8.3%)
Non-mastitis: 0	148	15 (10.1%)	133 (89.9%)
Total	449	**(276 + 133) / 449 * 100 = 91.09%**	

The table shows the numbers of correct and incorrect classifications for each group. Of 301 cases of mastitis group, 276 (91.7%) were predicted correctly to be the members of that group, while 25 (8.3%) were assigned incorrectly to non-mastitis group. Similarly, 133 (89.9%) out of 148 of the non-mastitis group were identified correctly and 15 (10.1%) were misclassified. Hence, the overall percentage of cases correctly classified was 91.09 percent (i.e., 409 out of 449). Overall, the discriminant model so developed could discriminate 91 percent of mastitic and non-mastitic animals correctly, by analyzing some of the animal and environmental factors/attributes. Thus, this model could very well be used in the field conditions to predict the milch animals more susceptible to mastitis and to make necessary management alterations to prevent mastitis.

11.5 Cox Regression

Cox regression is used in survival time analysis to determine the influence of different variables on survival time. The variables can be any mixture of continuous, binary, or categorical data. The Cox hazard model is then used to determine the effect on survival time. Cox Regression allows us to determine the effects of multiple independent variables on a time-to-event outcome, either to test hypotheses about the independent variables or to build a predictive model. In 1972, Sir David Cox wrote an article to incorporate patients' baseline characteristics, such as age, clinical history or exposure to certain factors, and time [Cox, 1972]. The Cox regression model is also known as proportional hazards regression analysis.

11.5.1 Survival Time Analysis

In survival time analysis, the survival times of the animals that have a particular disease are recorded. We would then know how many of the animals studied remain alive over time. This survival time analysis considers a variable that has a start time and an end time when a certain event (disease) occurs. The time between the start time and the event of death is considered in the analysis. This can be measured in days, weeks or months. There is a problem in this type of study that the study cannot last indefinitely. Because we have only limited time and financial resources, survival time analysis has to have a start date and an end date. If there is no clear event (death) date for a case, then it is referred to as censoring.

If we want to analyze the survival time after the detection of a disease, we are not interested in the survival time alone, but also in what influences the survival time. So, we want to know if the survival time depends on one or more factors, called predictors or independent variables. This regression is then used to evaluate the effect of each predictor on the survival time.

11.5.2 Assumptions of a Cox Regression

Constant effect of predictor variables: The effect of the predictor variables on the hazard function is assumed to be constant over time.

Independence of survival times: Cox regression assumes that the survival times of individuals are independent of each other, given the values of the predictor variables. This means that the survival time of one animal does not influence the survival time of another animal.

Linearity: Cox regression assumes that the relationship between the predictor variables and the log of the hazard rate is linear. This assumption implies that the effect of a continuous predictor is constant over its entire range.

No Multicollinearity: Cox regression assumes that there is no multicollinearity among the predictor variables. Multicollinearity occurs when two or more predictor variables are highly correlated, making it difficult to separate their individual effects on the outcome.

No Outliers: Cox regression assumes that there are no outliers that can significantly affect the results. Outliers are observations that deviate substantially from the overall pattern of the data and can distort the estimated coefficients.

No Interaction Between Predictor Variables: Cox regression assumes that there is no interaction between the predictor variables.

11.5.3 Cox Hazard Functional Model

The survival time after diagnosis of a disease in animals depends on a few predictor variables such as the type of the disease, severity of the disease, age of the animal affected, treatment given, etc. Multiple linear regression cannot be used for analyzing the time-to-event data, since there is no way to handle censored observations. Censored cases are those for which the event has not occurred. However, this cannot be ignored, but must be incorporated into the analysis. A special type of regression model namely the Cox regression model is used to analyze such data that contain censored observations. The Cox regression model is:

$$h(t) = [h_0(t)]\, e^{(b_1x_1 + b_2x_2 + \ldots + b_px_p)}$$

where x_1 to x_p are the independent variables (covariates).

From the above model, we can see that for any values of the independent variables, the proportion of getting into a hazard at time 't' depends on two quantities. The first, designated as $h_0(t)$ in the equation, is called the baseline hazard function. The baseline hazard function is similar to the constant term in multiple regression. That is, it is the reference value that is increased or decreased depending on the values of the independent variables and their relationship with the dependent variable. The second part of the equation, $e^{(b_i x_i)}$, in the model, depends not on time but on the values of the independent variables (covariates) like x_1 to x_p and the regression coefficients b_i.

To examine the effects of independent variables on hazard, we fit a Cox regression model with death time as the dependent variable and the independent variables as the covariates. One important statistic that is calculated here is the Wald statistic which is the ratio of the coefficient to its standard error. For large samples, the Wald statistic has a χ^2 distribution. The letter 'R' measures the partial correlation of each independent variable with the dependent variable. R ranges from -1 to +1. R is 0 if the Wald statistic is less than twice the degrees of freedom for the variable.

In sheep farming, there are at least two economically important diseases *viz.*, sheep pox and enterotoxaemia which cause very high mortality in the affected animals. Hence, Senthilkumar *et al.* (2006) attempted to assess the survival times in sheep affected by these diseases. It will be useful to understand the models fitted by them and to comprehend the predictor variables chosen, coefficients estimated and other measures assessed.

11.5.4 Cox Hazard Functional Model fitted for Sheep Pox

The results of the Cox hazard functional model fitted for sheep pox are presented in the table below. While the 'B' column presents the coefficients estimated, the standard errors of the coefficients are shown in the next column. The square of the ratio of the coefficient to its standard error is given in the column labelled 'Wald stat'. The degree of freedom associated with the statistic is 1. From column `Sig', it can be seen that the coefficients for age, breed, vaccination, and veterinary care are significantly different from 0, while the coefficients for others are not. The column 'Exp (B)' indicates the percentage change in the hazard rate for a unit increase in the covariate. For example, a unit increase in the breed and veterinary care indicators would increase the hazard rate by 10.49 and 15.61 percent respectively. Since the ratio of the hazard rates are 1.1049 and 4.1561. Similarly, a unit increase in age and vaccination would decrease the hazard rate by 66.40 and 67.23 percent respectively.

Cox hazard functional model for sheep pox

Variable	B	SE	Wald stat	df	Sig	R	Exp (B)
Age	-0.4095	0.1004	16.6448	1	0.0000	-0.0394	0.6640
Sex	0.0319	0.1077	0.0877	1	0.7671	0.0000	1.0324
Breed	0.0997	0.0456	4.7927	1	0.0286	0.0172	1.1049
Season	0.0972	0.0796	1.4914	1	0.2220	0.0000	1.1020
Vaccination	-0.3971	0.1013	15.3480	1	0.0001	-0.0376	0.6723
Veterinary Care	1.4246	0.1037	188.8740	1	0.0000	0.1407	4.1561

[Note: Age – 1 if adult, 0 if young; Sex – 1 if female, 0 if male; Breed – 3 if Trichy Black, 2 if Mandya, 1 if Mecheri), Season - (4 if winter, 3 if northeast monsoon, 2 if summer, 1 if southwest monsoon); Vaccination – 1 if unvaccinated, 0 if vaccinated); Veterinary Care – 1 if not given, 0 if given)]

Further, for the dichotomous significant variables (age, vaccination, and veterinary care), the Exp (B) value is called as the Relative Risk (RR) associated with the variable. If RR is one, the variable concerned does not influence survival. But if RR is less than one, a positive value for the variable is associated with increased survival, since the hazard rate is decreased. The RR for the non-provision of veterinary care is 4.16, which indicates that the estimated risk of dying is 4.16 times higher in an animal not provided any veterinary care, than the one which received veterinary attention.

11.5.5 Cox Hazard Functional Model fitted for Enterotoxaemia

From column `Sig', it can be seen that the coefficients for breed, deworming and veterinary care are significantly different from 0, while the coefficients for others are not. The column Exp (B), which is the relative risk, indicates that a unit increase in breed and veterinary care indicators would increase the hazard rate by 78.00 and 2.43 percent respectively, since the ratio of the hazard rates are 1.7800 and 3.0243. Similarly, a unit increase in deworming would decrease the hazard rate by 36.01 percent. It can also be seen that the relative risk for the non-provision of veterinary care is 3.02 which indicates that the estimated risk of succumbing to the disease is 3.02 times higher in an animal not provided any veterinary care, than the one which received veterinary care.

Cox hazard functional model for Enterotoxaemia

Variable	B	SE	Wald stat	df	Sig	R	Exp (B)
Age	-0.1183	0.5269	0.0504	1	0.8224	0.0000	0.8885
Sex	-0.0431	0.2068	0.0435	1	0.8348	0.0000	0.9578
Breed	0.5766	0.2974	3.7581	1	0.0526	0.0359	1.7800
Season	0.0070	0.5018	0.0002	1	0.9888	0.0000	1.0071
Deworming	-1.0213	0.4721	4.6796	1	0.0305	-0.0443	0.3601
Veterinary Care	1.1067	0.2111	27.4783	1	0.000	0.1365	3.0243

[Note: Age – 1 if young, 0 if adult; Sex – 1 if male, 0 if female; Breed – 3 if Mecheri, 2 if Trichy Black, 1 if Mandya), Season - (4 if Southwest monsoon, 3 if Northeast monsoon, 2 if Winter, 1 if Summer); Deworming – 1 if not done, 0 if done); Veterinary Care – 1 if not given, 0 if given)]

12

Programming Techniques for Animal Health Economics

Programming techniques are used the mathematical tools by the scientists, economists, and planners to specify the optimum combination of resources and enterprises in farms and firms, to identify the profit maximizing mixes of commodities to be produced, to specify the cost minimizing methods of production and transportation of goods, to identify the least cost locations from which raw materials can be purchased, to determine the locations of production at which a particular commodity should be produced and the consumption centres to which it should be shipped, and to specify the least cost ingredients of a feed or ration which must meet the specified nutritional requirements. Programming techniques can be either linear or non-linear. Although several non-linear programming techniques (like quadratic, integer, separable, dynamic programming, etc., which are very complex to work with) are available, we will largely deal with linear programming technique and to a certain extent will brief the theory of dynamic programming.

12.1 LINEAR PROGRAMMING

Linear Programming (popularly abbreviated as LP) is a mathematical procedure used to solve a wide range of management problems from compounding of a chick mash to the logistics of a milk transport system. It is defined as a mathematical procedure to allocate scarce resources to competing production activities in an optimal way if the problem can be expressed as a linear objective function and linear inequality constraints. This tool has application opportunities in any type of problems for which an objective can be defined in quantitative terms. Ordinarily, the objective will be one of maximising or minimising quantities. The quantity to be maximized can be profits, revenues, total output, etc. The quantity to be minimized may be the cost of a good or service, the cost of transportation between the origins and destinations of a product, the cost of storage facilities or the amount of labour required to do a particular work.

12.1.1 Advantages of LP

1. The result obtained through LP is the best possible plan that can be formulated for the data used. That is, no other more profitable production system or transportation system can be developed without either altering some of the assumptions or violating some of the constraints imposed.
2. Problems of any dimension can be solved by this technique.

12.1.2 Disadvantages of LP

1. LP can be used only when the constraints and objective function of the problems are linear in relationship. However, in real situations, the constraints or objective functions are not linear.
2. This technique often gives an optimal solution with decimal points of objective function values, although the values of labour or machine cannot be in decimal values. But we may use the nearest whole number.
3. Access to a computer is needed to carry out the calculation of the problems of bigger dimensions.
4. It requires a certain amount of expert knowledge and a good deal of practice.

12.1.3 Components of an LP Problem

An LP problem has three quantitative components, *viz.*, 1. an objective; 2. a few alternate methods to achieve the objective; and 3. two or more restrictions or constraints to achieve the objective. A problem, which has all these three components, in any farm, firm, factory, industry, etc. can be expressed as an LP problem.

The Objective

For a typical farm management problem, the objective will be maximum income or minimum cost. For instance, the farmer may be interested in maximizing his farm income. The objective must be clearly specified, if the result obtained from LP is to be sensible. The objective of an LP study may be expressed in physical or monetary.

Alternate methods of attaining the objective

Given the objective, it is obvious that, unless it can be attained in more than one way, there is no problem to be analyzed. If a farmer can produce only milk and that too in only one way, then the solution to the problem of maximizing farm income is unimportant. He can produce as much milk as possible using the only technique available. But, given several methods or processes by which the objective can be attained, we choose from them the method or process that is the most efficient in converting resources into the objective.

Restrictions or Constraints

An LP problem does not exist unless resources are restricted or limited. A firm / farm may have a given amount of land, fixed space for buildings, and a given amount of machinery, labour, and capital. In a nutrition problem, the restrictions are the minimum amounts of vitamins, calories, minerals etc. necessary for a healthy diet. In a transportation problem, the restrictions are the supplies of commodities at production centres and the quantities demanded at consuming centres.

12.1.4 Formulating an LP Problem

A butcher traditionally makes meatloaf by combining beef and pork. Beef contains 80% lean meat and 20% fat and costs Rs.240/- kg. Pork contains 68% lean meat and 32% fat and costs Rs.400/- kg. In addition, he also must keep the fat content of the meatloaf to no more than 25%. How much of each kind of meat should be used in each kg of meatloaf if the butcher wants to minimize the cost of 1 kg of meatloaf?

Identification of decision variables to be optimized

Decision variables: X_B = Quantity of Beef in kg; and X_P = Quantity of Pork in kg. Expression of these variables in mathematical form as an objective function:

Objective function: Minimize Z (or Min. Z) = $240\ X_B + 400\ X_P$

where 240 is the price of Beef per kg, and 400 is the price of Pork per kg

Identification of all resource requirements and resource restrictions

Subject to

$0.20\ X_B + 0.32\ X_P \leq 0.25$ ......Constraint 1

(Inequality - less than or equal to – constraint, because you have <)

(where 0.20 = 20% fat in Beef and 0.32 = 32% fat in Pork; '≤' indicates less than or equal to constraint, i.e. the fat content in the meatloaf made should be no more than 25%)

$X_{B+} X_P = 1$ ......Constraint 2

(Equality constraint because we have =)

(indicates both Beef and Pork are to be used for making meatloaf)

$X_{B,}\ X_P \geq 0$ ......Constraint 3

(This is called the non-negativity constraint, indicating that the quantity of Beef and the quantity of Pork cannot be used in negative quantities. This constraint will be there in all the LP problems.)

Rewriting this LP problem, we will have:

Objective function

Min. $Z = 240\ X_B + 400\ X_P$

Subject to the constraints,

$0.20\ X_B + 0.32\ X_P \leq 0.25$

$X_B + X_P = 1$

$X_B, X_P \geq 0$

General Form of the LP Problem

Hence, the general form of the minimization LP problem will be:

Min. $Z = C_1\ X_1 + C_2\ X_2$

Subject to

$a_{11}\ X_1 + a_{12} X_2 \leq b_1$

$a_{21} X_1 + a_{22} X_2 \leq b_2$

$X_1, X_2 \geq 0$

Similarly, the general form of the maximization LP problem will be:

Max. $Z = C_1\ X_1 + C_2\ X_2$

Subject to

$a_{11}\ X_1 + a_{12} X_2 > b_1$

$a_{21} X_1 + a_{22} X_2 > b_2$

$X_1, X_2 \geq 0$

Look at the differences in the objective function and the constraints of a maximization problem and a minimization problem. In the objective function, we have Min. for the minimization problem and Max. for the maximization problem. In the constraints, we have less than or equal to (≤ inequality) constraint for the minimization problem and greater than or equal to (> inequality) constraint for the maximization problem. However, the latter one is not a universal rule, as sometimes, you may have one or two greater than or equal to constraint(s) for a minimization problem and less than or equal to constraint(s) for a maximization problem. An equality (=) constraint may also be there in maximization / minimization problems, as we have seen in our example.

Hence, more generally,

$$z = \sum_{j=1}^{n} CjXj$$

(j = 1, 2, 3, ..., n)

Subject to

$$\sum_{i=1}^{n} aijXj \lesseqgtr bi$$

(i = 1, 2, 3, ..., n)

$X_j > 0$

where Cj are the coefficients representing the per unit contribution of decision variable Xj to the value of the objective function;

aij's are the technological coefficients or input-output coefficients; may be positive, negative, or zero; and bi's are the total availability of the resources.

Matrix form of the LP problem is:

$Z = C'X$

Subject to

$$AX \gtreqless B$$

$X \geq 0$

Where,

$C' = (C_1, C_2, \ldots, C_n)$

$B = (b_1, b_2, \ldots, b_m)$

$$X = \begin{pmatrix} x_1 \\ x_2 \\ \cdot \\ x_n \end{pmatrix} \quad A = \begin{pmatrix} a_{11} & a_{12} & \ldots a_{1n} \\ a_{21} & a_{22} & \ldots a_{2n} \\ \cdot & & \\ a_{m1} & a_{m2} & \ldots a_{mn} \end{pmatrix}$$

12.1.5 Solving LP Problems

LP problems can be solved by two methods: 1) Graphical Method and (2) Simplex Method. Though the graphical method is simple, it can be applied only to problems which have at most 3 decision variables. But, by simplex algebraic method, we can solve any LP problem with more than two decision variables too. In simplex problems, we transform the verbal expression of the problems into a mathematical form (algebraic form) and further into standard form by removing the inequalities in the constraints. What is being done in graphical approach is that all the constraints are plotted on a graph, a feasible region is being outlined depending on the direction shown by the constraints and an optimal solution point is being searched and obtained using the objective function line.

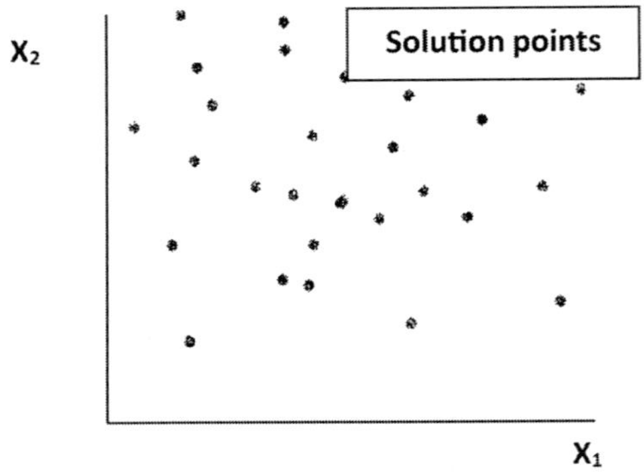

E.g., Max $Z = 10\ X_1 + 9\ X_2$

Subject to:

$7/10\ X_1 + X_2 \leq 630$

$½\ X_1 + 5/6\ X_2 \leq 600$

$X_1 + 2/3\ X_2 \leq 708$

$1/10\ X_1 + ¼\ X_2 \leq 135$

$X_{1,}\ X_2 \geq 0$

12.1.5.1 Graphical Method of Finding Solution to LP Problem

Step 1: Formulate the LP problem.

Step 2: Construct an X - Y coordinate graph.

Step 3: Plot all the constraint lines on the graph.

Step 4: Determine the valid side of each constraint line.

Step 5: Identify the feasible solution region.

Step 6: Plot the objective function on the graph.

Step 7: Move the objective function line parallel, upward or downward, as the case may be.

Step 8: Find the optimum solution point by locating the point of tangency between the objective function line and the boundary of the feasible region.

By choosing the upper right-hand quarter of the graph, we ensure that the non-negativity constraint is taken care of. Each point (each combination of X_1 and X_2) in the graph is known as the solution point, but not the optional point that we are interested in. To satisfy the constraints being imposed, we separate the whole graph space into a feasible region or zone or area and an infeasible zone or zone or area, with regard to the constraints.

To find the value of one variable, we equate the other variable to zero and find the value. For e.g., in the constraint b_1,$7/10\ X_1 + X_2 \leq 630$, X_2 is made equal to zero and the value of X_1 is calculated. i.e., $7/10\ X_1 + 0 = 630$ and so $X_1 = 900$ and by making X_1 equal to 0, we find that $X_2 = 630$. We plot these two values on the graph in their respective axes and connect these two points ($X_1 = 900$ and $X_2 = 630$) to obtain the line of b1 constraint, which separates the whole graphical space into feasible and infeasible zones with respect to b1 constraint.

The triangle OAB is called as the feasible region, which accommodates all the feasible points of production. Beyond this region, the zone is infeasible. Because, production of any levels of products of X_1 and X_2 within the feasible zone OAB will use the resource b_1 lesser than or equal to the available 630 units and any point of production beyond this zone will need b_1 resource something in excess of the available 630 units of b_1.

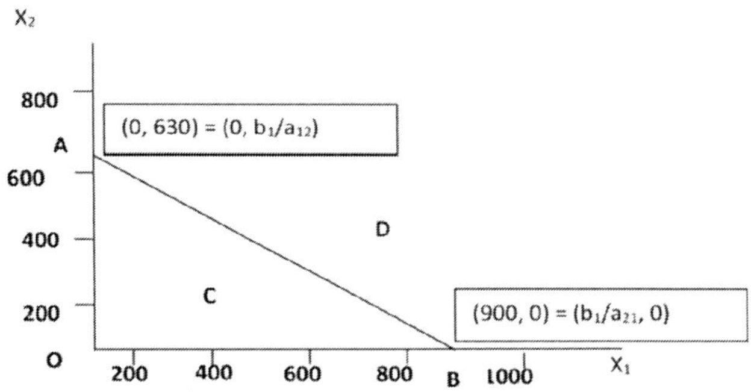

For e.g., at point C,

$7/10\ X_1 + X_2 \leq 630$; $7/10 \times 400 + 1 \times 200 \leq 630$; $280 + 200 =$ **480 < 630**

(**feasible**, because this point satisfies b1 constraint. It requires only less than the available b1 constraint or resource of 630 units)

However, at point D,

$7/10\ X_1 + X_2 \leq 630$; $7/10 \times 800 + 1 \times 400 \leq 630$; $560 + 400 =$ **960> 630**

(**infeasible**, because this point does not satisfy b1 constraint. This point violates the b1 constraint, as it requires more than the available b1 constraint of 630 units)

Similarly, all other constraints can also be plotted on the same graph, as below. Now, look at point E and find that this solution point is feasible for the constraints b_2 and b_3, but infeasible for b_1 and b_4. Feasible solution points are called the solution points which are bounded by the constraints. The area is called the feasible region, which consists of all the potential feasible solution points. However, the optimal solution point will be a unique one. The solution points within or on the boundary line of the feasible region are the feasible solution points. All of these feasible solution points have the potential to become the optimal solution point. The optimal solution point can be defined as the feasible solution point, which provides the best possible value for the objective function.

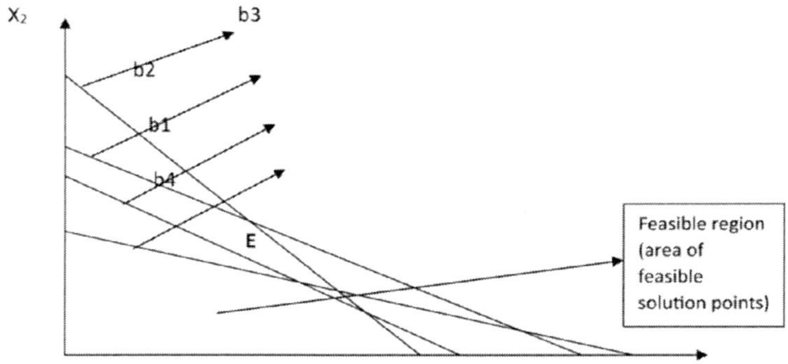

Finding the Best Possible Value (Optimal Solution Point) for Objective Function

Moving the Objective function method

By this method, we pick up an arbitrary level of Z value, for e.g., 900 (any number you can choose!). Hence, the objective function (in our example) will now become:

$10X_1 + 9X_2 = 900$

Now, keep $X_1 = 0$, and we can find $X_2 = 100$

Similarly, keep $X_2 = 0$, and we can find $X_1 = 90$

Now, draw the objective function line with the above X_1 and X_2 values of 90 and 100, respectively. Keep on moving this objective function line, until this line becomes tangent to the boundary line of the feasible region. The objective function line would move parallel, since the coefficients (10 and 9) are constant. So long as the objective function line intersects the feasible region or is away from the feasible region, then there exists a higher level of objective function value to the preceding one with the imposed constraints. Hence, maximum profit is given by the objective function line at a point of production, where it is tangent to the boundary of the feasible region. This would be the upper line of the objective function value that can be obtained with the given objective function and constraints. Depending on the accuracy with which the objective function line and the constraints are drawn in the graph, we can get the optimal values for X_1 and X_2. Those optimal values in this problem will be $X_1 = 540$ and $X_2 = 252$.

Other useful information obtained from the graphical solution

By plugging in the values of X_1 and X_2 at the optimal point of production in the constraints, we can know what resources are fully utilized for producing these optimal levels of X_1 and X_2 and what resources are not fully utilized. Now, plug in the values of X_1 (=540) and X_2 (=252) in the constraints, we will get:

- Constraint b_1, 7/10 (540) + 252 < 630; 630 = 630 (fully utilized, because by producing 540 units of X_1 and 252 units of X_2, we will be fully utilizing the 630 units of b1 resource available)
- Constraint b_2, ½ (540) + 5 (252) < 600; 480 < 600 (not fully utilized, because by producing 540 units of X_1 and 252 units of X_2, we will be utilizing only 480 units of b2 resource from the available 600 units)
- Constraint b_3, 540 + 2/3 (252) < 708; 708 = 708 (fully utilized, because by producing 540 units of X_1 and 252 units of X_2, we will be fully utilizing the 708 units of b3 resource available)
- Constraint b_4, 1/10 (540) + ¼ (252) ≤ 135; 117 < 135 (not fully utilized, because by producing 540 units of X_1 and 252 units of X_2, we will be utilizing only 117 units of b2 resource from the available 135 units)

Therefore, there is an oversupply of b2 and b4 by 120 and 18 units respectively that can be either sold out or diverted to some other production processes to improve the efficiency of production. This information is useful for management. It could be further seen from the graph that the optimal solution is restricted by only two constraints b_1 and b_3, which are fully utilized. Hence, it can be inferred that whichever constraints restrict optimal solution will be fully utilized. That is, they would be used at their maximum capacity. b_2 and b_4 are not restricting the optimal solution and hence they are not fully utilized. The constraints which restrict the optimal solution are called as the binding constraints and those which do not restrict the optimal solution are called non-binding constraints. Hence, in this problem, b1 and b3 are the binding constraints, and b2 and b4 are the non-binding constraints.

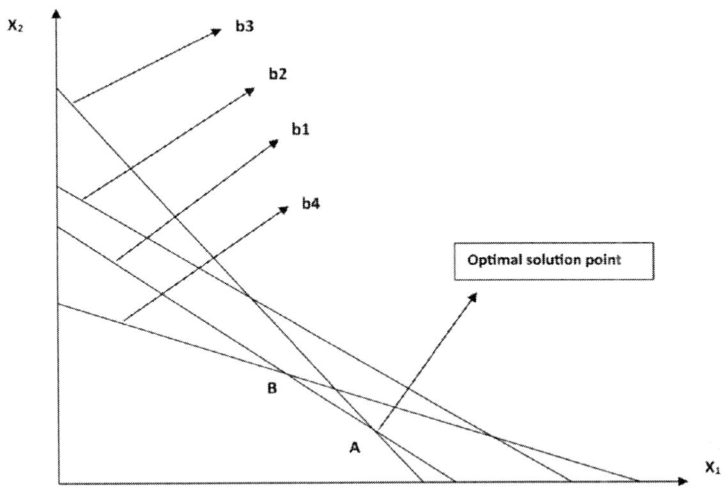

Redundant constraint

The constraint, that does not limit the feasible region, is called the redundant constraint. In the above example, the redundant constraint is b_2. Look at that b_2 constraint line, it is far away from the feasible region and hence, does not limit the feasible region. In other words, the resource b_2 is not restricting even the boundary of the feasible region. It means that we do not have to have that constraint in calculating the optimal solution. This situation exists because the capacity of the available resource b_2 is so much that it can accommodate any production level set by the other resource constraints. Naturally, it (redundant constraint) does not affect the final optimal solution either. It indicates that we can even drop this constraint from the LP problem, without affecting the final solution.

Corner Points or Extreme Points

The objective function shifts parallelly only when the coefficients are constant. When we change one of the coefficients, then the slope of the line will change ending with a different optional solution.

For e.g., $10X_1 + 9X_2 = Z0$

New objective function line $5X_1 + 9X_2 = Z1$

Now, the optional solution point will change from A to B (See the figure above). However, in both cases, optional solutions occur only at a corner, i.e., where two or more constraint lines intersect each other. This is the important point to be noted. These corner points are also called the extreme points which are the feasible solution points occurring only at the corner points of the feasible region. The extreme points are determined by the intersection of two or more constraint lines. An important property of the corner points is that the optional solution to an LP problem always occurs only at a corner.

In the above example, we have got five corner points. We can now evaluate all these five different corner points by plugging in the corresponding values of X_1 and X_2 in the objective function and looking for the maximum value of the objective function. Another important point is that the constraints of a maximization problem form the convex shaped feasible region, while that of a minimization problem form a concave feasible region.

Exercise: Solve the following minimization LP Problem by graphical method:

Minimize $Z = 20X_1 + 40X_2$

Subject to constraints

$36X_1 + 6X_2 \geq 108$

$3X_1 + 12X_2 \geq 36$

$20X_1 + 10X_2 \geq 100$

$X_1, X_2 \geq 0$

Solution

Represent the first constraint $36X_1 + 6X_2 \geq 108$. We set $36X_1 + 6X_2 = 108$; When $X_1 = 0$ in this constraint, we get $36 \times 0 + 6X_2 = 108$ and hence, $X_2 = 108/6 = 18$. Similarly, when $X_2 = 0$, we get $36X_1 + 6 \times 0 = 108$ and hence, $X_1 = 108/36 = 3$. Now, represent the second constraint $3X_1 + 12X_2 \geq 36$. We set $3X_1 + 12X_2 = 36$; When $X_1 = 0$ in this constraint, we get $3 \times 0 + 12X_2 = 36$ and hence, $X_2 = 36/12 = 3$. Similarly, when $X_2 = 0$, we get $3X_1 + 12 \times 0 = 36$ and hence, $X_1 = 36/3 = 12$.

Lastly, represent the third constraint $20X_1 + 10X_2 \geq 100$. We set $20X_1 + 10X_2 = 100$; When $X_1 = 0$, we get $20 \times 0 + 10X_2 = 100$ and hence, $X_2 = 100/10 = 10$. Similarly, when $X_2 = 0$, we get $20X_1 + 10 \times 0 = 100$ and hence, $X_1 = 100/20 = 5$.

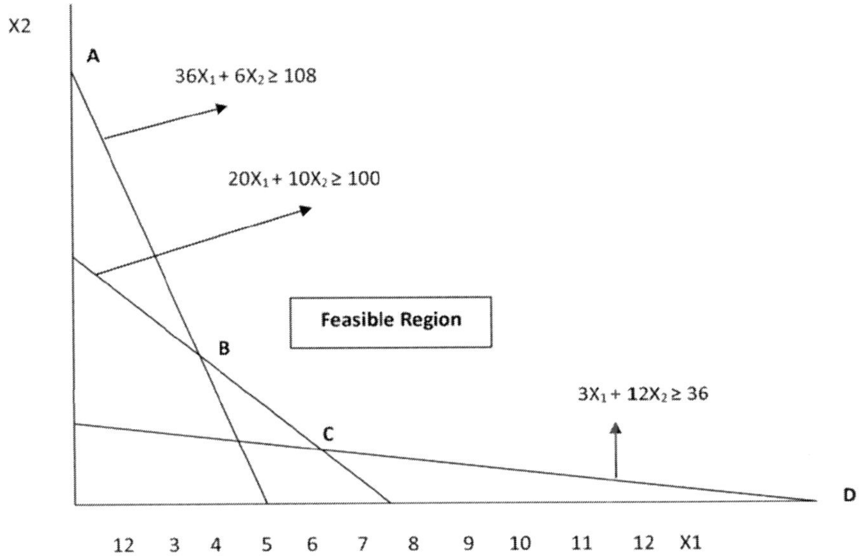

Look at the feasible region in this minimization problem. The feasible region in any minimization problem will be concave in shape (as opposed to convex in the maximization problem). This is a good point to remember. Evaluating the corner points, we will get:

Extreme or Corner Points	X1	X2	Z = 20X1 + 40X2
0	0	0	0
A	0	18	Z = 20 x 0 + 40 x 18 = 720
B	2	6	Z = 20 x2 + 40 x 6 = 280
C	**4**	**2**	**Z = 20 x 4 + 40 x 2 = 160; Minimum**
D	12	0	Z = 20 x 12 + 40 x 0 = 240

The minimum cost is at point C, when $X_1 = 4$ and $X_2 = 2$; Z = 160.

12.1.5.2 Simplex Method of Solution of LP Problems

Before the application of the simplex method to solve any LP problem, the mathematical or algebraic form of the problem must be transformed into a standard form. Because solving a system of equations needs equality for solutions. Hence, algebraic forms of the LP problem which are generally inequality constraints need to be transformed into equality constraints by some standard procedures, and the transformed set of equations is called as the standard form of the LP problem.

E.g. $7/10\ X_1 + 1\ X_2 \leq 630$

Here, the < sign indicates that the Right-Hand Side (RHS) of the equation, i.e., 630 is greater than (or equal to) the Left-Hand Side (LHS) of the equation, i.e., $7/10\ X_1 + 1\ X_2$. We have to add something to the LHS to make up the difference between these two and make them (LHS and RHS) equal. Since the LHS of the constraint varies with the value of X_1 and X_2 which are variables, we have to add a variable to the LHS. This added variable is called as the Slack variable (S1) which will change the inequality constraint into an equality constraint. Hence, we now add slack variables to all the less than or equal to constraints, as below:

$7/10\ X_1 + 1X_2 + 1S_1 = 630$ ---------1

$½\ X_1 + 5/6\ X_2 + 1S_2 = 600$ ---------2

$1X_1 + 2/3\ X_2 + 1S_3 = 708$ ---------3

$1/10\ X_1 + 1/4\ X_2 + 1S_4 = 135$ ---------4

Since we have added four (4) new variables to the constraints, these variables should also enter into the objective function. At the beginning, Cj values of those variables are zeros, since the opportunity costs of the resources are zeros before the start of the production process as they do not have any opportunities to be employed other than the present production process at least at present. So, at the beginning of the production process when no production occurs ($X_1 = 0$, $X_2 = 0$), the objective function becomes,

Max. $Z = 10X_1 + 9X_2 + 0S_1 + 0S_2 + 0S_3 + 0S_4$ ---------5

$S_1 = 630$, $S_2 = 600$, $S_3 = 708$, and $S_4 = 135$ ---------6

Also, these slack variables should enter into the non-negativity constraint:

$X_1, X_2, S_1, S_2, S_3, S_4 \geq 0$ ---------7

These equations 1, 2, 3, 4, 5, 6, and 7 are together called the standard form of that particular LP problem.

Let us now take up a minimization problem, where one of the greater than or equal to constraint may be $1X_1 + 2X_2 \geq 80$. Here, LHS is greater than RHS. Hence, we add a Surplus variable to the LHS to ensure equality as follows:

$1X_1 + 2X_2 - 1S_1 = 80$ ---------1

where S_1 is a surplus variable

Similarly, for ½ X_1 + 2/3 $X_2 \geq 50$, we will have ½ X_1 + 2/3 $X_2 - 1S_2 = 50$-------2

The objective function will be: Min. $Z = 10X_1 + 5X_2 + 0S_1 + 0S_2$ ---------3

$X_1, X_2, S_1, S_2 \geq 0$

The physical interpretation of the value of the surplus variable is that it is the extra amount of resource over and above the available level of b1, i.e., 80 units required to produce 1 unit of X_1 and 2 units of X_2.

Having obtained the standard form for the LP problem, the next step is to solve the problem. To solve a set of linear equations, we need the number of variables and number of equations to be equal. But in LP problems, we usually have more number of variables than the number of equations, i.e., there are 'n' number of variables and 'm' number of equations, where $m < n$. If this is the case, this form of equations is called the canonical form. In this type of situation, the solution can be obtained by setting $n - m$ variables equal to 0 and solving for m variables using the m constraint equations, and such a solution is referred to as the basic solution. The solved variables are called the basic variables (BV) and the unsolved as the non-basic variables (NBV).

The simplex procedure, otherwise known as the simplex algorithm, can be explained by an example below:

Max. $Z = 10X_1 + 20X_2$

Subject to,

$2X_1 + 2X_2 \leq 18$

$2X_1 + 1X_2 \leq 10$

$X_1, X_2 \geq 0$

The standard form of the LP problem

Max. $Z= 10X_1 + 20X_2 + 0S_1 + 0S_2$

Subject to,

$2X_1 + 2X_2 + 1S_1 + 0S_2 = 18$

$2X_1 + 1X_2 + 0S_1 + 1S_2 = 10$

$X_1, X_2, S_1, S_2 \geq 0$

Here, there are 4 variables and 2 constraint equations. i.e., the number of variables is greater than the number of equations. If we try to solve this characteristic system of equations, then it will lead to the following implications (or complications):

1. It can lead to an infinite number of solutions. This is against the principle of LP.
2. There is a chance that it can have a negative value (i.e., it may not satisfy the non-negativity condition).

The special procedure to solve this peculiar problem is called as the simplex procedure or simplex algorithm.

Properties or Characteristics of Simplex Procedure

1. It enables to form the Basic Feasible Solution (BFS) which is consistent with the given system of equations.
2. It can eliminate all the negative solutions.
3. It can choose the optimal solution among the positive ones.

Definition of Simplex Algorithm

The simplex algorithm is an efficient iterative procedure that will identify the basic feasible solution in such a way that each new solution is at least as good as the previous one, in terms of optimizing the objective function.

Let us now consider the problem. The solution to such a system can be found by assigning zero values to any two variables and solving for the remaining two variables. For e.g., we set X_1 equal to and $S_2 = 0$. Therefore, the new system will be:

$2X_2 + 1S_1 = 18\ [b_1]$ ---------1

$1X_2 \quad = 10 \quad [b_2]$ ---------2

Eqn. 2 x (-2) => $- 2X_2 = - 20$ ---------3

Eqn. 3 + Eqn. 1 => S1 = - 2

i.e., $0X_2 + 1S_1 = -2$ ---------4

and $1X_2 + 0S_1 =10$ ---------5

This procedure is called the Gauss-Jordan method.

The last two equations can be written in a matrix form as below:

$$\begin{pmatrix}0\\1\end{pmatrix}^{X_2}+\begin{pmatrix}1\\0\end{pmatrix}^{S_1}=\begin{pmatrix}-2\\10\end{pmatrix}$$

$\begin{pmatrix}S1\\X2\end{pmatrix} \begin{pmatrix}-2\\10\end{pmatrix}$ is called as the Basic Solution (BS).

S_1 and X_2 are called the basic variables and X_1 and S_2 are called the non-basic variables. Note that each basic variable has got coefficient of 1 in one equation and 0 in other equation(s) and each equation has exactly one basic variable with a coefficient of 1. This particular basic solution is not a basic feasible solution, since it violates the non-negativity constraint, because S_1 = -2. It is only an infeasible solution. Therefore, we will work it out in another way. i.e., set X_1 = 0 and X_2 = 0. The new system of equations will be as follows:

$1S_1 = 18$; i.e., $1S_1 + 0S_2 = 18$

$1S_2 = 10$; i.e., $0S_1 + 1S_2 = 10$

This is the Basic Feasible Solution (BFS). This BFS is exactly on the extreme or corner point. This particular BFS is called the Initial Basic Feasible Solution (IBFS), as it represents the situation before the start of the production process where X_1 = 0 and X_2 = 0. This IFBS is located at the origin of the graph, indicating no production is taking place.

After forming the standard form, the next step is to obtain this Initial Basic Feasible Solution in a tableau form. Transferring the standard form into the tableau (this table is called the tableau in the simplex algorithm) form would ensure the Initial Basic Feasible Solution. The tableau would contain all the necessary information about the objective function and all the constraints and it would move from one Basic Feasible Solution to another better Basic Feasible Solution. This tableau is as follows:

Basis	**Decision variables**	**X1**	**X2**	**...**	**Xn**	**S1**	**...**	**Sm**	**bi**	**bi/ aij**
	Cj	**C1**	**C2**	**...**	**Cn**	**Cn+1**	**...**	**Cm**		
S1	Cn+1	a11	a12	...	...	...	...	a1n	b1	
.	.	a21	a22	...	...	...	...	a2n	b2	
.	.	.	.	...	...	...	...	.	.	
.	.	.	.	...	...	...	...	.	.	
Sm	Cm									
		am1	am2	...	...	...	...	amn	bm	
Zj										
Cj-Zj										

where,

Cj - objective function coefficient for the variable j

bi - RHS value of the constraint i

aij - coefficient associated with variable j in constraint i

When we move from (0, 0) in the IBFS to another corner solution, some non-basic variable may enter the basis and become a basic variable and some basic variable may make an exit. To keep track of the entry and exit of the basis, a profit change or price change row is to be added which is done by finding Cj – Zj. The Zj row implies the total Z value at each iteration.

Properties of the Tableau

1. To find the basic solution. i.e., m of the variables must have a co-efficient of 1 in exactly one equation and appear with 0 co-efficient in all other equations. Each basic variable will have a unit column.

   $$\begin{pmatrix} 1 \\ 0 \\ 0 \\ 0 \end{pmatrix}$$

   If these m variables are made basic by setting n - m = 0, the value of the basic variable can be read from the RHS column (i.e., b column).

2. To find the Basic Feasible Solution, i.e., the value of the RHS of the constraint equation should be non-negative.

IBFS Tableau

Max. $Z = 10X_1 + 20X_2 + 0S_1 + 0S_2$

$2X_1 + 2X_2 + 1S_1 + 0S_2 = 18$ --------------b_1

$2X_1 + 1X_2 + 0S_1 + 0S_2 = 10$ --------------b_2

$X_1, X_2, S_1, S_2 \geq 0$

$Z = 10(0) + 20(0) + 0S_1 + 0S_2 = 0$ ----------→

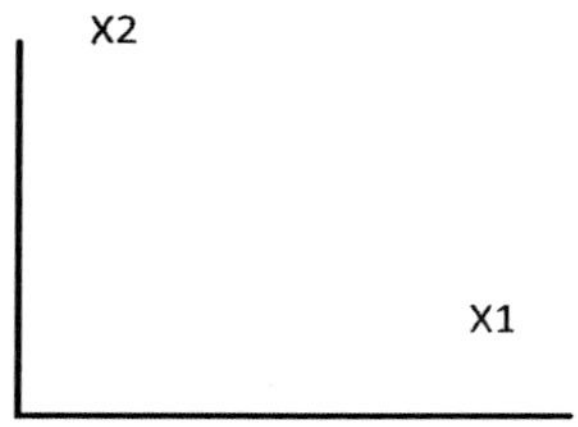

This is the IBFS, where X_1=0 and X_2=0. This IBFS can be represented in the form of a Tableau as below:

Basis	**Decision Variables**	**X1**	**X2**	**S1**	**S2**	**bi**
	Cj	**10**	**20**	**0**	**0**	
S1	0	2	2	1	0	18
S2	0	2	1	0	1	10
Zj		0	0	0	0	0
Cj - Zj		10	20	0	0	0

IBFS is one of the possible BFSs. Hence, S_1 and S_2 are the basic variables, and X_1 and X_2 are the non-basic variables. Tableau form of the LP problem is otherwise called the Initial Basic Feasible Solution. Our aim now is to find a new basic feasible solution. To find this, we have to obtain a new set of basic variables. From the Initial Basic Feasible Solution, it is known that the basic variables are S_1 and S_2 and non-basic variables are X_1 and X_2. So, the non-basic variables X_1 and X_2 have the potential to become the basic variables. Among them, one will become the basic variable and one of the current basic variables will get eliminated as the non-basic variable. The problem is how to select the non-basic variable to become the basic variable.

Criterion for Selection of Non-Basic Variable to become Basic Variable

Select a non-basic variable so that the replacement of such a variable for a current basic variable provides a new solution for which the objective function is greater than or at least as good as the one corresponding to the present or current solution. This is done by looking for the variable that has the biggest possible Cj - Zj value, which would indicate the increase / decrease in the Zj for every unit of the variable introduced into the basis. Therefore, the non-basic variable that contributes the greatest per unit increase / decrease in the objective function must be selected to become a basic variable.

For e.g., Assume that one unit of X_1 is introduced into the Initial Basic Feasible Solution:

b1 => $2X_1 + 2X_2 + 1S_1 + 0S_2 = 18$

$2(1) + 2(0) + 1S_1 + 0S_2 = 18$

$2 + 1S_1 = 18; S_1 = 18 - 2 = 16$

i.e., Production of one unit of X_1 will utilize 2 units of b1 resource of the existing 18 units.

b2 => $2X_1 + 1X_2 + 0S_1 + 0S_2 = 10$

$2(1) + 1S_2 = 10; S_2 = 10 – 2 = 8$

i.e., Production of one unit of X_1 utilizes 2 units of b2 resource of the available 10 units. Therefore, by introducing 1 unit of X_1 into the production process, we are not violating constraints.

$Z = 10(1) + 20(0) + 0S_1 + 0S_2 = 10$

Let us now consider X_2. In the Initial BFS, we introduce 1 unit of X_2.

$S_1 = 18 - 2X_2 = 18 – 2 = 16$

$S_2 = 10 - 1X_2 = 10 – 9 = 9$

This also does not violate the constraints.

$Z = 10(0) + 20(1) + 0S_1 + 0S_2 = 20$

Introduction of one unit of X_2 gives 20 units of revenue or profit, while that of X_1 is only 10. Hence, it is worth introducing one unit of X_2, because X_2 gives relatively better increase in the objective function. Therefore, we can select X_2 to enter the basic variable set. However, we do not know how many units of X_2 can enter into the basis.

From the b_1 constraint, it is clear that the production of one unit of X_2 needs 2 units (coefficient attached to X_2 in b1 constraint) of b1 resource. It means that 18/2 = 9 units of X_2 can be produced with the available 18 units of b1 resource. Similarly, 10/1 = 10 units of X_2 can be produced with the available 10 units of b2 resource. To satisfy both cases, we can produce only 9 units. Because the production of 10 units of X_2, though satisfies the constraint b_2, would not satisfy the b_1 constraint as it can allow only 9 units of X_2. Therefore, b1 dictates the level of production of X_2 as it is the most restrictive constraint. We can thus conclude that 9 units of X_2 must be produced to maximize Z, at the same time, without violating any of the constraints.

Let us now look at the b_1 constraint.

$2X_1 + 2X_2 + 1S_1 + 0S_2 = 18$

$2 \times 0 + 2 \times 9 + 1S_1 + 0S_2 = 18$

$0 + 18 + 1S_1 + 0 = 18; S_1 = 18 - 18 = 0$

It implies that in the solution where 9 units of X_2 are produced, $S_1=0$ which means that the resource b1 is fully exhausted or fully used up. This also gives additional information that the variable S1 which was in the basis before X_2 enters the basis, now becomes a non-basic variable in the new basic feasible solution. i.e., the outgoing basic variable is also identified in the process of determining to which level the new basic variable is to be produced. At this level, we know two things. $X_2=9$ units and $S_1=0$ in the new basic feasible solution. To complete the new basic feasible solution, we have to apply the Gauss-Jordon elimination process to the equations in the initial tableau. The new set of equations generated by this process should result in a unit column for X_2 variable, since it has been chosen to become a basic variable. The column and the row corresponding to the new basic variable X_2 are called the pivot column and pivot row, respectively, and the element where the pivot row and column intersect is called the pivot element.

Pivot Column
X2
20
2
1

Pivot Row						
			X2			
S1	0	2	**2**	1	0	18
			↑ **Pivot Element**			

To make the pivot element as 1, divide the first constraint b1 by 2 (pivot element). Then we get a new equation as follows:

$b_1 => 1X_1 + 1X_2 + ½ S_1 + 0S_2 = 9$

Basis	Decision Variables	X1	X2	S1	S2	bi
	Cj	10	20	0	0	
X2	20	1	1	½	0	9
S2	0	1	0	- ½	1	1

Similarly, $b_2 => 2X_1 + 1X_2 + 0S_1 + 1S_2 = 10$

In the equation b2, the coefficient of X_2 must be made as 0. For that, the following mathematical manipulations are done:

Deduct new row from b2,

$2X_1 + 1X_2 + 0S_{1+} 1S_2 = 10$ minus $1X_1 + 1X_2 + ½ S_1 + 0S_2 = 9$ equals $1X_1 + 0 - ½ S_1 + 1S_2 = 1$

Basis	Cj	X1	X2	S1	S2	bi
		10	20	0	0	
X2	20	1	1	½	0	9
S2	0	1	0	- ½	1	1
Zj		20	20	10	0	180
Cj-Zj		-10	0	-10	0	

This row is the new b_2 constraint after producing 9 units of X_2. Now the new basic feasible solution is:

$$\begin{pmatrix} X_1 \\ X_2 \\ S_1 \\ S_2 \end{pmatrix} = \begin{pmatrix} 0 \\ 9 \\ 0 \\ 1 \end{pmatrix}$$

where Z = 10(0) + 20(9) + 0(0) + 0(1) = 180 [profit / revenue / output]

Now, let us look for some other non-basic variable to be introduced. As already discussed, the new basic variable which corresponds to the biggest positive Cj - Zj value deserves to enter into the basis. However, in this tableau, there is no positive element yet. All Cj - Zj's are either zeros or negative elements. The variables that are already in the basis (X_2 and S_2) have the Cj - Zj values of 0 which indicate that they are already in the basis and that further increase in the production of such variables would not result in any more improvement in Zj. This is because per unit increase in Zj of such variable would only be zero as indicated by Cj - Zj.

Other variables X_1 and S_1 have the Cj-Zj values of –10 and –10 respectively which indicate that the introduction of one unit of these variables would result in a decrease of Zj by 10 units. i.e., the introduction of any of these two would only cause a drop in revenue, profit, or output as the case may be. Hence, it can be concluded that no more variable deserves to be included in the basis, as they would not maximize the objective or optimize the level of the production anymore.

Thus, the endpoint of the process of the simplex procedure of solution of LP problem is that all the Cj - Zj values are less than or equal to zero, indicating the possibility of no further improvement in Z.

Interpretation of Results obtained through Simplex Algorithm

The final tableau of a maximization problem is as below:

Basis	Cj	X1	X2	X3	S1	S2	S3	bi
		2	4	5/2	0	0	0	
X1	2	1	0	- 6/5	3/5	0	- 12/5	**12**
S2	0	0	0	3	-1	1	7/3	**10**
X2	4	0	1	21/15	- 3/5	0	27/45	**6**
Zj		2	4	48/15	6/5	0	36/45	**48**
Cj-Zj		**0**	**0**	**-21/30**	**-6/5**	**0**	**-36/45**	

Profit is 48 units. It can be concluded that this is the maximum possible profit level in this particular production process with the available resources (bi), the current prices (Cj), and the present technology (aij), as all the Cj - Zj's are either zeros or negative. Even a minor change in any one of the above three or two or all can bring about a change in the optimal solution. The optimal production levels of the basic variables (X_1 and X_2) are 12 units and 6 units, respectively. Product X_3 (the non-basic variable) is kept out of the production process in the current situation of the resource base, price levels, and technology, as production of this product would bring about a drop of 21/30 units in profit for every unit of X_3 produced.

The resources b_1 and b_3 are called the fully utilized resources or exhausted resources or binding resources, since they are the ones which limit the optimal solution point. Since the present optimal production level fully utilizes these resources, the present availability of these resources must be there to exploit the profit of 48 units. Any reduction in the resource levels of these binding constraints may lead to a drop in the level of production of X_1 and X_2 as they (reduced b_1 and b_3 resources) would not be enough to carry out the production process. That is, every unit reduction in the availability of these b_1 and b_3 resources would make the profit to decline by 6/5 and 36/45 units respectively, as indicated by Cj - Zj. However, the b2 resource otherwise called as non-binding resource or the resource not fully utilized would remain 10 units in excess of the quantity demanded by the optimal production level, the diversion of which may increase the efficiency by the process.

12.1.6 Minimization Problems

In the minimization problems, after transforming them into the standard forms, we just transform the objective function as follows and do the rest as done for maximization problems. i.e., Min. Z subject to the constraints is identically equal to Max. (-Z), subject to the constraints.

$$\begin{pmatrix} \text{Min.}Z = CX \\ \text{s.t.}, AX \geq B \\ X \geq 0 \end{pmatrix} = \begin{pmatrix} \text{Max.}(-Z) = -CX \\ \text{s.t.} AX \geq B \\ X \geq 0 \end{pmatrix}$$

E.g., Min. $Z = 3X_1 + 1X_2 + 2X_3$

Subject to,

$8X_1 + 2X_2 + 3X_3 \geq 5$

$4X_1 + 5X_2 + 6X_3 \geq 5$

$X_1, X_2, X_3 > 0$

Standard form

Min. $Z = 3X_1 + 1X_2 + 2X_3 + 0S_1 + 0S_2 + Ma_1 + Ma_2$

Subject to,

$8X_1 + 2X_2 + 3X_3 - 1S_1 + 0S_2 + 1a_1 + 0a_2 = 5$

$4X_1 + 5X_2 + 6X_3 + 0S_1 - 1S_2 + 0a_1 + 1a_2 = 5$

$X_1, X_2, X_3, S_1, S_2, a_1, a_2 \geq 0$

Transforming the objective function

Max. $(-Z) = -3X_1 - 1X_2 - 2X_3 + 0S_1 + 0S_2 - Ma_1 - Ma_2$

Subject to,

$8X_1 + 2X_2 + 3X_3 - 1S_1 + 1a_1 = 5$

$4X_1 + 5X_2 + 6X_3 - 1S_2 + 1a_2 = 5$

$X_1, X_2, X_3, S_1, S_2, a_1, a_2 \geq 0$

Initial tableau   Pivot element

Basis	Cj	X1	X2	X3	S1	S2	a1	a2	bi	bi/aij
		-3		2	0	0	-m	-m		
a1	-m	**8**	[illegible]	2	-1	0	1	0	5	5/8
a2	-m	4	5	6	0	-1	0	1	5	5/4
Zj		-12m	-7m	-9m	m	m	-m	-m	-10m	
Cj-Zj		12m-3	7m-1	9m-2	-m	-m	0	0		

First iteration (divide b1 by 8)

Pivot element

Basis	Cj	X1	X2	X3	S1	S2	a1	a2	bi	bi/ aij
		-3	-1	-2	0	0	-m	-m		
X1	-3	1	¼	3/8	-1/8	0	1/8	0	5/8	5/3
a2	-m	0	4	**9/2**	½	-1	-1/2	1	5/2	5/9
Zj		-3	-3/4 –4m	-9/8–9m/2	3/8-m/2	m	-3/8+m/2	-m	-15/8– 5m/2	
Cj-Zj		0	-1/4 + 4m	-7/8+ 9m/2	-3/8+m/2	-m	3/8-m/2	0		

b_2 – (New row x 4) =>

$4X_1 + 5X_2 + 6X_3 + 0S_1 - 1S_2 + 0a_1 + 1a_2 = 5$

$4X_1 + 1X_2 + 3/2X_3 - 1/2 S_1 + 0S_2 + 1/2a_1 + 0a_2 = 5/2$

$0X_1 + 4X_2 + 9/2X_3 + 1/2 S_1 - 1S_2 - 1/2a_1 + 1a_2 = 5/2$

Second iteration (divide b2 by 9/2)

$0X_1 + 8/9X_2 + 1X_3 + 1/9S_1 - 2/9S_2 - 1/9a_1 + 2/9a_2 = 5/9$

Basis	Cj	X1	X2	X3	S1	S2	a1	a2	bi	bi/aij
		-3	-1	-2	0	0	-m	-m		
X1	-3	1	-1/12	0	-1/6	1/12	1/6	-1/12	5/12	-5
X3	-2	0	**8/9**	1	1/9	-2/9	-1/9	2/9	5/9	5/8
Zj		-3	-55/36	-2	1/9	7/36	-5/8	-7/36	-95/36	
Cj-Zj		0	19/36	0	-1/9	-7/36	-m+5/8	-m+7/36		

b_1 – (new row x 3/8)

$1X_1 + 1/4X_2 + 3/8X_3 - 1/8S_1 + 0S_2 + 1/8a_1 + 0a_2 = 5/8$

$0X_1 + 1/3X_2 + 3/8X_3 + 1/24S_1 - 1/12S_2 - 1/24a_1 + 1/12a_2 = 5/24$

$1X_1 - 1/12X_2 + 0X_3 - 1/6S_1 + 1/12S_2 + 1/6a_1 - 1/12a_2 = 5/12$

Third iteration (divide b3 by 8/9)

Basis	Cj	X1	X2	X3	S1	S2	a1	a2	bi	bi/ aij
		-3	-1	-2	0	0	-m	-m		
X1	-3	1	0	3/32	-15/96	3/48	15/96	-3/48	45/96	
X2	-1	0	1	9/8	1/8	-1/4	-1/8	¼	5/8	
Zj		-3	-1	-45/32	11/32	1/16	-1132	-1/16	**-195/96**	
Cj-Zj		**0**	**0**	**-19/32**	**-11/32**	**-1/16**	**-m+11/16**	**-m+1/16**		

b_1 – [new row x (-1/2)] =>

$1X_1 - 1/12X_2 + 0X_3 - 1/6S_1 + 1/12S_2 + 1/6a_1 - 1/12a_2 = 5/12$

$0X_1 - 1/12X_2 - 9/96X_3 - 1/196S_1 + 1/48S_2 + 1/96a_1 - 1/4a_2 = -5/96$

$1X_1 + 0X_2 + 9/96X_3 - 15/96S_1 + 3/48S_2 + 15/96a_1 - 3/48a_2 = 45/96$

12.1.7 Duality in LP

Each original LP problem (which is called a primal LP problem) will have an alternate form, which will be called a dual LP problem. The dual LP problem will be almost like a mirror image of the primal problem, which is because the nature of the dual problem depends on the nature of the primal problem. Therefore, the solution obtained in dual is basically related to the solution of primal. i.e., we can read the primal solution from the dual and vice versa.

Primal	**Dual**
Max. Z = CX	Min. W = BY
AX ≤ B	AY ≥ C
X ≥ 0	Y ≥ 0

12.1.7.1 Primal-Dual Relationship

- The objective function coefficients of the primal problem become the Right-Hand Side values of the constraints of the dual problem.
- Similarly, the Right-Hand Side values of the constraints of the primal problem become the objective function coefficients of the dual problem.
- The inequalities in the primal problem become reversed in the dual problem. That is, the objective function changes from Max. in primal problem to Min. in dual problem.
- Each column in the primal problem corresponds to the constraints (rows) in the dual problem. Thus, the number of dual constraints is equal to the number of primal variables.
- Each row (constraint) in the primal problem corresponds to the column in the dual problem. Hence, there is one dual variable (Y) for every primal constraint.

- The dual of the dual problem is the primal problem [Dual (dual) = primal].
- In both primal and dual problems, the variables are non-negative and the constraints are in-equal.

Primal Problem

Max. $Z = C_1X_1 + C_2X_2 + \dots + CnXn$

Subject to,

$a_{11} X_1 + a_{12}X_2 + \dots + a_{1n}Xn \leq b1$

$a_{21} X_1 + a_{22}X_2 + \dots + a_{2n}Xn \leq b2\dots$

$a_{m1} X_1 + a_{m2}X_2 + \dots + a_{mn}Xn \leq bm$

$X_1, X_2, \dots, Xn \geq 0$

Corresponding Dual Problem

Min. $W = b_1 Y_1 + b_2 Y_2 + \dots + b_m Y_m$

Subject to,

$a_{11}Y_1 + a_{12}Y_2 + \dots + a_{1m}Y_m > C_1$

$a_{21}Y_1 + a_{22}Y_2 + \dots + a_{2m}Y_m > C2$

$a_{n1}Y_1 + a_{n2}Y_2 + \dots + a_{nm}Y_m > Cn$

$Y_1, Y2, \dots, Ym \geq 0$

In short,

$$z = \sum_{j=1}^{n} Cj\,Xj = -w = -\sum_{i=1}^{n} bi\,Yi$$

Primal Corresponding Dual

Example

Primal LP Problem	Corresponding dual LP Problem
Max. $Z = 10X_1 + 9X_2$ Subject to, $7/10X_1 + 1X_2 \leq 630$ $½ X_1 + 5/6X_2 \leq 600$ $1X_1 + 2/3X_2 \leq 708$ $1/10X_1 + 1/4X_2 \leq 135$ $X_1, X_2 \geq 0$	Min. $W = 630Y_1 + 600Y_2 + 708Y_3 + 135Y_4$ Subject to, $7/10Y_1 + 1/2Y_2 + 1Y_3 + 1/10Y_4 \geq 10$ $1Y_1 + 5/6Y_2 + 2/3Y_3 + 1/4Y_4 \geq 9$ $Y_1, Y_2, Y_3, Y_4 \geq 0$

More generally,

Primal (Maximize)	Dual (Minimize)
i^{th} constraint $\leq$	i^{th} variable ≥ 0
i^{th} constraint $\geq$	i^{th} variable ≤ 0
j^{th} variable ≥ 0	j^{th} constraint $\geq$
j^{th} variable ≤ 0	j^{th} constraint $\leq$

The final tableau of the primal problem and reading dual results from it

Basis	Cj	X1	X2	S1	S2	S3	S4	bi
		10	9	0	0	0	0	
X2	9	0	1	15/8	0	-21/16	0	252
S2	0	0	0	-15/16	1	25/160	0	120
X1	10	1	0	-10/8	0	15/8	0	540
S4	0	0	0	-11/32	0	9/32	1	18
Zj		10	9	70/16	0	111/16	0	**7668**
Cj-Zj		0	0	-70/16	0	-111/16	0	
				Y1	**Y2**	**Y3**	**Y4**	
				Dual variables				

X_1 and X_2 are primal variables; $Y_{!}$, Y_2, Y_3 and Y_4 are the dual variables.

Zp = 7668

Wd = 630 (-70/16) + 708 (-111/16) = -7668

The above table indicates that we can read dual values from the results of a primal problem itself.

Let us find the solution for the dual problem of the above primal problem using the Simplex method (Big M method, because it becomes the minimization problem):

Min Z = 630y1 + 600y2 + 708y3 + 135y4

Subject to

7/10y1 + 1/2y2 + 1y3 + 1/10y4 > 10

1y1 + 5/6y2 + 2/3y3 + 1/4y4 > 9

y1, y2, y3, y4 >= 0

Solution

The problem can be converted into:

Min. $Z = 630y1 \ + 600y2 \ + 708y3 \ + 135y4$

Subject to

$0.7y1 + 0.5y2 + 1y3 + 0.1y4 \geq 10$

$1y1 + 0.833y2 + 0.667\,y3 + 0.25y4 \geq 9$

$y1, y2, y3, y4 \geq 0$

Converting this objective function of the minimization problem into that of the maximization problem, we get:

Max. $Z = -630y1 - 600y2 - 708y3 - 135y4$

Converting the constraints into to canonical form by adding slack, surplus, and artificial variables as appropriate, we get,

1. As the constraint - 1 is of type '≥', we should subtract surplus variable $S1$ and add artificial variable $A1$;
2. As the constraint - 2 is of type '≥', we should subtract surplus variable $S2$ and add artificial variable $A2$.

After introducing surplus and artificial variables, we get:

Max $Z = -630y1\ -600y2\ -708y3\ -135y4\ +0\,S1 + 0\,S2 - M\,A1 - M\,A2$

Subject to

$0.7y1\ \ +0.5y2 + 1y3 + 0.1y4 - 1S1 + 0S2 + 1A1 + 0A2 = 10$

$1y1 +\ 0.833y2 +\ \ 0.667y3 + 0.25y4 + 0S21 - 1S2 + 0A1 + 1A2 = 9$

$y1, y2, y3, y4, S1, S2, A1, A2 \geq 0$

Iteration-1

Basis	***Cj***	***y1***	***y2***	***y3***	***y4***	***S1***	***S2***	***A1***	***A2***	**bi**	**bi/aij**
		-630	-600	-708	-135	0	0	-*M*	-*M*		
*A*1	-*M*	0.7	0.5	1	0.1	-1	0	1	0	10	14.286
***A*2**	-*M*	**(1)**	0.833	0.667	0.25	0	-1	0	1	9	**9**
Zj		-1.7*M*	-1.333*M*	-1.667*M*	-0.35*M*	*M*	*M*	-*M*	-*M*	**19M**	
Cj - Zj		**1.7*M* - 630**	1.333*M* - 600	1.667*M* - 708	0.35*M* - 135	- *M*	- *M*	0	0		

The negative minimum *Zj-Cj* is $-1.7M+630$ and its column index is 1. So, the entering variable is $y1$. The minimum ratio is 9 and its row index is 2. So, the leaving basis variable is $A2$. Therefore, the pivot element is 1.

Entering = $y1$, Departing = $A2$, Key Element =1.

$R2$ (new) = $R2$ (old)

$R1$ (new) = $R1$ (old) - $0.7R2$ (new)

Iteration-2

Basis	Cj	*y*1	*y*2	*y*3	*y*4	*S*1	*S*2	*A*1	*A*2	bi	bi / aij
		-630	-600	-708	-135	0	0	-*M*	-*M*		
***A*1**	-*M*	0	-0.083	0.533	-0.075	-1	**(0.7)**	1	-0.7	3.7	**5.286**
*y*1	-630	1	0.833	0.667	0.25	0	-1	0	1	9	-9
Zj		-630	0.083*M* -525	-0.533*M* -420	0.075*M* -157.5	*M*	-0.7*M* +630	-*M*	0.7*M* -630	**-3.7*M* -5670**	
Cj - Zj		0	-0.083*M* -75	-0.533*M*+ 288	- 0.075*M* +22.5	- *M*	**0.7*M* -630**	0	-1.7*M* +630		

The negative minimum *Zj-Cj* is -0.7*M*+630 and its column index is 6. So, the entering variable is *S*2**.** The minimum ratio is 5.2857 and its row index is 1. So, the leaving basis variable is *A*1. Therefore, the pivot element is 0.7.

Entering = *S*2, Departing = *A*1, Key Element = 0.7

*R*1 (new) = *R*1 (old) ÷ 0.7

*R*2 (new) = *R*2 (old) + *R*1 (new)

Iteration-3

Basis	*Cj*	*y*1	*y*2	*y*3	*y*4	*S*1	*S*2	*A*1	*A*2	bi	bi / aij
		-630	-600	-708	-135	0	0	-*M*	-*M*		
***S*2**	0	0	-0.119	**(0.762)**	-0.107	-1.429	1	1.429	-1	5.286	**6.938**
*y*1	-630	1	0.714	1.429	0.143	-1.429	0	1.429	0	14.286	9.997
Zj		-630	-450	-900	-90	900	0	-900	0	**-9000**	
Cj - Zj		0	-150	**192**	-45	-900	0	-*M*+900	-*M*		

The negative minimum *Zj-Cj* is -192 and its column index is 3. So, the entering variable is *y*3. The minimum ratio is 6.9375 and its row index is 1. So, the leaving basis variable is *S*2. Therefore, the pivot element is 0.7619.

Entering = *y*3, Departing = *S*2, Key Element = 0.7619

*R*1 (new) = *R*1 (old) ÷ 0.7619

*R*2 (new) = *R*2 (old) - 1.4286 *R*1 (new)

Iteration-4

Basis	*Cj*	*y*1	*y*2	*y*3	*y*4	*S*1	*S*2	*A*1	*A*2	bi
		-630	-600	-708	-135	0	0	-*M*	-*M*	
*y*3	-708	0	-0.156	1	-0.141	-1.875	1.313	1.875	-1.313	6.938 **(=111/16)**
*y*1	-630	1	0.938	0	0.344	1.25	-1.875	-1.25	1.875	4.375 **(=70/16)**
Zj		-630	-480	-708	-117	540	252	-540	-252	**-7668**
Cj - Zj		0	-120	0	-18	**-540**	**-252**	-*M*+540	-*M*+252	

Since all Cj – $Zj<0$, optimal solution is arrived at with values of variables as $y1=4.375$, $y2=0$, $y3=6.938$ and $y4=0$. Max Z = -7668. Therefore, Min Z = 7668. Look at the Cj – Zj values of S1 and S2 (-540 and -252) which were in the primal solution as the optimal quantities of X1 and X2 to be produced. The bi values of 111/16 and 70/16 for y3 and y1 were represented as negative Cj – Zj values of S1 and S3 in the primal solution. So, it is clear that we can read the primal solution from the dual results and the dual solution from the primal results.

12.1.7.2 Diagrammatic Representation of Primal-Dual Relationship

Dual end (Here feasibility is missing; hence we move towards feasibility)

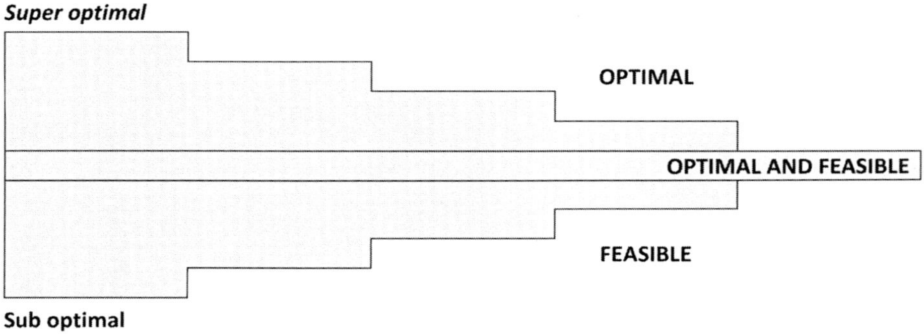

Primal end (Here, optimality is missing; hence, we move towards optimality)

The above diagram explains primal and dual LP problems more explicitly. In a primal LP problem, we are very much in the feasible region and hence try to reach the optimal end (Sub-optimal to optimal and feasible point). Meanwhile, in a dual LP problem, we are very much in the optimal zone and hence try to reach the feasible end (Super-optimal to optimal and feasible point).

Christiansen and Carpenter (1983) and Habtemarian *et al.* (1984) used linear programming as a tool in animal disease control studies. As Rich *et al.* (2005) put it, LP can even be adapted to assess risk in decision-making. For e.g., portfolio theory has evolved to address the problem of finding a mix of activities that maximize expected returns while minimizing risk (or variance in returns); such problems are known as mean-variance problems (Mangen *et al.,* 2003). An application of portfolio theory in animal disease can include an evaluation of a mix of various veterinary interventions with known costs and improvements in production efficiency. The Minimization of Total Absolute Deviations (MOTAD) approach has also been adopted in farm applications as a linear approximation to portfolio models (McCarl and Spreen, 2003). Rich *et al.* (2005) presented some selected applications of LP to animal diseases:

Author(s)	Level	Time	Parameters	Disease
Habtermariam *et al.* (1984)	Herd aggregated to sub-region	Five-year simulation period	Benefits of disease control efforts	Trypanosomiasis
Galligan and Marsh (1988)	National	Five-year simulation period	Costs of alternative veterinary programmes	Multiple diseases (Portfolio theory)
Bicknell *et al.* (1999)	Farm aggregated to nation	Changing disease over time	Costs of different disease prevention policies	Bovine Tuberculosis
Stott *et al.* (2003)	Farm	Ten-year simulation period, discounted over time	Costs of different disease prevention policies	Bovine viral diarrhoea (MOTAD)

12.2 DYNAMIC PROGRAMMING

Dynamic programming (DP) is a mathematical optimization method, developed by Richard Bellman (1920-1984) in 1950s, who is known as the father of DP. It has very many applications in different fields, from engineering to economics. It is a technique for solving a complex problem by first breaking the problem into a collection of simpler subproblems, solving each subproblem just once, and then storing their solutions to avoid repetitive computations. This optimization technique speeds up the process, when we repeatedly solve the same problem.

12.2.1 Recursion

A recursive function solves a particular problem by solving smaller subproblems of the original problem. Recursion is a remarkable technique with the help of which we can reduce the length of solution process and make it easier to read and write. It has some advantages over the iteration technique. A task that can be defined with its similar subtasks, recursion is one of the best methods for finding solutions for it. The properties of recursion are:

- Repeating the same operations many number of times with different inputs.
- At each step, smaller inputs are tried so as to make the problem smaller.
- Base condition is required to end the recursion at some stage, else infinite loop will result.

Wherever we see a recursive solution that has repeated calls for same inputs, we can optimize it using DP. The logic is that the results of subproblems are stored, avoiding the necessity to re-compute them if required later. This simple optimization reduces time required efficiently.

12.2.2 DP more efficient than recursion

Essentially, DP is an efficient recursive algorithm, making sure it does not have to solve the same subproblem twice. It stores the results of subproblems, so we do not have to re-compute those results next time when they are needed. That is, it is an alternative to plain recursion, which requires repeating the solution process every time the subproblem is encountered. In this way, it makes it easier to use past knowledge to solve a future problem, thus saving calculating time.

It uses the principle of optimality, in the sense that if all the steps of a process are optimized, then the result is also optimized. It means that it takes the least amount of time, as it requires fewer new computations. In other words, instead of recomputing the shared steps, DP allows to simply store the results of each step the first time and reuse it each subsequent time. DP is a special case of larger category of recursive programming, but, not all recursive cases can use DP.

When both recursive programs and Dynamic Programming are closely intertwined, why Dynamic Programming is favored? This is because recursive programs often repeat the works if there are overlapping steps, spending extra time and resources in the process. Dynamic Programming solves this issue by ensuring that each identical step is only completed once, storing that step's results in an array to call whenever it is needed again. In doing so, Dynamic Programming allows for less repeated works, resulting in better time efficiency.

12.2.3 Tabulation vs Memoization

To reuse the values of a sub-problem, the values are stored in two different ways. These two patterns are 1. Tabulation: Bottom Up and 2. Memoization: Top Down.

Memoization is an excellent way for computationally expensive programs and it is the process of storing the results of a sub-problem in a top-down approach. Since top-down approaches solve problems as needed, memoization will store data in a non-sequential / unordered way. Rather than understanding the required techniques, we focus on simply memoizing as many solutions as we can. Memoizing gives us a quick and easy win. When we focus on memoizing, our strategy becomes very simple. We just go through as many problems as we can. During the process, we will see a problem which we have already studied. There are only some which we can actually memoize, but the number of problems we may be asked may be large.

This approach may prevent us from actually being able to achieve our target. Imagine learning a new language (let's say Tamil). We decide that we are going to create a massive deck of flashcards and simply memoize individual words. This is our plan to get to fluency.

So, we start memoizing. Here's one sample set of words: "*Naan*", "*Nee*", "*Aval*", "*Naam*", "*Neerellaam*", "*Avarkal*". What is the connection between these words? We will not understand at once. So, we will be memoizing 6 discrete words. However, there is a close connection between these words.

If we look at the translations, we see:

- "*Naan*" – "I am"
- "*Nee*" – "You are"
- "*Aval*" – "She is"
- "*Naam*" – "We are"
- "*Neerellaam*" – "You all are"
- "*Avarkal*" – "They are"

This is easier now, because we have connected them in some way useful to us.

Tabulation Method – Bottom-Up Dynamic Programming

As the name implies, it is about starting from the bottom and accumulating answers to the top. Let's describe a state for a DP problem to be dp[x] with dp[0] as base state and dp[n] as our destination state, meaning that we need to find the value of destination state i.e dp[n]. If we start the transition from the base state, i.e., dp[0] and follow the state transition relation to reach the destination state dp[n], it is called as the bottom up approach, since it is clear that we started the transition from the bottom base state and reached the topmost desired state.

Memoization Method – Top-Down Dynamic Programming

If we need to find the value for some state say dp[n] and instead of starting from the base state, i.e., dp[0], we try to ask our answer from the states that can reach the destination state dp[n], following the state transition relation, then it is the top-down fashion of DP. Here, we start from the top most destination state and compute its answer by taking into account the values of states that can reach the destination state, till we reach the bottom-most base state. That is, we store the most recent value to a limit, so that if next time, we have a call from the same state, we simply return it from the memory. So, this is why we call it memorization, as we are storing the most recent state values.

	Tabulation (Bottom-Up DP)	Memoization (Top-Down DP)
State transition relation	Difficult to think	Easy to think
Code	Gets complicated, especially when lot of conditions are required	Easy and less complicated
Speed	Fast, as we directly access previous states from the table	Slow, due to lot of recursive calls and return statements
Subproblem solving	If all subproblems must be solved atleast once, a bottom-up DP algorithm usually outperforms a top down memoized algorithm by a constant factor	If some subproblems need not be solved, the memoized solution has the advantage of solving only those subproblems that are essentially required
Table entries	Starting from the first entry, all entries are filled one by one	All entries are not necessarily filled in memoized version

12.2.4 Solving a DP Problem

As detailed above, to dynamically solve a problem, we need to check two necessary conditions:

1. **Overlapping Subproblems:** This is where the actual optimization comes in. If the problem has overlapping subproblems, it means that we are using the same function with same inputs multiple times. So, we are doing repetitive works for no reason. If we can memoize the results, we will be able to save a lot of time. When the solutions to the same subproblems are needed repetitively for solving the actual problem, the problem is said to have overlapped subproblems property.
2. **Optimal Substructure Property:** The first criterion is that the problem must have optimal substructure. Technically, this means that we must be able to find an optimal solution to a problem by solving for its subproblems. That is, we must be able to solve the problem recursively. If we already found a recursive problem, then we can safely assume we have optimal substructure. If an optimal solution can be obtained for the problem by using optimal solutions of its subproblems, then the problem is said to possess optimal substructure property.

   If we meet these two criteria, then we can optimize our solution using DP.

12.2.5 Steps to solve a DP Problem

This part was implored from Kumar, who contributed the article (in *https://www.linkedin.com/in/nk17kumar/ and https://www.geeksforgeeks.org/solve-dynamic-programming-problem/*), as this particular manuscript is meant for learning purpose and his excellent effort in effectively explaining the steps is gratefully acknowledged.

1. **Identify if it is a DP problem:** All the problems that require **maximizing or minimizing** certain quantities or counting problems, for e.g., counting the arrangements under certain conditions or certain probability problems can be solved by using DP. All DP problems satisfy the **overlapping subproblems** property and most of the DP problems also satisfy the **optimal substructure** property. Once we observe these properties in a given problem, it can be solved using DP.
2. **Decide a state expression with the least parameters:** DP problems are all about the state and its transition. This is the most basic step which must be done carefully because the state transition depends on the choice of state definition we make. A state is defined as the set of **factors** *that can exclusively identify a position in* a given problem. This set of factors should be as small as possible to reduce the state space.
3. **Formulate state and transition relationship:** This is the difficult stage of solving a DP problem and hence requires a lot of insight, observation, and practice. For e**xample, g**iven 3 numbers (1, 3, 5), the task may be to tell the total number of ways we can form a number **N** using the sum of these three numbers (allowing repetitions and different arrangements):

   Total number of ways to form 6 is 8.

   1+1+1+1+1+1

   1+1+1+3

   1+1+3+1

   1+3+1+1

   3+1+1+1

   3+3

   1+5

   5+1

   The steps to solve the given problem are:

   - Decide a state for the given problem.
   - Take a parameter N to decide the state, as it can uniquely identify any subproblem.
   - DP state will look like state (N), meaning the total number of arrangements to form N by using (1, 3, 5) as elements. Derive a transition relation between any two states.
   - Now, we need to compute state (N).

How to compute the state?

We use 1, 3, or 5 to form a given number N and assume that we know the result for N = 1, 2, 3, 4, 5, 6. We now know the result for state (n = 1), state (n = 2), state (n = 3), … and state (n = 6). Now, let us know the result of the state (n = 7). We can add 1, 3, and 5 and we get a total of 7 in 3 ways:

1. ***Adding 1 to all possible combinations of state (n = 6)***

   [(1+1+1+1+1+1) + 1]

   [(1+1+1+3) + 1]

   [(1+1+3+1) + 1]

   [(1+3+1+1) + 1]

   [(3+1+1+1) + 1]

   [(3+3) + 1]

   [(1+5) + 1]

   [(5+1) + 1]

2. ***Adding 3 to all possible combinations of state (n = 4)***

   [(1+1+1+1) + 3]

   [(1+3) + 3]

   [(3+1) + 3]

3. ***Adding 5 to all possible combinations of state (n = 2)***

   [(1+1) + 5]

It is sufficient to add only on the right side, as all the additions from the left side cases are covered, either in the same state, or another. E.g. [1+ (1+1+1+3)] is not needed in state (n=6), because it is covered by state (n = 4) [(1+1+1+1) + 3]). Now, the above three cases are covering all possible ways to form a sum total of 7. Therefore, we can say that result for state (7) = state (6) + state (4) + state (2) OR state (7) = state (7-1) + state (7-3) + state (7-5). In general, state (n) = state (n-1) + state (n-3) + state (n-5). So, we just need to add memoization.

12.2.6 Solving DP Problems using FAST Method

FAST method is a repeatable strategy for solving any DP problem, whether we have seen the problem before or not. The FAST method is an acronym for 4 steps we need to solve any DP problem:

1. Find the First Solution
2. Analyze the First Solution
3. Identify the Subproblems
4. Turn around the solution

Following these 4 steps, we can find the optimal DP solution for any problem.

1. **Find the First Solution:** The first important step for any DP problem is to find an initial basic solution to the problem. The goal is to just get something written on the paper without any concern for efficiency. There are several keys to go about while doing this step:
   i. The solution should be recursive. Otherwise, the problem need not be solved by DP.
   ii. Each recursion must be self-contained. This means that we cannot store our results or insert a variable into our function.
   iii. It is important that we minimize the number of variables that we are using in our recursive function.
2. **Analyze the First Solution:** This is the step where we decide whether we can actually use DP to solve a problem. To do this, we are going to look at a couple of specific things. First, we should determine what is the actual time complexity currently. One mistake we may do is attempting to optimize something that doesn't need to be optimized. If our solution is already efficient, spending time for optimizing is a wasteful exercise.
3. **Identify the subproblems:** If we find that we are able to use DP, the next step is to identify and define the subproblems. Once we have identified the subproblems, we can also memoize the recursive solution to make it more efficient. That is, we add an array that stores all the values that we have previously computed. Whenever we want to make a function call, we will look into the array of results to check if a result has already been computed for the current inputs. If so, then we can return it without actually computing anything. If it is not available, we can compute it and save it into our array.
4. **Turn around the solution:** We will notice that the majority of the DP solution are iterative, not recursive. That is, up to this point in the FAST Method, we only generate recursive solutions. In this optional final step, we take our recursive solution and make it into an iterative solution.

12.2.7 Bellman's Principle of Optimality

Solution for DP is here based on Bellman's principle of optimality, where a problem is broken down into several stages, and after the first decision all the remaining decisions must be optimal (Bellman, 1952). The decisions at each stage are found by either working forward or backward at each stage. An optimal policy has the property that whatever may be the initial state and decisions, the remaining decisions will constitute optimal policy for the state which resulted from the first decision.

Mathematically, this can be written as:

$$f_N(x) = \max. [r(d_n) + f_N - 1T(x, d_n)]d_n \square x$$

where

$f_N(x)$ = optimal return from an N-stage process, when initial state is x

$r(d_n)$ = immediate return due to decision d_n

$T(x, d_n)$ = the transfer function which gives the resulting state

$\{x\}$ = set of admissible decisions

This equation is also known as a DP equation. It represents a necessary condition for optimality associated with the optimization method (DP). It writes the value of a decision problem in time in terms of the payoff from some initial choices and the value of the remaining decision problem resulting from initial choices. This breaks a DP optimization problem into simpler sub-problems.

Examples

Example 1

Imagine you want to go to a new grocery store a few streets away, but you don't know how to get there. To solve the sub-problem of the route to the store, we look for directions on our phone's map and then make our way there. In a recursive program, we will have to take time to look for the directions again, each time we want to go to the store. Instead in DP, we remember the directions to the store from when we first looked for it. As a result, we don't need to spend time looking for directions when we want to go to the store in the future. This is in essence how DP functions.

Example 2

Given a list of currency notes, you are required to count the number of ways in which you can represent a certain amount. For example, if you have only two kinds of notes, Rs.10 and Rs.20, and you want to represent Rs.30, there are only two ways:

- 3 bills of Rs.10
- 1 bill of Rs.20 and 1 bill of Rs.10

While designing the algorithm, we have to take care that we do not over-count. Rs.30 can be represented with Rs.20+ Rs.10 as well as Rs.10+ Rs.20, but these are the same thing. Therefore, we should not count both cases. A simple recursive solution will timeout for large inputs; thus, you should try to write a dynamic programming algorithm. Start with a recursive solution and build up to a dynamic solution.

Example 3

Imagine we have a bag of coins where each coin is of value 5 Rs. and we have to find the total amount of money available in that bag, what will we do to find the total amount in the bag? We count the number of coins and multiply it with 5 *Rs*. So, if the number of coins is 100, then, we have 500 *Rs*. amount of money. Now if we add 10 more coins of 5 *Rs*. in that bag, how much is the amount now? The answer is 550 Rs. How we calculated this answer. Did we count all the number of coins in the bag and multiply it with 5 *Rs*.? No, we already knew that the bag had 100 coins and by adding 10 more coins, the total number of coins is 110 and when we multiply 110 with 5 *Rs*. we get 550 *Rs*. This approach to problem-solving is called DP. We store the answer to a subproblem in memory and use that to solve the future problem.

12.2.8 Disadvantages of DP

Both Tabulation (Bottom-Up) and Memoization (Top-Down) approaches give the same complexity. However, many prefer the bottom-up approach, because recursive code tends to execute slower than iterative code that does the same work. The key to find a bottom-up solution is to look for the smallest subproblems. This is why we need to carefully identify and define the subproblems. We can start with computing the base case. Then we need to determine how to compute a given subproblem, assuming all the smaller subproblems have already been computed. We will save all of these subproblem solutions into an array so that we can easily look them up.

In short, DP is a challenging topic. We cannot magically become a master overnight. However, it is also not something we should be afraid of. If we know recursion skills and understand the solution steps, even the most challenging DP problems can be easily solved.

Another challenge with DP is that it is counterintuitive (we have to go north first, if we want to go south). When we try to solve DP problems, all the steps that we would normally take actually pull us further away from the correct solution:

- Want to find the optimal solution? We actually need to start with the basic approach.
- Want to find an iterative solution? We have to start with recursion (a process of defining a function or calculating a number by repeated application of an algorithm).
- Want to solve the problem quickly? We need to slow it down and go step by step.

13

Economics of Animal Disease Control

There are three types of disease occurrence namely, endemic, epidemic and outbreaks. Martin *et al.* (1993) described the term endemic as the disease occurrence in a predictable pattern. There can be low, moderate or high levels of endemicity. Although many times the terms epidemic and outbreak are used synonymously, the term epidemic is used when there is an unexpected incidence of a disease. Thrusfield (1995) defined an outbreak as the occurrence of a disease involving one or more animals. An outbreak can result in an epidemic and subsequently, it may even become an epidemic. OIE (1996) defined outbreak as an occurrence of one of the diseases in list A or B:

<table>
<tr><th>List A Diseases</th><th colspan="2">List B Diseases</th></tr>
<tr><td colspan="3">Transmissible animal diseases characterized by</td></tr>
<tr><td>Serious and rapid spread, having serious socio-economic and public health consequences, and affecting international trade</td><td colspan="2">Serious socio-economic and public health consequences within countries, besides affecting international trade</td></tr>
<tr><td>• Foot and Mouth Disease
• Vesicular Stomatitis
• Swine Vesicular Disease
• Rinderpest
• Peste des Petits Ruminants
• Contagious Bovine Pleuro Pneumonia
• Lumpy Skin Disease
• Rift Valley Fever
• Bluetongue
• Sheep Pox and Goat Pox
• African Horse Sickness
• African Swine Fever
• Classical Swine Fever
• Fowl Plaque
• Newcastle Disease</td><td>Multiple Species
• Aujeszky's Disease
• Leptospirosis
• Johne's Disease
• Rabies
Cattle
• Bovine Brucellosis
• Infectious Bovine Rhinotracheitis
• Bovine Spongiform Encephalopathy</td><td>Pigs
• PEARS (Mystery Swine Disease)
• Atrophic Rhinitis
• Transmissible Gastro Enteritis
Poultry
• Infectious Bursal Disease
• Marek's Disease
• Salmonella enteritidis
• Salmonella typhimurium</td></tr>
</table>

Animal disease prevention and control activities offer valuable benefits for food production, food security and safety, animal and human welfare, and alleviation of poverty. The effectiveness of disease prevention and control policies depends on the good governance and quality of the veterinary services, in compliance with OIE standards and guidelines on animal disease control. The apex body in each country is the core system that takes care of the prevention and control of animal diseases. This body is responsible for early detection of diseases and rapid response to outbreaks. The veterinary services in developing countries require adequate human and financial resources and capacity building to carry out the tasks of disease prevention and control and to protect animal health and thus public health, including food security and food safety.

Disease prevention and control strategies may differ from disease to disease. However, the following are some possible actions that can be done:

- Doing nothing
- Restrictions on the movement of affected animals
- Quarantine of affected animals
- Vaccination of non-affected animals, either preventive or strategic
- Treatment of affected animals
- Improved husbandry practices
- Disinfection of sheds, pathways, and surrounding areas
- Stamping out / culling affected animals and their safe disposable
- Monitoring and surveillance

13.1 STRATEGIES IN DISEASE PREVENTION AND CONTROL

Effective Surveillance

There must be effective active (planned) or passive (event-based) surveillance. The OIE defines surveillance as the systematic ongoing collection, collation, and analysis of data, and the timely dissemination of information to the stakeholders to enable them to take action. This strategy requires optimal communication and collaboration between all stakeholders at all levels of the animal production chain, from the animal producers, veterinary staff, and laboratory, to the top national-level veterinary authorities.

Early Detection of Disease

An early detection system enables the timely detection and identification of the emergence or re-emergence of a disease or infection in a country, zone, or region. It must follow the relevant OIE standards and should include the following characteristics:

- Representative coverage of target animal populations, by field services throughout the territory in cooperation with farmers and stakeholders;
- Ability to undertake effective epidemiological investigations and reporting;

- Access to laboratories capable of diagnosing and differentiating diseases;
- Training programmes for veterinarians, para-veterinarians, and other stakeholders for detecting and reporting animal health incidents;
- Legal obligation for private veterinarians to report to the veterinary authorities;

Collection of Samples

To ensure a rapid and effective diagnosis of any new disease occurrence, the veterinary authorities must have a mechanism for sample collection and laboratory analysis of samples.

Diagnosis

Once a disease outbreak is identified, the veterinary authorities must ensure that the national and international community is alerted at the earliest and that a final confirmation and characterization of the pathogen is determined, if necessary, in an OIE Reference Laboratory for the specified disease. OIE has a global network of Reference Laboratories and Collaborating Centres covering all relevant animal diseases.

Notification of Animal Disease to the OIE

The OIE strives to ensure the transparency of the world's animal health situation. On becoming an OIE Member, each country undertakes to report the animal health situation in its territory in a timely and transparent manner. The OIE Member Countries can connect to the OIE server at any time to fulfill their obligation to provide information, on time, on any relevant domestic or wild animal disease detected within their territory.

Vaccination

Vaccination is a very useful strategy in the prevention and control of many diseases, if it conforms to an existing disease control programme. A vaccination programme should be a part of an integrated disease control strategy utilizing a combination of other disease control measures. If it is determined that vaccination is an option, before launching a specific vaccination policy Member Countries should make sure that the preconditions like ensuring the quality of vaccine and following the conditions under which any vaccination policy must eventually be stopped (exit strategy). Vaccines produced should have followed the guidelines prescribed in the OIE Manual of Diagnostic Tests and Vaccines for Terrestrial Animals. For most vaccines, ensuring an effective cold chain is critical to the successful implementation of a vaccination campaign.

Animal Identification and Traceability

Animal identification and traceability are useful tools in the effective control of animal diseases. In case of outbreaks, such measures will make it easier to identify animals and animal products exposed to the pathogen and allow them to be traced, so that the appropriate control measures can be implemented. Again, the application of animal identification and traceability should also comply with OIE standards.

Biosecurity

Biosecurity measures should be followed to protect human and animal health from biological risks. In the case of a disease outbreak in a non-endemic area, depopulation (by the humane killing of infected and in-contact animals following OIE standards), followed by disinfection of farm sheds, equipment, and vehicles, with a temporary ban or control of movements of animals are required to prevent the spread of the pathogen. Appropriate biosecurity measures must be implemented by ensuring that all those involved are properly trained and by providing them with the necessary material and human resources.

Zoning and Compartmentalization

To make it possible for countries with areas that are partially infected with diseases to access international markets without placing importers at risk, the OIE has defined several concepts in the Terrestrial Code:

- Zoning allows a country to isolate parts of its territory that are free from certain diseases from other areas that are still infected.
- Compartmentalization is a procedure implemented to pursue trade from an animal disease-free subpopulation of animals within a country or zone not free of the disease.

A compartment means an animal subpopulation in one or more areas under a common biosecurity management system with a distinct health status concerning a specific disease for which required surveillance, control, and biosecurity measures have been applied for the purpose of international trade. All compartments need to be approved and audited by the national veterinary authorities.

13.2 USE OF ECONOMICS IN ANIMAL DISEASE CONTROL PROGRAMMES

The project appraisal which is the economic analysis of a disease control programme before it is undertaken (called *ex-ante* analysis), and the project evaluation which is the assessment of a control programme after it has been undertaken (called *ex-post* analysis) are the two fundamental applications of economic principles applied to decision-making for animal disease control. Both involve setting out costs and benefits over a period of time and comparing them to determine whether the disease control programme would be economically viable.

For any animal disease control project, economic theory can help to provide a framework for ranking different disease control alternatives and making a decision whether to implement the control programme or not, based on the cost-effectiveness of the programme to the sector or the society. Of course, decisions cannot be taken based on economic considerations alone. The technical feasibility of any proposed project must first be examined by the concerned veterinarians and experts. Next, its overall compatibility with the policies and goals of the sector must be ensured, and thirdly its feasibility from the organisational and social points of view needs to be ascertained.

As we have seen in an earlier chapter, the following economic methods can be used to evaluate the cost-effectiveness of disease control projects, as detailed below (partly derived from Otte and Chilonda, 2002):

Method	Level	Concept	Choice Indicator
Gross Margin Analysis	Farm / herd	Gross margin; Fixed Costs not included	Gross margin = Output – Variable Costs
Enterprise Budget	Farm / herd	Enterprise budget; Fixed Costs also included	Profit = Output – Total Costs
Partial Budget Analysis	Farm / herd	Costs and benefits of a new intervention	Net effect on the income
Cost-Benefit Analysis	Sector / Region / Nation	Comparison of benefits and costs of the project usually for a year or more	Net Present Value (NPV), Benefit - Cost Ratio (BCR) and Internal Rate of Return (IRR),
Decision Tree Analysis	Farm / Sector / Region / Nation	Computing the values of different courses of action by incorporating probabilities of revenues and losses	Optimum output based on the expected value of the benefit
Linear Programming	Farm	Finding the best solution from competing activities subject to constraints	Optimal solution
Dynamic Programming	Farm	Searching for optimal solution	Optimal solution

13.3 Costs and Benefits of Animal Disease Control Programmes

When assessing the costs and benefits of an animal disease control programme, we must identify the additional costs incurred and new benefits reaped. An investment in the disease control programme is deemed worthwhile if the benefits arising out of the programme are able to offset the additional costs invested in the programme. This is normally measured using a cost-benefit analysis, which measures the economic profitability of the control programme.

Costs of Controlling a Disease

The costs of animal disease control will vary not only with the disease and the type of control policy adopted, but also with the region in which the programme is implemented. In examining and comparing different disease control policies, two aspects should be emphasized:

- Overall costs and their relation to the funds available.
- Timing of expenditures over the years. Treatments and prophylaxis involve costs over a number of years, while eradication demands a higher level of expenditure for a shorter period.

Components of Disease Control Costs

While working out the costs of disease control measures, it is essential to distinguish clearly between variable costs and fixed costs.

Variable costs include the costs of:

- Drugs for treatments, vaccinations, insecticides, etc.;
- Syringes, needles, and other small equipment; and
- Staff travel expenses and allowances.

Fixed costs include the costs of:

- Vehicle expenses;
- Salaries to permanent staff;
- Expenses at the office for administration;
- Depreciation of vehicles, equipment, and buildings; and
- Office rents, water, and electricity charges.
- Depreciation of vehicles, equipment, and buildings; and
- Office rents, water, and electricity charges.

13.4 ECONOMIC WORTH OF ANIMAL DISEASE CONTROL OR PREVENTION

The economic viability of a decision to control or prevent diseases in animals is vital to the government to justify its use of public resources or an individual to decide whether to invest in a disease control measure like vaccination. The methods to assess the economic worth of an intervention usually compare the expected benefits (positive economic impacts) that may arise with the expected costs (negative economic impacts) of control that may accrue. An economically viable initiative is one in which the benefits are at least equal to the costs, if not higher.

13.4.1 Sources of Benefits within Livestock Sector

Increased output and asset value

Increased output and herd values are the most obvious benefits of controlling disease and the easiest to estimate, which may result from reduced disease incidence, encouraging livestock owners to consume more and or sell more livestock and livestock products in the market. Since methods such as cost-benefit analysis and cost-effectiveness analysis use discounted values (present values of future costs and benefits), benefits realized early carry more weight in the estimate of economic viability than those realized later.

An evaluation of the economic impact of Rinderpest control by the PAN African Rinderpest Campaign between 1989-90 and 1996-97 concluded that the benefit resulting from avoided losses in the value of cattle outputs in ten countries amounted to ECU99 179 (Tambi *et al.*, 1999a). An ex-ante assessment of the economics of CBPP control in herds in Western Uganda found that about 95 percent of the benefit would come from increased output and asset value (Twinamasiko, 2002).

Reduced prevention costs and treatment costs

A disease control programme reduces the need for preventive vaccination or clinical treatment.

Benefit to Public Health

Benefits to public health from the control of a zoonotic disease can be saving human lives or life-years and reduced costs to the public health system when fewer people need to be treated.

13.4.2 Sources of Cost within Livestock Sector

Prevention costs

Prevention costs include animal health intelligence, biosecurity, & vaccination.

Animal health intelligence

Animal health intelligence, as defined by FAO [2010] covers all the activities related to the identification of potential hazards that may represent a risk to animal health which include surveillance activities, animal health information system development for disease reporting, and collection and analysis of disease and non-disease data.

Costs include the costs of active surveillance (i.e. surveys and monitoring in farms, markets, and abattoirs), passive surveillance (reporting of disease by farmers), investigation of disease reports, and maintenance of the national information system.

Biosecurity

The best way to protect a herd or flock from a disease is to prevent disease agents from crossing the farm boundary (FAO, 2008). This requires good biosecurity practices: restricting access to animals by people who do not normally live and work on the farm, and cleaning the footwear and vehicles of anyone who enters the farm, including the farm family and employees. Simple biosecurity measures such as soap and water, cheap rubber footwear for animal handlers, and management routines to minimize the chance that people and animals will carry disease agents from infected to uninfected herds.

Vaccination

All the infectious of the concern are caused by viruses (with the exceptions of CBPP and CCPP, caused by mycoplasmas). The most common preventive measure applied at the level of individual animals is vaccination. Vaccines are available for many diseases (except African Swine Fever). Vaccination may be a high recurrent cost, because of which governments are reluctant to commit to long-term programmes, except for FMD. Since vaccination protects their livestock assets, individual farmers in risk areas may be willing to bear vaccination costs. There may also be good food security for protecting the livestock of the poor through vaccination. However, countries free of specific diseases choose not to allow preventive vaccination. For e.g., in the European Union, vaccination against FMD is only used as a temporary measure in case of outbreaks, if any, and not a routine measure.

The cost per protected animal of vaccination varies enormously depending on:

- The number of vaccinations needed in an animal's life.
- The ability of the vaccine to protect against multiple strains of the disease agent.
- The cost of delivery of vaccine to livestock farmers.
- The capacity (human and equipment) of the public and private veterinary service to produce or import, test, and deliver vaccines whenever needed in good quality.

Outbreak control costs

Outbreak control costs include:

- Operational costs of disease confirmation, movement control, culling of animals, disposal of carcasses, and disease tracing.

- The loss of animals culled.
- Loss of production value through delayed sales or delays in restocking.

Quantifying operational costs and the value of lost animals is straightforward, but that of the effects of quarantine and delayed restocking are not easy. In countries that have a strong motivation to control diseases, compensation is paid to livestock owners for animals culled and feed destroyed within the outbreak control programmes.

The cost of vaccinating a bovine against FMD in the EU in 1987 was estimated to vary from US$ 0.74 in Greece to US$ 2.66 in the UK (Horst *et al.*, 1999b). The cost of vaccinating a broiler chicken against Newcastle Disease was estimated to be approximately US cents 4.1 per bird in Cambodia in 1994, and US cents 1.5 in the Netherlands in 1997 (Horst *et al.*, 1999b).

13.5 METHODS OF ANALYSIS OF ANIMAL DISEASE CONTROL PROGRAMMES

13.5.1 Cost-Benefit Analysis

Cost-benefit analysis (CBA) is perhaps the best-known method for the economic analysis of animal health programmes and projects. It is suitable for sector-wide or nationwide analysis, and also for farm-level interventions where the effects of changes will develop over several years. CBA constructs the benefit flows minus the cost flows year by year and uses this to estimate the Net Present Value (NPV) of the project (the total discounted profit from the project), the Benefit – Cost Ratio (BCR), the ratio of the total discounted benefits to the total discounted costs, and the Internal Rate of Return (IRR), the rate of return on the investment made in the project. An NPV of zero or greater, or a BCR of greater than one, or an IRR equal to or greater than the opportunity cost of the investment indicates an economically viable investment. A detailed note on how to work out NPV, BCR and IRR is given in Section 10.4 of Chapter 10. A CBA can be used for appraisal (estimating the economic viability of a proposed project, also known as ex-ante analysis) or evaluation (estimating the economic viability of a project that is partly or fully completed, also known as ex-post analysis).

Many studies on the economic viability of disease control interventions use CBA. A few examples include:

- The first study to apply the CBA technique to an animal disease was conducted by Ellis (1972) for the CSF eradication programme in the UK in 1972. The success of this study led to the interest in applying CBA to animal diseases of zoonotic importance such as anthrax and brucellosis. Mcleod *et al.* (2003) used CBA to analyze the economic potential of CSF control in Vietnam.

- James and Ellis (1978) published one of the earliest papers on the CBA of FMD. Perry *et al.* (1999) and Randolph *et al.* (2002) analyzed the economic viability of FMD control in Southeast Asia, while Perry *et al.* (2003) did the same for Southern Africa. McLeod (2010) estimated the costs and benefits of the Southeast Asia FMD Campaign.
- Tambi *et al.* (1999a) retrospectively analyzed the economic impact of the Pan African Rinderpest Campaign. Omiti and Irungu (2010) carried out a cost-benefit analysis of Rinderpest eradication in Kenya and Ethiopia.
- Taylor *et al.* (2003) analyzed the economic viability of FMD and CSF-free zones in Vietnam. McLeod and Honhold (2012) reviewed the viability of setting up an FMD disease-free zone in Zambia.

13.5.2 Cost-Effectiveness Analysis

Cost-Effectiveness Analysis (CEA) has many similarities to CBA but measures the benefits differently. Like CBA, it is suitable for sector-wide or nationwide initiatives or interventions on a smaller scale. Like CBA, it can be used for appraisal or evaluation. Similarly, figures are discounted in CEA. Unlike CBA, which estimates both costs and benefits in monetary terms, CEA does not monetize benefits, instead, it expresses them as units of an effectiveness measure. The result of CEA is the cost per unit of the chosen outcome. CEA may be used to compare the cost of achieving the same level of outcome in different ways or the cost of achieving different levels of a particular outcome. Krupnik (2004) and Abelson (2008) provided a more complete discussion on CEA. CEA is useful for assessing the economic viability of projects to control zoonotic diseases whose impacts are on human health as well as animal health. CAE has the limitation that it only allows for one type of outcome, for e.g., the number of lives saved. When the control of a zoonotic disease results in improved human health and increased livestock outputs, a CEA cannot fully express the potential benefits.

Examples of CEA applied to disease control include analysis of brucellosis control in Mongolia (Roth *et al.*, 2003), estimation of the cost-effectiveness of Rinderpest vaccination in Africa, and using the cost per animal vaccinated as the measure of effectiveness (Tambi *et al.*, 1999a), and estimation of the cost-effectiveness of avian influenza virus surveillance in Switzerland (Häsler *et al.*, 2011).

13.5.3 Other Methods

Both CBA and CEA are the most commonly used methods for economic analysis of animal disease control programmes. However, both have a few limitations. While they can indicate whether a control intervention is economically viable, they cannot suggest what might be the best intervention. Further, they do not deal effectively with intangible losses. McInerney (1991) and Tisdell (1994) pointed out the theoretical and practical limitations of CBA, like the danger inherent in extrapolating the result from a small livestock population to a national estimate, and the wrong interpretation of results. The drawback of the use of CBA in animal health was also highlighted by Howe and Christiansen (2004).

A few examples of alternatives to CBA and CEA are:

1. ***Optimization models*** – These models are used to estimate the best combination of limited resources to achieve an outcome. . Kobayashi *et al.* (2007) used a dynamic optimization model to analyze the economic impacts of controlling an FMD outbreak affecting part of California, USA. They ran the model firstly to minimize disease incidence and then to minimize pre-emptive culling. They are data-demanding and generally used for analyses at the local or farm level. Carpenter *et al.* (2011) used an optimization model to estimate the impact of an FMD outbreak in California, the USA and examined the effect of delayed disease detection. Assuming a detection delay of 21 days, it was estimated that for every additional hour of delay, there would be an additional economic loss of $565 million. Optimization models are well suited to analysis at the farm level or within a limited geographic area.
2. ***Decision tree analysis*** can provide a framework for decision-making about disease control. It uses a sequence of decisions, each of which has two possible answers, to provide a step-by-step guide to a final choice. Tomassen *et al.* (2002) used a decision tree as the framework to estimate the benefits and costs of FMD control. Rushton and Upton (2006) described a generic decision-tree framework for making choices about the balance of active and passive measures to control an outbreak.
3. ***Contingent valuation and choice models*** are used in environmental economics, to place a value on attributes such as biodiversity, landscapes, or conservation of natural habitat (Winpenny, 1991, Moran, 1994 and Hanley *et al.*, 1998). Contingent valuation has also been used to evaluate Economic analysis of animal diseases. Junker *et al.* (2009) compared FMD control strategies by analyzing the potential impacts of a trade ban following an FMD outbreak on the economies of the USA, Canada, and the Netherlands. Costs associated with the outbreak were compared under four different control scenarios: stamping-out or vaccination, with or without regionalization (movement control confined to a defined geographic region rather than affecting the whole country). In the 1997-

98 epidemic of CSF in the Netherlands, farmers were compensated for the value of destroyed herds, but not for lost production from idle facilities (Horst *et al.*, 1999b). Contingent valuation can also be used to evaluate the willingness of farmers to pay for the disease control measures undertaken on their farms (Ahuja and Sen, 2006). For e.g., it has been used to assess farmer willingness to contribute to the cost of brucellosis vaccination in Tajikistan (Ahuja *et al.*, 2009). Choice models can be used to guide the design of disease control programmes based on the choices made by stakeholders about animal health control.

4. **Regression analysis** - Chilonda and Van Huylenbroeck (2001) described the use of regression analysis to analyze choices that livestock keepers make about animal health services or measures. They attempted to produce a mathematical equation that described the relationship between one or more causes (explanatory variables) and an effect (dependent variable), and also provided information on how well the set of data.
5. **Logistic regression techniques** suitable for explanatory variables with only two possible values include Probit, Logit, and Tobit analysis, all of which had been used to analyze farmers' choices about animal health care in African countries (Tambi *et al.*, 1999b, Chilonda, 1999 and Mutambara *et al.*, 2013).
6. **Partial budget analysis** - There are many descriptions of partial budget analysis in published documents. The simplest and most practical are found in agricultural extension and farm management publications, for e.g., Tigner (2006). Gari *et al.* (2011) used partial budget analysis to assess the economic viability of vaccinating against Lumpy Skin Disease in the Oromo region of Ethiopia and found a net benefit of USD1 per animal for local zebus and USD19 for exotic and crossbred cattle. Young *et al.* (2013) used partial budget analysis to assess the economic viability of vaccinating Cambodian smallholder cattle against FMD and estimated a net benefit of USD31 per animal.
7. **Decision trees**, a tool to guide a decision through a series of choices, can be used by a farmer, trader, dairy processing plant, or slaughterhouse owner to analyze decisions about investment in animal health. One example of use for disease control was described by Onono (2014), analyzing CBPP control in Kenya and he used decision tree analysis to analyze the net benefit of vaccination compared with no action for a single herd.

14

Animal Disease Information System

14.1 NEED FOR ANIMAL DISEASE INFORMATION SYSTEMS

Once the animal disease data are gathered, a few things need to be done with the data so collected. First, they must be managed and quality checked; Secondly, they must be analyzed to be understandable; and thirdly, they must be acted upon. For data to be analyzable and useful for decision-making, they need cautious management and quality control. An information system is the collection of data, people, procedures, hardware, software, files, and data required to accomplish an organized set of functions.

The constituents of an information system are:

- People – those who gather data, those responsible for data input and those responsible for data analysis
- A storage / retrieval / analysis system – which consists of computer hardware and appropriate software
- A feedback delivery system – mechanisms to ensure that processed data are fed back to data gatherers

Managing the Information System

A System Manager will manage the system, by carrying out the following functions:

- Monitor data flow into the system
- Check data quality – Cross-checking with data from other sources and providing feedback to data suppliers
- Data analysis and making the analyzed data (information) reach the decision makers.
- Feedback to the field

When designing an animal disease information system, it is important to know which disease would occur, which species would get affected, etc. The system in the process of conception should build on the system already there to show what kind of information is not used, and what could be done to make it more useful. In developing countries, it is better to start too small than too big. While designing an information system, it is important to build a flow diagram of how data flow is foreseen. Data quality control is an integral part of an information system at different like the field, the district office, the epidemiology unit, and the state state-level office.

14.2 OUTPUTS OF AN ANIMAL DISEASE INFORMATION SYSTEM

1. **Improve the collection of animal health data**

   Passive Surveillance

   - *Training of state and district veterinary staff*
   - *Provision of specimen collection kits*
   - *Monitoring staff activity*
   - *Support for specimen transport and feedback systems*
   - *Public awareness campaigns for livestock owners and traders*
   - *Establish links with village-level workers*

   Active Surveillance

   - *Training of staff in survey techniques*
   - *Implementing field disease surveillance*
   - *Use active surveillance to support disease control programs*

2. ***Ensure sustainable laboratory support***

   Effective laboratory support for field activities

   - *Provision of specimens to national and international reference laboratories*
   - *Provision of diagnostic reagents to laboratories*
   - *Sustainable local production of key diagnostic reagents*
   - *Train laboratory staff in new diagnostic techniques*

3. ***Implement an information management system***

   Efficient management of animal health information

   - *User needs analysis and database designs*
   - *Development of users' manuals*
   - *Training of staff in the use of systems*
   - *Phased implementation*

4. ***Establish National and Regional Analysis and Reporting Systems***

Improved ability of staff to analyze and interpret animal health information

- *Training of staff in data analysis*

Improved regional communication and coordination of disease control activities

- *Establishment of a regional disease outbreak database*
- *Regional data analysis*
- *Coordinators' meetings*

5. ***Control Program Formulation, Implementation and Monitoring***

- *Training*
- *Formulate disease control options*
- *Evaluate options to identify optimal strategies*
- *Implement priority disease control activities*

14.3 ACTIVITIES IN AN ANIMAL DISEASE INFORMATION SYSTEM

Regional	• Participation in regional meetings • Establishment of standard rules for disease reporting and control • Links with appropriate regional bodies • Analysis of disease and livestock movement patterns • Development of regional disease outbreak databases
National	• Improved passive surveillance systems • Effective active surveillance systems • Structured disease control programs for priority diseases • Improve laboratory capabilities
State level	• Training in active and passive surveillance • Improving skills in disease outbreak investigation
District	• Training in active and passive surveillance • Improved reporting of livestock demographics • Improved reporting of livestock movement
Village	• Increased awareness of the need to report and control diseases

14.4 NATIONAL ANIMAL DISEASE INFORMATION SYSTEM

Large numbers of staff with computer networks are there in developed countries, but in developing countries, it is better to start small than big. If one takes a convenient number of 20 to 25 veterinary districts to one computer, then it is quite practical to say that in large countries, a small computer unit at regional/ state level could handle the inputs from those administrative divisions and then pass the data on to the central unit. The easiest way to handle this would be for each station to post all of its inputs regularly (fortnightly; monthly) to its computer unit, and to keep duplicates of all questionnaires in reserve.

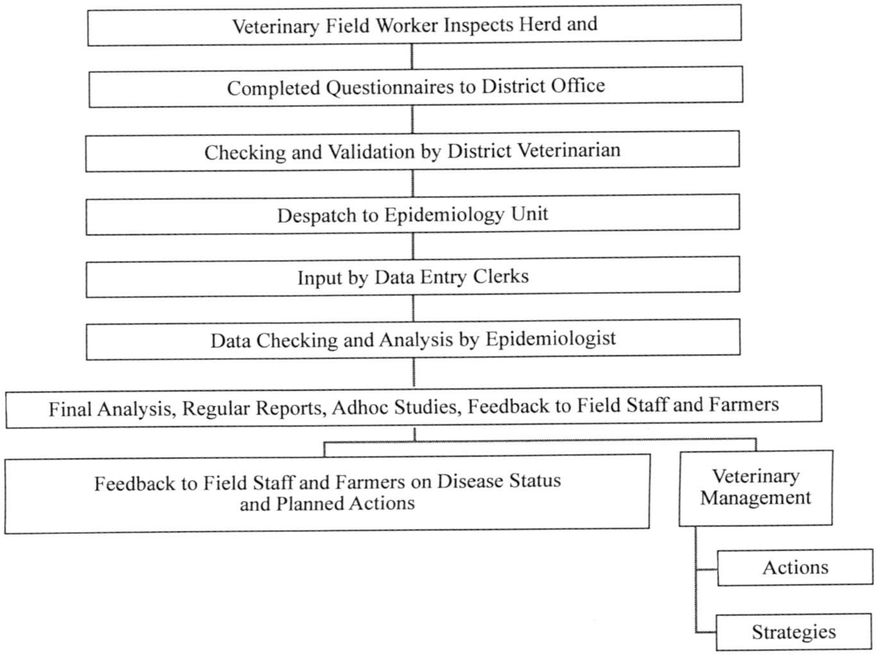

Managing the flow of information

When designing an information system, it is important to construct a flow diagram of how data flow in the system is envisaged, and what the various control points will be. In general, the flow of data in the case of visual surveillance will be: Farmer→ Animal Health Worker → Veterinarian → Epidemiology Unit → Analysis & Feedback → Management Decisions. In the case of sero-surveillance, it will be slightly different: Farmer/animals → Samples & Info → Laboratory → Results → Epidemiology Unit → Analysis & Feedback → Management Decisions.

Having determined the route of flow, the next important step is to determine exactly what will happen at each step. Sending data straight from the field to the Epidemiology Unit, and then typing it directly into a computerised database would be unwise. Checking and validation mechanisms must be built along the path to the database. There are a number of lines of defence in data protection. The first is the person collecting the data. Such people should have clear handwriting, an ability to work with people and extract information from them. They should be clearly briefed on what they are doing and why they are doing it. Obviously, if the person collecting the information is a veterinarian, the foregoing points should not be a problem, however, in many cases, the data collection staff will be community animal health workers or veterinary assistants.

The next line of defense is the veterinary district office. Here, the form must be carefully checked by the district veterinarian. He is the most familiar person with the district situation. This is the last opportunity to go back to the field and re-check the data before it is transferred to the epidemiology unit. If any suspicion of a disease is detected and reported, the district veterinarian must act immediately.

Items to be checked by the district veterinarian include:

- Legible writing on the questionnaire form and ensuring readability would save expensive phone calls from input clerks later.
- If geographic coordinates of places are included, these must also be checked.
- Data must be realistic. If 100 animals are reported sick in an area where herd sizes average only 40, the farmer has probably exaggerated his problem to the field worker or the field worker has not visited the farmer and has fabricated the data.

Only when the district veterinarian is fully satisfied that everything possible has been done to check and verify the data, he should submit the forms for computerisation. The next line of defense is the data input clerk. The most important person here is, of course, the epidemiologist. His job will involve preliminary analyses to see what is in the database, follow-up communications to field veterinarians, and the detection of fabricated data. Additionally, he will be on the lookout for trends in disease spread, and for unusual occurrences that will alert him to possible problems brewing in the field.

Data backup

Any information system must have a data backup capacity. Backups are kept in a variety of ways:

- Duplicate copies of completed questionnaires at field offices.
- Original copies of completed questionnaires, sorted according to district and month at the data input centre.
- Electronic backups of data that has been stored on the computer. Data may be backed up on compact disks or pen drives.

Data checking

- **In the field:** Careful questioning of the farmer to capture true epidemiological data is required. Leading and misleading questions should be avoided. If data comes from farmer's recall, it is worth to cross-check data with other family members or with the nearby farmers.
- **At the district office:** Completed questionnaires are evaluated for legibility, correctness (eg. place names, code usage) and accuracy. What is written must be clear, neat and make sense. Where a query arises, the district supervisor (preferably a veterinarian) must first contact the interviewer concerned to clarify the issue with him. If necessary, and if possible, a return should be made to the original data source (the farmer) to follow up.
- **At the epidemiology unit:** The data entry clerks will detect and complain about poor handwriting. The epidemiologist will do spot checks on individual questionnaires before data entry, and also cross-check data entered into the database with the questionnaires from which the data came on a random basis. Data input staff will need good training and careful monitoring. Where possible, data entry should be interspersed with other tasks, such as the sorting and filing of questionnaires, doing data backups, sending enquiries to the field about data quality, etc.

An important task of the epidemiologist is the detection of fabricated data. It is helpful to carry out a preliminary analysis of data and look for tendencies. First, simply view recently entered data in its raw form in the table, and then carry out a few simple statistical procedures, such as calculation of range, mean, and standard deviation, and construct histograms and look for the following:

- Repetition of the same, or similar values (eg. herd sizes, or numbers of animals affected by a particular disease).
- Variables having a small standard deviation, with many values clustered around the mean.
- A very homogenous disease/clinical signs pattern in a particular area.
- Many values ending in zeros or fives.
- Herd size distributions that are vastly different in adjacent and very similar areas.
- Details given for a visit to a particular place may be identical to another visit to the same place six months previously, i.e., the previous visit's questionnaire was copied.

- A particular disease being widespread in one worker's area while being absent from an adjacent area where prevailing conditions are very similar.

All the above are reasons to be suspicious about data. Where there is a pattern of repetition in a particular worker's data, then his data are suspect. Where there are vast disparities between data of two adjacent field worker's areas, it will be difficult to say exactly which of the two is at fault. In general, however, it may be necessary to send an independent team into the field to conduct random inspections in the areas from which doubtful data have come as a verification study.

Routine surveillance is very often not randomized, but pre-programmed, and anomalies may arise:

- Field workers might not reach more remote areas.
- Field workers are usually male and they will not interview women.

Errors done by data input staff may be minimized through:

- Thorough staff training;
- Creating strong farmer awareness and gaining their cooperation;
- Good planning of data collection, and routine surveillance; and
- Having a vigilant epidemiologist.

14.5 ANIMAL DISEASE INFORMATION SYSTEM AS A MANAGEMENT TOOL

From the point of view of an epidemiologist, having a strong flow of analyzable data can be good. Using information from a system for research and retrospective studies may be exciting, but day-to-day management is the aim. Regular preparation of month-by-month incidence graphs of the main diseases can be very informative. Doing such work for one or two years may reveal important seasonal tendencies, particularly as far as vector-borne diseases are concerned, but possibly with others, as well. This may give good indicators for planning of strategic controls and regular reminders to farmers.

Longitudinal studies will be of value in monitoring progress with eradication efforts, or to change from visual surveillance for a particular disease to sero-surveillance or abattoir surveillance. Spatial analyses using a GIS are extremely useful for monitoring disease spread, and for noting the association a disease may have with weather conditions, ecological zones or geographic features such as rivers or roads. Areas under particular threat can be noticed early in the development of a disease, enabling more rational deployment of resources, planning for staff distribution, transport arrangements and vaccine purchases.

Long-term studies of disease data will also reveal cyclical tendencies, association with long-term climate changes, and so on. It may be possible to build reliable models of some diseases which enable predictions of spread to be made with greater accuracy. An important fact about disease information systems is the ability to link them with economic data, and make inferences regarding economic impacts of diseases and the costs and benefits of control measures.

References

Abelson, P. (2008), Establishing a monetary value for lives saved: issues and controversies, Working papers in CBA 2008-02. Paper prepared for the conference on Delivering better-quality proposals through better CBA, Office of Best Practice and Regulation, Department of Finance and Deregulation, Government of Australia.

Ahuja, V., R. Rajabova, D. Ward and A. McLeod (2009), Willingness to pay for disease prevention: Case of brucellosis control in Khatlon Oblast of Tajikistan, Report of the European Commission Project, 'Enhancing individual incomes and improving living standards in Khatlon, Tajikistan', Reference: EuropAid/125-743/L/ACT/TJ.

Ahuja. V. and A. Sen (2006), Willingness to pay for veterinary services: Evidence from poor areas in rural India. PPLPI Research Report RR Nr. 06-03. Rome, FAO.

Atkinson, A.C. (1990), A note on the generalized information criterion for choice of a model, Biometrika, 67: 413 – 418.

Awa, D.N., A. Njoya and A.C. Ngo Tama (2000), Economics of Prophylaxis against PPR and gastrointestinal helminthiasis in small ruminants in North Cameroon, Tropical Animal Health and Production, 32: 391 – 403.

Bar, D. and E. Ezra (2005), Effects of common calving diseases on milk production in high-yielding dairy cows, Israel Journal of Veterinary Medicine, 60 (4).

Barasa, M., A. Catley, D. Machuchu, H. Laqua, E. Puot, D. Tap Kot, and D. Ikiror (2008), FMD vaccination in South Sudan: Benefit-cost analysis and livelihoods impact, Transboundary and Emerging Diseases, 55: 339 – 351.

Bates, T.W., T.E. Carpenter and M.C. Thurmond (2003), Benefit-cost analysis of vaccination and pre-emptive slaughter as a means of eradicating FMD, American Journal of Veterinary Research, 64 (7): 805 – 812.

Bendixen P.H., B. Vilson, I. Ekesbo and D.B. Astrand (1987), Disease Frequencies in dairy cows in Sweden: IV. Ketosis, Preventive Veterinary Medicine, 5: 99 - 109.

Berentsen, P.B.M., A.A. Dijkhuizen, and A.J. Oskam (1990), FMD and export, Wageningen Economic Studies nr. 20 Pudoc, Wageningen, pp. 89.

Bicknell, K.B., J.E. Wilen and R.E. Howitt (1999), Public policy and private incentives for livestock disease control, Australian Journal of Agricultural Resource Economics, 43 (4): 501 – 521.

Blake, A., M.T. Sinclair and G. Sugiyarto (2003), Quantifying the impact of FMD on tourism and the UK economy, Tourism Economics, 9 (4): 449 – 465.

Box, G.E.P., J.S. Hunter and W.G. Hunter (2005), Statistics for Experiments: Design, Innovation and Discovery, Wiley Interscience, John Wiley & Sons Publication, New Jersey.

Boxall, A.B. (2004), The environmental side effects of medication, EMBO Reports, 5 (12): 1110 – 1116.

Carpenter, T.E., J.M. O'Brien, A.D. Hagerman and B.A. McCarl (2011), Epidemic and economic impacts of delayed detection of foot-and-mouth disease: A case study of a simulated outbreak in California, Journal of Veterinary Diagnostic Investigation, 23 (1): 26 – 33.

Chilonda, P. (1999), Health management and uptake of veterinary services by small scale cattle farmers in Eastern Province of Zambia, PhD thesis, University of Ghent, Belgium.

Chilonda, P. and G. Van Huylenbroeck (2001), A conceptual framework for the economic analysis of factors influencing decision-making of small-scale farmers in animal health management. Rev. sci. tech. (OIE), 20 (3): 687 – 700.

Christiansen, K.H. and T.E. Carpenter (1983), Linear programming as a planning tool in the New Zealand brucellosis eradication scheme, In Proceedings of the Third International Symposium on Veterinary Epidemiology and Economics, 6 – 10, 1982, Arlington, VA, Veterinary Medicine Publishing Company, Edwardsville, KS, 369 – 379.

Cox, D.R. (1972), Regression models and life-tables, Journal of the Royal Statistical Society: Series B (Methodological), 34 (2): 187 – 202.

Dijkhuizen, A.A. (1983), Economic aspects of diseases and disease control in dairy cattle, Unpublished PhD Thesis submitted to State University of Urecht, Urecht (in Dutch, English summary), 192 pp.

Dijkhuizen, A.A. (1988), Modelling to support health programs in modern livestock farming, Netherlands Journal of Agricultural Science, 37: 1 – 12.

Dijkhuizen, A.A. (1992), Modelling animal health economics, Inaugural speech delivered upon entering the post of Professor in Animal Health Economics in the Dept. of Farm Management at Wageningen Agricultural University on Feb. 27, 1992.

Dijkhuizen, A.A., R.B.M. Huirne and A.W. Jalwingh (1995), Economic analysis of animal diseases and their control, Preventive Veterinary Medicine, 25 (2): 135 – 149.

Disney, W.T., J.W. Green, K.W. Forsythe, J.F. Wiemers and S. Weber (2001), Benefit-cost analysis of animal identification for disease prevention and control, In: Traceability of animals and animal products (H.A. MacDaniel and M.K. Sheridam, eds), Res. Sci. tech (OIE), 20 (2): 385 – 405.

Dohoo, I.R. and S.W. Martin (1984), Subclinical ketosis: Prevalence and associations with production and disease, Canadian Journal of Comparative Medicine, 48: 1 - 5.

Dyke, G.V. and H.D. Patterson (1992), Analysis of factorial arrangements when the data are proportions, Biometrics, 8: 1 – 12.

Ellis, P. (1972), An economic evaluation of the swine fever eradication programme in Great Britain using cost-benefit analysis techniques, Study No. 11, 1972. Department of Agriculture, University of Reading, UK.

Ellis, P.R. and S.N. Putt (1981), The epidemiological and economic implications of FMD vaccination programme in Kenya. Consultancy report.

Erb, H.N. and S.W. Martin (1978), Age, breed and seasonal patterns in the occurrence of 10 dairy cow diseases: A Case-control study, Canadian Journal of Comparative Medicine, 42: 1 - 9.

Erb, H.N. and Y.T. Grohn (1988), Epidemiology of metabolic disorders in the periparturient dairy cow, Journal of Dairy Science, 71: 2557 - 2571.

Eyduran, E., T. Ozdemir, B. Cak and E. Alarslan (2005), Using of logistic regression in animal science, Journal of Applied Sciences, 5 (10): 1753 – 1756.

FAO (1997), Prevention and control of transboundary animal diseases, FAO Animal Production and Health Paper 133, FAO, Rome.

FAO (1999), Manual on Livestock Disease Surveillance and Information Systems (www.fao.org/3/x3331e/X3331E01.htm)

FAO (2008), Biosecurity for highly pathogenic Avian Influenza. FAO Animal Production and Health Paper 165. Rome.

FAO (2010), Animal disease intelligence. Emergency Centre for Transboundary Animal Diseases. Rome (http://www.fao.org/docrep/012/ak729e/ak729e00.pdf).

Fisher, R. A. (1935), The design of experiments, Oliver & Boyd.

Galligan, D.T. and W.E. Marsh (1988), Application of portfolio theory for the optimal choice of dairy veterinary management programmes, Preventive Veterinary Medicine, 5 (4): 251 – 261.

Gari, G., P. Bonnet, F. Roger and A. Waret-Szkuta (2011), Epidemiological aspects and financial impact of lumpy skin disease in Ethiopia, Preventive Veterinary Medicine, 102 (4): 274 - 283.

Grohn, Y., H.N. Erb, C.E. McCulloch and H.S. Saloniemi (1989), Epidemiology of metabolic disorders in dairy cattle: association among host characteristics, disease and production, Journal of Dairy Science, 72: 1876 - 1885.

Habtemariam, T., R. Howaitt, R. Ruppanner and H.P. Reimann (1984), Application of linear programming model to the control of African Trypanosomiasis, Preventive Veterinary Medicine, 3 (1): 1 – 14.

Hanley, N., D.C. MacMillan, R.E. Wright, C. Bullock, I. Simpson, D. Parsisson and B. Crabtree (1998), Contingent valuation versus choice experiments: Estimating the benefits of environmentally sensitive areas in Scotland, Journal of Agricultural Economics, 49 (1): 1 – 15.

Häsler, B., K.S., Howe, R. Hauser K.D.C. Stärk (2011), A qualitative approach to measure the effectiveness of active avian influenza virus surveillance with respect to its cost: A case study from Switzerland, Preventive Veterinary Medicine, 105 (3): 209–222.

Horst, H.S., A.A. Dijkhuizen, R.B.M. Huirne and M.P.M. Meuwissen (1999a), Monte Carlo Simulation of virus introduction into the Netherlands, Preventive Veterinary Medicine, 41 (2-3): 209 – 229.

Horst, H.S., C.J. de Vos, F.H. Tomassen, and J. Stelwagen (1999b), The economic evaluation of control and eradication of epidemic livestock diseases, Rev. Sci. Tech. (IOE), 18:2, 367 - 379.

Houben, E.H.P., A.A. Dijkhuizen, J.A.M. van Arendonk and R.B.M. Huirne (1993), Short and long-term production losses and repeatability of clinical mastitis in dairy cows, Journal of Dairy Science, 76: 2561 – 2578.

Howe, K. and K.H. Christiansen (2004), The State of Animal Health Economics: A Review. Proceedings of the Society for Veterinary Epidemiology and Preventive Medicine, pp. 68 – 80.

Jadhav, K.L., V.N. Tripathi and M.M. Kale (1995), Economics of health disorders in Holstein X Sahiwal crossbreds, Indian Journal of Animal Sciences, 65 (8): 949 – 951.

Jadhav, K.L., V.N. Tripathi and M.M. Kale (1996), Incidence and economics of various health disorders in crossbred cows, Indian Journal of Animal Production and Management, 12 (1): 45 – 50.

Jalvingh, A.W. (1993), Dynamic livestock modelling for on-farm decision support, PhD Thesis, Wageningen Agricultural University, 164p.

James, A.D. and P.R. Ellis (1978), Benefit-cost analysis in FMD control programmes, British Veterinary Journal, 134 (1): 47 - 52.

Jeyakumari, M. (2000), An economic analysis of post-partum reproductive disorders in bovines, Unpublished MVSc thesis submitted to Tamil Nadu Veterinary and Animal Sciences University, Chennai.

Jeyakumari, M., M. Thirunavukkarasu and G. Kathiravan (2003a), Epidemiological measures of association between the incidence of postpartum reproductive disorders in dairy animals and their predisposing factors, Indian Journal of Animal Sciences, 73 (8): 992 – 994.

Jeyakumari, M., M. Thirunavukkarasu and G. Kathiravan (2003b), Economic impact of postpartum reproductive disorders in dairy farms, Indian Journal of Animal Sciences, 73 (12): 1360 – 1362

Jeyakumari, M., M. Thirunavukkarasu and G. Kathiravan (2006), Factors influencing the incidence of postpartum reproductive disorders in bovines, Tamil Nadu Journal of Veterinary and Animal Sciences, 2 (5): 188 - 190.

John Christy R. and M. Thirunavukkarasu (2006), Emerging importance of animal health economics – A note, Indian Journal Agricultural Economics, 2 (3): 113 - 117.

Junker F., J. Komorowska and F.V. Tongeren (2009), Impact of Animal Disease Outbreaks and Alternative Control Practices on Agricultural Markets and Trade, OECD Food, Agriculture and Fisheries Working Papers, No. 19, OECD Publishing.

Kauppinen, K. (1983), Prevalence of bovine ketosis in relation to number and stage of lactation, Acta Veterinary Scand., 24: 349 - 361.

Knight-Jones, T.J.D. and J. Rushton (2013), The economic impacts of foot and mouth disease – What are they, how big are they and where do they occur? Preventive Veterinary Medicine, 112: 161 - 173.

Kobayashi, M., T.E. Carpenter, B.F. Dickey and R.E. Howitt (2007a), A dynamic, optimal disease control model for FMD: I. Model description, Preventive Veterinary Medicine, 79 (2-4): 257 – 273.

Kobayashi, M., T.E. Carpenter, B.F. Dickey and R.E. Howitt (2007b), A dynamic, optimal disease control model for FMD: II. Model results and policy implications, Preventive Veterinary Medicine, 79 (2-4): 274 - 286.

Kumar (year unknown) in https://www.linkedin.com/in/nk17kumar/ and https://www.geeksforgeeks.org/solve-dynamic-programming-problem/

Kristula, M.A., C.R. Curtis, D.T. Galligan and R.O. Bartholomew (1992), Use of a repeated measures logistic regression model to predict chronic mastitis in dairy cows, Preventive Veterinary Medicine, 14: 57 – 68.

Krupnik, A.J. (2004), Valuing health outcomes: policy choices and technical issues, Washington D.C., Resources for the Future (http://www.rff.org/files/sharepoint/WorkImages/Download/RFF-RPT-ValuingHealthOutcomes.pdf).

Mangen, M.J.J. and A.M. Burrel (2003), Who gains, who loses? Welfare effects of CSF epidemics in the Netherlands, European Review of Agricultural Economics, 30 (2): 125 - 154

Martin, S.W., A.H. Meek and P. Willeberg (1993), Veterinary Epidemiology: Principles and Methods, Lucknow: International Book Distributing Co.

Martins, S.B., B. Häsler, and J. Rushton (2014), Economic aspects of zoonoses: Impact of zoonoses on the food industry, In: Sing, A. (eds) Zoonoses - Infections Affecting Humans and Animals. Springer, Dordrecht, pp. 1107-1126 (https://doi.org/10.1007/978-94-017-9457-2_45).

McDermott, J., D. Grace and J. Zinsstag (2013), Economics of brucellosis impact and control in developing countries, Rev. Sci. Tech. (OIE), 32 (1): 249 – 261.

McInerney, J. P. (1995), Economic aspects of disease in poultry production, Poultry Adviser, 28: 65 – 71.

McInerney, J.P. (1988), The economic analysis of livestock disease: the developing framework. Proceedings of the 5th International Symposium on Veterinary Epidemiology and Economics, 1988, Copenhagen, 18 – 27.

McInerney, J.P. (1991). Cost-benefit analysis of livestock disease: A simplified look at its economic foundations. Proceedings of the 6th International Symposium on Veterinary Epidemiology and Economics.

McInerney, J.P., K.S. Howe and J.A. Schepers (1992), A framework for the economic analysis of disease in farm livestock, Preventive Veterinary Medicine, 13 (2): 137 – 154.

McLeod, A. and J. Leslie (2001), Socio-economic impacts of freedom from livestock disease and export promotion in developing counties, Livestock Policy Discussion Paper No. 3, Rome: FAO.

Mcleod, A. and N. Honhold (2012), Livestock development and animal health project Zambia: Cost-benefit analysis of disease-free zone establishment and maintenance, Final report to the Government of Zambia.

McLeod, A., N. Honhold and H. Steinfeld (2010), Responses on emerging livestock diseases, In H. Steinfeld, H. Mooney, F. Schneider and L. Neville, eds. Livestock in a changing landscape, Vol. 1: Drivers, consequences, and responses. Washington, DC: Island Press.

McLeod, A., N. Taylor, N.T. Thuy and L.T.K. Lan, (2003), Control of CSF in the Red River Delta of Vietnam: A stakeholder analysis and assessment of potential benefits, costs and risks of improved disease control in three provinces. Phase 3 report, June 2003.

Meuwissen, M.P., S.H. Horst, R.B. Huirne and A.A. Dijkhuizen (1999), A model to estimate the financial consequences of classical swine fever outbreaks: Principles and outcomes, Preventive Veterinary Medicine, 42 (3&4): 249 – 270.

Moran, D. (1994), Contingent valuation and biodiversity conservation in Kenyan protected areas, CSERGE Working Paper GEC 94-16, Centre for Social and Economic Research on the Global Environment, University College, University of East Anglia, London (http:// cserge.ac.uk/sites/default/files/gec_1994_16.pdf).

Morris, R.S. (1969), Assessing the economic value of veterinary services to primary industries, Australian Veterinary Journal, 45: 295 – 300.

Mutambara, J., I. Dube, E. Matangi and F. Majeke (2013), Factors influencing the demand of the service of community-based animal health care in Zimbabwe, Preventive Veterinary Medicine, 112 (3–4): 174 – 182.

Ngategize, P.K. and J.B. Kaneene (1985), Evaluation of the economic impact of animal diseases on production: A review, Veterinary Bulletin, 55: 153 – 161.

Nielen, M., A.W. Jalvingh, M.P.M. Meuwissen, S.H. Horst and A.A. (1999), Spatial and stochastic simulation to evaluate the impact of events and control measures on the 1997-98 CSW epidemic in the Netherlands. II. Comparison of control strategies, Preventive Veterinary Medicine, 42 (3-4): 297 – 317.

Nielen, M., Y.H. Schukken, A. Brand, H.A. Deluyker and K. Mallje (1995), Detection of subclinical mastitis from online milking parlour data, Journal of Dairy Science, 78 (5): 1039 – 1049.

OIE (1996), International Animal Health Code, Office International des Epizooties, 1996.

Omiti, J. and P. Irungu (2010), Socio-economic benefits of rinderpest eradication from Ethiopia and Kenya, Report to the African Union Inter-African Bureau for Animal Rescurces.

Onono, J.O. (2014), Economics of CBPP control in Kenya, A presentation made at Ahmadu Bello University, Zaria, Nigeria.

Onono, J.O., B. Wieland and J. Rushton (2014), Estimation of impact of contagious bovine pleuropneumonia on pastoralists in Kenya, Preventive Veterinary Medicine, 115 (3&4): 122 – 129.

Otte, J., R. Nugent and A. McLeod (2004), Transboundary animal diseases: Assessment of socio-economic impacts and institutional responses. Livestock Policy Discussion Paper No. 9, Livestock Information and Policy Branch, FAO, Rome.

Otte, M.J. and P. Chilonda (2002), Animal Health Economics: An Introduction, FAO Policy Paper (https://openknowledge.fao.org/server/api/core/bitstreams/2ebc7da1-b842-48d5-b7d2-4e000e930c74/content)

Paarlberg, P.L., J.G. Lee and A.H. Seitzinger (2002), Potential revenue impact of an outbreak of FMD in the United States, Journal of American Veterinary Medical Association, 220 (7): 988 – 992.

Parsons, T.D., G. Smith and D.T. Galligan (1986), Economics of porcine parvovirus vaccination assessed by decision analysis, Preventive Veterinary Medicine, 4: 199 – 204.

Pendell, D.L., J. Leatherman, T.C. Schroeder and G.S. Alward (2007), The economic impacts of FMD outbreak: A regional analysis. Journal of Agricultural and Applied Economics, 39 (Special): 1 – 15.

Perry, B.D., J.J. McDermott and T. Randolph (2001), Can epidemiology and economics make a meaningful contribution to national animal-disease control? Preventive Veterinary Medicine, 48: 231 – 260.

Perry, B.D., T.F. Randolph, J.J. McDermott, K.R. Sones and P.K. Thornton (2002), Investing in animal health research to alleviate poverty, ILRI, Nairobi, Kenya, 140 pp.

Perry, B.D., T.F. Randolph, S. Ashley, R. Chimedza, A. Forman, J. Morrison, C. Poulton, L. Sibanda, C. Stevens, N. Tebele, and I. Yngstrom (2003), The impact and poverty reduction implications of foot and mouth disease control in southern Africa, Proceedings of the 10th International Symposium on Veterinary Epidemiology and Economics.

Perry, B.D., W. Kalpravidh, P.G. Coleman, H.S. Horst, J.J. McDermott, T. Randolph and I.J. Gleeson (1999), The economic impact of FMD and its control in South-east Asia: A preliminary assessment with reference to Thailand. In the economics of animal disease control (B.D. Perry ed.). Rev. sci. tech. (OIE), 18 (2): 478 – 497.

Pritchett, J., D. Thilmany and K. Johnson (2005), Animal disease impacts: A survey of literature and typology of research approaches, International Food and Agribusiness Management Review, 8 (1): 1 – 23.

Randolph, T.F., B.D. Perry, C.C. Benigno, I.J. Santos, A.L. Agbayani, P. Coleman, R. Webb and I.J. Gleeson (2002), The economic impact of FMD control and eradication in the Philippines, In FMD facing the new dilemmas (G.R. Thomson, ed.), Rev. sci. tech. (OIE), 21 (3): 645 – 661.

Rasmussen L.K., B.L. Nielsen, J.E. Pryce, T.T. Mottram and R.F. Veerkamp (1999), Risk factors associated with the incidence of ketosis in dairy cows, Journal of Animal Sciences, 68: 379 - 386.

Renkema, J.A. (1980), Economic aspects of disease in animals, with special reference to the assessment of losses, Bulletin OIE, 92: 443 - 458.

Renkema, J.A. and J. Stelwagen (1979), Economic evaluation of replacement rates in dairy herds: I. Reduction of replacement rates through improved health, Livestock Production Science, 6: 15 - 27.

Rich, K.M., G.Y. Miller and A. Winter-Nelson (2005), A review of economic tools for the assessment of animal disease outbreaks, Rev. sci. tech. (OIE), 24 (3): 833 – 845.

Rodrigues, A.C., I.A. Gardner and T.E. Carpenter (1990), Financial analysis of pseudorabies control and eradication in swine, Journal of American Medical Association, 197 (10): 1316 – 1323.

Roth, F., J. Zinsstag, D. Orkhon, G. Chimed-Ochit, G. Hutton, O. Cosivi, G. Carrin, and J. Otte (2003), Human health benefits from livestock vaccination for Brucellosis: Case study, Bulletin of the World Health Organization, 81 (12): 867 - 876.

Rushton, J. and M. Upton (2006), Investment in preventing and preparing for biological emergencies and disasters: Social and economic costs of disasters versus costs of surveillance and response preparedness, Rev. sci. tech. (OIE), 25 (1): 375 – 388.

Rushton, J., R. Viscarra, J. Otte, A. Mcleod and N. Taylor (2007), Animal health economics – where have we come from and where do we go next? CAB Reviews: Perspectives in Agriculture, veterinary science, nutrition and natural resources, 1(31) (http://www.cababstractsplus.org/cabreview).

Saini, S.S., J.K. Sharma and M.S. Kwatra (1994), Prevalence and etiology of subclinical mastitis among crossbred cows and buffaloes in Punjab, Indian Journal of Dairy Science, 47 (2): 103 – 106.

Saxena, R. (1994), Economic value of milk loss caused by FMD in India. Working Paper No. 60, Institute of Rural Management, Anand, 20 pp.

Schepers, J.A. and A.A. Dijkhuizen, A.A. (1991), The economics of mastitis and mastitis control in dairy cattle: A critical analysis of estimates since 1970, Preventive Veterinary Medicine, 10: 213 - 224.

Selvam, S. (2000), Economic analysis of certain poultry diseases, Unpublished PhD thesis submitted to Tamil Nadu Veterinary and Animal Sciences University, Chennai.

Selvam, S., M. Thirunavukkarasu and G. Kathiravan (2003), Measuring disease frequencies in commercial layer farms, Cheiron, 32 (5&6): 100 – 106.

Selvam, S., M. Thirunavukkarasu and G. Kathiravan (2004), Factors influencing loss due to diseases in layer farms, Cheiron, 33 (1&2): 13 – 17.

Selvam, S., R. Prabaharan and M. Thirunavukkarasu (2006), Economic losses in layer farms due to diseases, Tamil Nadu Journal of Veterinary and Animal Sciences, 2 (4): 129 – 135.

Senthilkumar, V. (2003), An economic analysis of sheep pox and enterotoxaemia in sheep, Unpublished MVSc thesis submitted to Tamil Nadu Veterinary and Animal Sciences University, Chennai.

Senthilkumar, V. and M. Thirunavukkarasu (2010), Economic losses due to sheep pox in sheep farms in Tamil Nadu, Tamil Nadu Journal of Veterinary and Animal Sciences, 6(2): 88–94.

Senthilkumar, V., M. Thirunavukkarasu and G. Kathiravan (2006a), Factors influencing prevalence of sheep pox in Tamil Nadu, Indian Veterinary Journal, 83: 670 – 672.

Senthilkumar, V., M. Thirunavukkarasu and G. Kathiravan (2006b), Survival time in sheep affected by sheep pox and enterotoxaemia, Journal of Animal and Veterinary Advances, 5 (8): 647 – 650.

Senthilkumar, V., M. Thirunavukkarasu and G. Kathiravan (2008), Economic losses due to Enterotoxaemia in sheep, Indian Journal of Science and Technology, 1 (6): 1 - 3.

Singh, B. and Shiv Prasad (2008), Modelling of economic losses due to some important diseases in goats in India, Agricultural Economics Research Review, 21: 297 - 302.

Singh, P.J. and P.B. Singh (1994), A study of economic losses due to mastitis in India, Indian Journal of Dairy Science, 47 (4): 265 – 272.

Sinha, M.K., N.N. Thombre, Biswajit Mondal and M.S. Meena (2017), Analysis of FMD in dairy animals: An assessment of cost and loss from sample farmers, Indian Journal of Animal Research, 52.

Stott, A.W., J. Lloyd, R.W. Humphry and G.J. Gunn (2003), A linear programming approach to estimate the economic impact of bovine viral diarrhoea at the whole-farm level in Scotland, Preventive Veterinary Medicine, 59 (1-2): 51 – 66.

Tambi, E.N., O.W. Maina, A.W. Mukhebi and T.F. Randolph (1999a), Economic impact assessment of rinderpest control in Africa, Rev. sci. tech. (OIE), 18 (2): 458 - 477.

Tambi, E.N., A.W. Mukhebi, O.W. Maina and H.M. Solomon (1999b), Probit analysis of livestock producers' demand for private veterinary services in the high potential areas of Kenya, Agricultural Systems, 59: 163 – 176.

Tambi, N.E., W.O. Maina and C. Ndi (2006), An estimation of the economic impact of contagious bovine pleuropneumonia in Africa, Rev. Sci. Tech. (OIE), 25 (3): 999–1012.

Taneja, V.K., V.K. Dwivedi, M.M. Saxena, A.E. Nivsarkar and L.P. Nautiyal (1989), Incidence of mastitis and production losses in crossbreds, Indian Journal of Animal Sciences, 59 (10): 1346 – 1348.

Taylor, N., A. McLeod, N.T. Thuy, M. Stone, V.T. Binh, L.T.K. Lan, D.H. Dung and F. Barwinek (2003), Examining the options for a Livestock disease-free zone in the Red River Delta of Vietnam, Strengthening of Veterinary Services in Vietnam (SVSV), ALA/96/20, Supported by the European Commission.

Thirunavukkarasu, M. (1996), An economic analysis of mastitis in dairy farms, Unpublished PhD thesis submitted to Tamil Nadu Veterinary and Animal Sciences University, Chennai.

Thirunavukkarasu, M. (2003a), An economic analysis of artificial breeding of bovines, ICAR funded project.

Thirunavukkarasu, M. (2003b), A model to discriminate mastitic and non-mastitis milch animals, Indian Veterinary Journal, 80: 890 – 894.

Thirunavukkarasu, M. (2004), An economic analysis of Foot and Mouth Disease in Tamil Nadu, University (TANUVAS) funded project.

Thirunavukkarasu, M. (2008), An economic analysis of metabolic disorders in bovines, ICAR funded project.

Thirunavukkarasu, M. and G. Kathiravan (2006a), Economic losses due to mortality and culling of FMD affected livestock, Tamil Nadu Journal of Veterinary and Animal Sciences, 2 (1): 13 – 17.

Thirunavukkarasu, M. and G. Kathiravan (2006b), Factors influencing economic losses due to conception failures in artificially inseminated bovines, Tamil Nadu Journal of Veterinary and Animal Sciences, 2 (6): 208 – 211.

Thirunavukkarasu, M. and G. Kathiravan (2006c), Economic losses due to conception failures in artificially inseminated bovines, Indian Veterinary Journal, 83: 196 – 199.

Thirunavukkarasu, M. and G. Kathiravan (2007), Monetary losses due to reproductive failures in FMD affected bovines, Indian Journal of Dairy Science, 60 (5): 364 – 368.

Thirunavukkarasu, M. and G. Kathiravan (2009), Factors affecting conception rates in artificially inseminated bovines, Indian Journal of Animal Sciences, 79 (9): 871 – 875.

Thirunavukkarasu, M. and R. Prabaharan (1998a), Factors influencing clinical mastitis in bovines – A study in Tamil Nadu, Indian Journal of Animal Production and Management, 14 (2): 110 – 114.

Thirunavukkarasu, M. and R. Prabaharan (1998b), Epidemiologic measures of association between the incidence of mastitis and some of its predisposing factors, Indian Veterinary Journal, 75: 718 – 722.

Thirunavukkarasu, M. and R. Prabaharan (1999a), Prevalence of clinical mastitis in bovines – A survey in Tamil Nadu, Cheiron, 28 (3): 55 - 61.

Thirunavukkarasu, M. and R. Prabaharan (1999b), Impact of mastitis on dairy farms – An economic analysis, Cheiron, 28 (6): 188 - 194.

Thirunavukkarasu, M. and R. Prabaharan (1999c), Estimating the probability of a milch animal going mastitic – A logistic approach, Proceedings the 2nd International Conference on Operations and Quantitative Management, Jan. 3 – 6, 1999, Ahmedabad, India.

Thirunavukkarasu, M. and R. Prabaharan (2000), Factors determining mastitis losses – The results from a regression analysis, Cheiron, 29 (5&6): 131 - 133.

Thirunavukkarasu, M., G. Kathiravan and A. Kalaikannan (2009), Epidemiological measures of association between factors predisposing and prevalence of ketosis, Paper presented in the International Summit on Advancing veterinary medical care: Challenges and strategies, Feb. 19 – 21, 2009, p.184.

Thirunavukkarasu M., G. Kathiravan, A. Kalaikannan and W. Jebarani (2010a), Prevalence of ketosis in dairy farms – A survey in Tamil Nadu, Tamil Nadu Journal of Veterinary and Animal Sciences, 6 (4): 193 - 195.

Thirunavukkarasu, M., G. Kathiravan, A. Kalaikannan and W. Jebarani (2010b), Quantifying economic losses due to milk fever in dairy farms, Agricultural Economics Research Review, 23: 77 - 81.

Thirunavukkarasu, M., G. Kathiravan, A. Kalaikannan and W. Jebarani (2010c), Factors influencing economic losses due to milk fever in dairy animals, Tamil Nadu Journal of Veterinary and Animal Sciences, 6 (5): 231 - 235.

Thirunavukkarasu, M., G. Kathiravan, A. Kalaikannan and W. Jebarani (2010d), Epidemiological measures of association between factors predisposing and prevalence of milk fever among dairy animals, Tamil Nadu Journal of Veterinary and Animal Sciences, 6 (3): 125 - 127.

Thirunavukkarasu, M., G. Kathiravan, A. Kalaikannan and W. Jebarani (2011a), Epidemiological measures on prevalence of ketosis in dairy farms, Indian Veterinary Journal, 88 (7): 91 -92.

Thirunavukkarasu, M., G. Kathiravan, A. Kalaikannan and W. Jebarani (2011b), Economic losses due to ketosis in dairy farms, Indian Veterinary Journal, 88 (8): 52.

Thirunavukkarasu, M., G. Kathiravan, A. Kalaikannan and W. Jebarani (2011c), Factors influencing ketosis in dairy farms, Indian Veterinary Journal, 88 (8): 48 - 49.

Thombre, N.N. Sinha and Mukesh Kumar (2009), Economic implications of PPR in sheep and goats: A sample analysis of District Pune, Maharashtra, Agricultural Economics Research Review, 22 (2): 319 – 322.

Thrusfield, M. (1995), Veterinary Epidemiology, 2nd Edition, Blackwell Science, Oxford.

Tigner, R. (2006), Partial budgeting: A tool to analyse farm business changes. Ag Decision Maker File C-150, Iowa State University Extension (http://www.extension.iastate.edu/agdm/wholefarm/pdf/c1-50.pdf).

Tisdell, C. (1994), Animal health and the control of diseases: Economic issues with particular reference to a developing country, Working Paper No. 2, Sep. 1994, University of Queensland, Australia, pp. 1 - 16.

Tomassen, F.H.M., A. de Koeijer, M.C.M. Mourits, A. Dekker, A. Bouma and R.B. Huirne (2002), A decision-tree to optimize control measures during the early stage of an FMD epidemic, Preventive Veterinary Medicine, 54 (4): 301 – 324.

Twinamasiko, E. K. (2002), Development of an appropriate programme for the control of contagious bovine pleuropneumonia in Uganda, PhD thesis, University of Reading, UK.

Van Arendonk, J.A.M. (1985), Studies on the replacement policies in dairy cows in cattle, PhD Thesis, Wageningen Agricultural University, 126p.

Whatford, L., S. van Winden and B. Häsler (2022), A systematic literature review on the economic impact of endemic disease in UK sheep and cattle using a One Health conceptualisation, Preventive Veterinary Medicine, 209: 105756.

Winpenny, J.T. (1991), Values for the environment: a guide to economic appraisal, London: HMSO.

Yadav, M.P. (2003), Foreword for the book – Foot and Mouth Disease: A Monograph, ICAR, New Delhi.

Yang, P.C., R.M. Chu, W.B. Chung and H.T. Sung (1999), Epidemiological characteristics and financial costs of the 1997 FMD epidemic in Taiwan, Veterinary Record, 145 (25): 731 – 734.

Young, J.R., S. Suon, C.J. Andrews, L.A. Henry and P.A. Windsor (2013), Assessment of financial impact of foot and mouth disease on smallholder cattle farmers in southern Cambodia, Transboundary and Emerging Diseases, 60 (2): 166 - 174.

Zinsstag, J., E. Schelling, F. Roth, B. Bonfoh, D. de Savigny, and M. Tanner (2007), Human benefits of animal interventions for zoonosis control, Emerging Infectious Diseases, 13 (4): 527 - 531.

Index